RON BAKER
10538 Concord Dr.
Berrien Springs, MI 49103

Musculoskeletal Physical Examination

An Evidence-Based Approach

Musculoskeletal Physical Examination

An Evidence-Based Approach

Gerard A. Malanga, MD

Associate Professor of Physical Medicine and Rehabilitation
University of Medicine and Dentistry of New Jersey
New Jersey Medical School
Newark, New Jersey

Scott F. Nadler, DO

Professor of Physical Medicine and Rehabilitation
University of Medicine and Dentistry of New Jersey
New Jersey Medical School
University Hospital
Newark, New Jersey

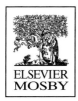

ELSEVIER
MOSBY

ELSEVIER
MOSBY

1600 John F. Kennedy Boulevard
Suite 1800
Philadelphia, PA 19103-2899

MUSCULOSKELETAL PHYSICAL EXAMINATION
An Evidence-based Approach

ISBN–13: 978–1–56053–591–1
ISBN–10: 1–56053–591–1

Notice

Knowledge and best practice in this field are constantly changing. As new research and experience broaden
our knowledge, changes in practice, treatment, and drug therapy may become necessary or appropriate.
Readers are advised to check the most current information provided (i) on procedures featured or
(ii) by the manufacturer of each product to be administered, to verify the recommended dose or
formula, the method and duration of administration, and contraindications. It is the responsibility of the
practitioner, relying on his or her own experience and knowledge of the patient, to make diagnoses,
to determine dosages and the best treatment for each individual patient, and to take all appropriate safety
precautions. To the fullest extent of the law, neither the Publisher nor the Authors assume any liability
for any injury and/or damage to persons or property arising out of or related to any use of the material
contained in this book.

Library of Congress Cataloging-in-Publication Data

Musculoskeletal physical examination: an evidence-based approach/ [edited by]
 Gerard A. Malanga, Scott F. Nadler.
  p. cm.
 Includes bibliographical references and index.
 ISBN-13: 978-1-56053-591-1   ISBN-10: 1-56053-591-1
  1. Musculoskeletal system–Examination. 2. Musculoskeletal system–Diseases–Diagnosis.
  3. Evidence-based medicine. 4. Physical diagnosis. I. Malanga, Gerard A. II. Nadler, Scott, 1964–

RC925.7.M876 2006
616.7′075–dc22   2005041575

Acquisitions Editor: Dolores Meloni
Developmental Editor: Louise Cook
Project Manager: Cecelia Bayruns

Printed in the United States of America.

Last digit is the print number: 9 8 7 6 5 4 3 2

Working together to grow
libraries in developing countries

www.elsevier.com | www.bookaid.org | www.sabre.org

ELSEVIER   BOOK AID International   Sabre Foundation

In memoriam

Scott F. Nadler, DO

whose spirit permeates the pages of this book.

Dedication

To those that bring meaning to my life: friends, family, and God.

GAM

To my wife Jodi, the love and inspiration in my life, you are and always will be my soulmate.

To my daughters, Sydni and Haley, you have taught me the meaning of living and have made me the happiest "daddy" in the world

To my family and friends, thanks for being there for me in times of good and bad.

To my coauthor, coeditor, and friend Gerry Malanga, you will always be my other brother.

SFN

Contents

Contributors

Thomas Agesen, MD
Assistant Clinical Professor, University of Medicine and Dentistry of New Jersey, New Jersey Medical School, Newark, New Jersey

Stephen Andrus, MD
Staff Physiatrist, Department of Orthopedics, Beth Israel Medical Center, New York, New York

Jay E. Bowen, DO
Assistant Professor of Physical Medicine and Rehabilitation, University of Medicine and Dentistry of New Jersey, Newark, New Jersey

Larry H. Chou, MD
Assistant Professor, Sports and Spine Rehabilitation, Department of Rehabilitation Medicine, University of Pennsylvania School of Medicine, Philadelphia, Pennsylvania; Medical Director, Physical Medicine and Rehabilitation Services, Penn Medicine at Radnor, Radnor, Pennsylvania

Diane Dahm, MD
Assistant Professor, Department of Physical Medicine and Rehabilitation, Mayo Clinic, Rochester, Minnesota

James Farmer, MD
Assistant Attending Orthopaedic Surgeon, Hospital for Special Surgery, New York, New York

Garrett S. Hyman, MD, MPH
Clinical Assistant Professor, Department of Rehabilitation Medicine, University of Washington, Seattle, Washington; Staff Physician, Overlake Hospital Medical Center, Bellevue, Washington and Evergreen Hospital Medical Center, Kirkland, Washington

Scott J. Jarmain MD
Medical Director, Physical Medicine and Rehabilitation, Coastal Spine, Morristown, New Jersey

Daniel Kim, MD
Comprehensive Sports and Spine, Wilmington, Delaware

Brian J. Krabak MD
Assistant Professor of Physical Medicine and Rehabilitation, Assistant Professor of Orthopedic Surgery, The Johns Hopkins Hospital, Baltimore, Maryland

Phillip Landes, MD
Assistant Professor, Department of Neurology, Uniformed Services University of the Health Sciences, Bethesda, Maryland; Clinical Assistant Professor, Department of Rehabilitation Medicine, University of Texas Health Center, San Antonio, Texas; Assistant Chief, Physical Medicine and Rehabilitation Service, Brooke Army Medical Center, Fort Sam Houston, Texas

Gerard A. Malanga, MD

Associate Professor of Physical Medicine and Rehabilitation, University of Medicine and Dentistry, New Jersey Medical School, Newark, New Jersey; Director, Sports Medicine, Mountainside Hospital, Montclair, New Jersey; Director, Pain Management, Overlook Hospital, Summit, New Jersey

Edward McFarland, MD

Associate Professor, Department of Orthopedic Surgery, Johns Hopkins Medicine; Director, Division of Sports Medicine and Shoulder Surgery, Baltimore, Maryland

Jeffrey Miller, MD

Clinical Instructor, University of Medicine and Dentistry of New Jersey, New Jersey Medical School; Newark, New Jersey; Attending Physician, Morristown Memorial Hospital, Overlook Hospital, Saint Barnabus Medical Center, New Jersey

Scott F. Nadler, DO†

Professor, Department of Physical Medicine and Rehabilitation, University of Medicine and Dentistry, New Jersey Medical School; University Hospital, Newark, New Jersey

Tutankhamen Pappoe, MD

Department of Rehabilitation Medicine, Mount Sinai Medical Center, New York, New York

Heidi Prather, DO

Assistant Professor of Physical Medicine and Rehabilitation, Washington University School of Medicine, St. Louis, Missouri

Joel Press, MD

Associate Clinical Professor, Department of Physical Medicine and Rehabilitation, Feinberg School of Medicine, Northwestern University, Chicago, Illinois; Medical Director, Spine and Sports Rehabilitation Center, Rehabilitation Institute of Chicago, Chicago, Illinois

Luke Rigolosi, MD

Director of Pain Management, Northeast Orthopedics, Albany, New York

Jennifer Solomon, MD

Assistant Attending Physiatrist, Hospital for Special Surgery, New York, New York; Clinical Instructor, Weill Medical College, Cornell University, New York, New York

Michael Stuart, MD

Professor, Mayo Clinic College of Medicine, Rochester, Minnesota; Vice-Chairman, Department of Orthopedics, Co-Director, Sports Medicine Center, Mayo Clinic, Rochester, Minnesota

John Wrightson, MD

Pain Management Specialist, Regional Anesthesia Associates, New Castle, Pennsylvania

---

†deceased

Foreword

To go back to tradition is the first step forward.

—African saying

Modern medicine is a technological marvel. Remarkable advances in diagnosis and management of disease and injury utilizing sophisticated biochemical and biophysical tools bring great hope. Yet the practice of medicine cannot be equated with the application of technology; indeed, viewing medical practice only in these terms guarantees the inevitable misuse of these scientific advances. This fact is particularly true in the area of musculoskeletal medicine.

It is the art of our profession to match the patient with the best treatment available. A cogent history and skilled physical examination still remain the cornerstones of patient care. This foundation allows the physician to rationally choose diagnostic tests and treatment strategies.

Drs. Nadler and Malanga, along with their contributors, have crafted a textbook focusing on the musculoskeletal physical examination that clearly delivers this message. *Musculoskeletal Physical Examination: An Evidence-based Approach* critically examines the reliability and validity of the musculoskeletal examination, reminding the reader of the facts often forgotten or never initially learned in their entirety. Such lessons strengthen our fundamentally important examination skills and thereby improve our ability to properly care for our patients. Revisiting the past indeed better prepares us for the future. This text is an important and useful resource for the new physicians interested in orthopedic problems and no less of a valuable reminder for the practitioner with many years of experience.

Stanley A. Herring, MD
Clinical Professor
Departments of Orthopedics and
Rehabilitation Medicine
University of Washington Medical Center
Swedish Medical Center
Puget Sound Spine and Sports Physicians
Seattle, Washington

P reface

The idea for this book arose after working with residents and fellows and discovering the confusion that existed when discussing various physical examination maneuvers. One of these literature reviews involved the Yergason test, which was rather challenging to perform. On review, the Yergason test was found to be based on a single case report dating back to 1931. No validation of this physical examination test has been performed in the subsequent 72 years since it was originally described, and yet it has remained as one of the standard physical examination tests for the evaluation of bicipital tendinitis.

It became clear in reviewing test descriptions presented in lectures and textbooks, that the originally described test maneuvers had been altered over time. More disturbing was the fact that these altered tests were being taught by instructors to their students. It is reminiscent of the childhood game "telephone" where an initial statement is whispered around a room and the final statement is completely different from the original one. One can only imagine the confusion that occurs when this happens in medicine, which is exactly what we have found. Not only is there confusion, there is also misinterpretation of the clinical significance of these test maneuvers, which is compounded when they are not standardized. This has resulted in confusion in the medical literature, especially when attempting to demonstrate the scientific validity of these tests. We therefore feel strongly that when using an eponym for a test, such as McMurray's test, it should be performed and interpreted as originally described. Those instructors deemed qualified to teach these tests should be fluent not just in the technique but in the science behind the maneuver. This text has been written with that purpose in mind, and as such the reader will find the original description of the various test maneuvers and the scientific literature (if any) to support the test.

In a time where musculoskeletal conditions remain one of the most common reasons for a patient to see a physician, it is clear that exposure to musculoskeletal education is lacking. We hope this textbook clears up some of the misunderstanding surrounding the musculoskeletal physical examination and improves the clinician's ability to properly perform and interpret what is found.

Gerard A. Malanga, MD
Scott F. Nadler, DO
EDITORS

Introduction

An Evidence-based Approach to the Musculoskeletal Physical Examination

SCOTT F. NADLER, DO • GERARD A. MALANGA, MD

Musculoskeletal complaints represent one of the most common reasons for patient encounters with physicians.[8] This trend is likely to increase secondary to societal changes in health and fitness which has led our aging population to be more physically active than in years past.

Musculoskeletal injuries are diagnosed following a comprehensive history and physical examination. A poor history or physical examination may lead to inappropriate diagnostic testing and will influence patient outcome.[18] The history can quickly produce a more discrete differential diagnosis and includes the mechanism of injury, the quality, location, referral of pain, and the associated functional deficits. The fact that physical examination is not performed in a vacuum but in conjunction with the history needs to be stressed. The information gained from the history helps to focus the physical examination, especially if the physician has a good understanding of the underlying anatomy and biomechanics. Unfortunately, there appears to be a deficiency in education and research regarding the focus of this text, the musculoskeletal physical examination. The advent of more advanced diagnostic imaging has led to a change in the perception of the physical examination. In particular, magnetic resonance imaging (MRI) now provides excellent delineation of musculoskeletal pathology.

With the advent of MRI, many utilize this test as a replacement for the physical examination with the false perception that it gives a true picture of clinical diagnosis. Significant research has been performed to validate the use of MRI in the diagnosis of common musculoskeletal injury. Unfortunately, this is not the case with the physical examination. Simel and Rennie[16] found the lack of investment in improving our understanding of the clinical examination ironic, as much of the diagnostic testing performed would be unnecessary if more attention was paid to the clinical examination.

1

Over-reliance on imaging and other diagnostic studies can additionally result in improper diagnosis and unnecessary treatment. Multiple studies have demonstrated the incidence of MRI abnormalities in *normal* subjects. This has been reported in the spine,[7] the shoulder,[12] knee,[9] and other areas. LaPrade et al.[9] noted that 24% of normal individuals have findings consistent with grade II meniscal tears on MRI, and they recommended that clinicians match clinical signs and symptoms with MRI findings prior to surgical intervention. O'Shea et al.[13] noted that the correct diagnosis was made in 83% of patients utilizing the history and physical examination alone in the diagnosis of knee injuries. This, along with the significant findings on MRI in asymptomatic individuals, brings into question the need for MRI as part of a standard screen for musculoskeletal injury. It also highlights the importance of a properly performed clinical examination.

The physical examination of the musculoskeletal system is befuddled by a lack of research into the sensitivity and specificity for the disease processes that these tests are used to assess. Sackett and Rennie[15] noted that studies have been limited in regards to the physical exam, though the capability of reporting sensitivity, specificity, and predictive power would be similar to commonly studied laboratory tests. Reliability or reproducibility in regards to the translation of skills between the same or different clinicians at various time points during the course of disease is also poorly defined. Finally, there is no true gold standard by which to assess the validity of the different maneuvers, as even reported surgical pathology may be a normal anatomic or age-related change in a variety of disease processes. This does not imply that physical examination maneuvers should be abandoned, but rather they need to be more completely understood and, ultimately, refined. Unfortunately, these issues are not understood by clinicians in various specialties and disciplines, leading to a promulgation of myths rather than facts.

Another issue arises when clinicians fail to recognize the importance of using more than one examination maneuver to make their diagnosis. Andersson and Deyo[2] identified improved sensitivity, specificity, and positive predictive value with the utilization of combinations of tests rather than tests in isolation. Although this makes the scientific validation of any particular test challenging, it reinforces the fact that, when properly performed and used in combination, it can be a powerful clinical tool.[1,10,17] Clearly, improved understanding of the science behind physical examination maneuvers should be part of the evaluation of all clinicians in training and should be initiated at the outset of training rather then when these skills become difficult to change habits.

Education becomes an important issue when considering musculoskeletal physical examination.[3] Medical students and residents, especially those choosing primary care as a specialty, are poorly trained in the basics of diagnosis and treatment of musculoskeletal problems.[4,5] Freedman and Bernstein examined the basic competency of internal medicine residents and found 78% failed to demonstrate basic competency on a validated musculoskeletal examination with a criterion set by their program directors.[4] These authors had previously noted deficiencies in musculoskeletal knowledge using this same competency examination and noted better scores in residents who had rotated through orthopedics while in medical school.[5] Those who had rotated through rheumatology, physical medicine and rehabilitation, or neurology unfortunately did not have scores significantly different from those who did not rotate in these specialties. Even those that rotated through orthopedics scored lower than the recommended passing score. This suggests that there may be a problem with course content in addition to musculoskeletal exposure in medical school and residency education. Exposure to an outpatient orthopedics or physical medicine and rehabilitation rotation would appear to be beneficial to medical students, residents, and fellows. Mazzuca and Brandt[11] surveyed 271 rheumatology fellows regarding their experience in various aspects of musculoskeletal care; 60% desired more experience in non-operative sports medicine and indicated that they would have opted for a three-year fellowship.[11]

In addition to exposure to musculoskeletal problems, there are issues regarding the knowledge and experience of those who teach these skills. These educators need to have a broad knowledge base, which should include an understanding of the techniques as originally described, test limitations, and educational strategies to relay this information. Overall, the lack of proper training in the diagnosis and treatment of musculoskeletal problems is distressing given the high incidence of patient visits to primary care physicians for musculoskeletal complaints.

Proficiency in physical examination skills has not been extensively evaluated. Clinical competency can be measured in many different ways – including the use of traditional multiple choice tests, bedside assessment, and the objective structured clinical examination (OSCE). When a physical examination skill is taught or performed inaccurately, the result is inaccurate information that is communicated to patients, and poor examination skills that are disseminated to clinicians in training. Multiple-choice examination questions do not capture the hands-on skills required during physical exam. Bedside evaluation is probably the best assessment of examining skills, but unfortunately changes in healthcare leading to increased paperwork and patient load have resulted in less time to evaluate these skills at the bedside. Utilizing an OSCE format, Petrusa et al.[14] demonstrated excellent agreement (0.80) in evaluation of resident physical examination skills between patient and faculty evaluators. Utilizing the OSCE to assess inter-rater reliability of physical examination skills of the ankle, hand, knee, shoulder, and lower back, excellent reliability was demonstrated for examination of the lower back (0.837), good reliability for the knee (0.582) and hand (0.622), with fair agreement for the ankle (0.460) and shoulder (0.463).[6] Of interest, physical examination skills were later compared with the existing gold standard, the board certification examination results, and scores on the test poorly correlated with the physical examination skills of the lower back (0.15) and ankle (−0.64) and only fair agreement was demonstrated with shoulder examination skills (0.44).[6] This tells us that we need better ways to assess examination skills of individuals we are training, and that the current means of verifying competency (board certifying examinations) do not currently assess these skills.

Physical examination skills remain a vital part of the art of medicine which must be supported by as much science as possible. As such, they require proper instruction, practice, and feedback to ensure that they are done correctly. We must take a thoughtful look at the physical exam and ask some important questions. How, why, and what are we doing, and where are we going in regards to the educational needs of those learning these skills? This book was undertaken with the goal of improving not only the competency of musculoskeletal physical exam skills, but also understanding of the current exams that we perform in order to make them more valuable in the decision-making process. We hope that this text spurs interest in elaborating upon the reliability and validity of the existing musculoskeletal physical exam maneuvers. Potentially, utilizing a scientific approach that is supported by anatomic, biomechanical, and clinical validation, we may be able to develop more sensitive, specific, and reliable tests for the musculoskeletal physical examination.

REFERENCES

1. Ahern MJ, Scultz D, Soden M, Clark M. The musculoskeletal examination: a neglected clinical skill. Aust NZ J Med 1991;21:303–306.
2. Andersson GB, Deyo RA. History and physical examination in patients with herniated lumbar discs. Spine 1996;21(suppl. 24):10–18S.
3. Branch VK, Graves G, Hanczyc M, Lipsky PE. The utility of trained arthritis patient educators in the evaluation and improvement of musculoskeletal examination skills of physicians in training. Arthritis Care Res 1999;12(1):61–69.
4. Freedman KB, Bernstein J. Educational deficiencies in musculoskeletal medicine. J Bone Joint Surg 2002;84A:604–608.
5. Freedman KB, Bernstein J. The adequacy of medical school education in musculoskeletal medicine. J Bone Joint Surg 1998;80A:1421–1427.
6. Jain SS, DeLisa JA, Eyles MY, et al. Further experience in development of an objective structured clinical examination for physical medicine and rehabilitation residents. Am J Phys Med Rehabil 1998;77:306–310.
7. Jensen MC, Brant-Zawadzki MN, Obuchowski N, et al. Magnetic resonance imaging of the lumbar spine in people without back pain. N Engl J Med 1994;331:69–73.
8. Karpman RR. Musculoskeletal disease in the United States. Clin Orthop Rel Res 2001;385:52–56.
9. LaPrade RF, Burnett QM, Veenstra MA, Hodgman CG. The prevalence of abnormal magnetic resonance imaging findings in asymptomatic knees, with correlation of magnetic resonance imaging to arthroscopic findings in symptomatic knees. Am J Sports Med 1994;22:739–745.
10. Lawry GV, Schulat SS, Kreiter CD, et al. Teaching a screening musculoskeletal examination: a randomized, controlled trial of different instructional methods. Academic Med 1999;74:199–201.
11. Mazzuca SA, Brandt KD. Clinical rheumatology training in an uncertain future: opinions of recent and current rheumatology fellows about an extended fellowship in musculoskeletal medicine. Arthritis Rheum 1994;37:329–332.
12. Miniaci A, Dowdy PA, Willits KR, Vellet AD. Magnetic resonance imaging evaluation of the rotator cuff tendons in the asymptomatic shoulder. Am J Sports Med 1995;23:142–145.

13. O'Shea KJ, Murphy KP, Heekin RD, Herzwurm PJ. The diagnostic accuracy of history, physical examination, and radiographs in the evaluation of traumatic knee disorders. Am J Sports Med 1996;24:164–167.

14. Petrusa ER, Blackwell TA, Rogers LP, et al. An objective measure of clinical performance. Am J Med 1987;83:34–42.

15. Sackett DL, Rennie D. The science of the art of the clinical examination. JAMA 1992;267:2650–2652.

16. Simel DL, Rennie D. The clinical examination: an agenda to make it more rational. JAMA 1997;277:572–573.

17. Smith MD, Henry-Edwards S, Shanahan EM, Ahern MJ. Evaluation of patient partners in the teaching of the musculoskeletal examination. J Rheumatol 2000;27:1533–1537.

18. Solomon DH, Simel DL, Bates DW, Katz JN, Schaffer JL. The rational physical exam. Does this patient have a torn meniscus or ligament of the knee? Value of the physical examination. JAMA 2001;286:1610–1620.

Chapter 1

Reliability and Validity of Physical Examinations

LARRY H. CHOU, MD

Introduction

In 1880, John Venn, a priest and lecturer in Moral Science at Caius College, Cambridge University, England, introduced and popularized Venn diagrams (Figure 1–1).[7] Each circle represents a distinct domain that interacts with and is overlapped by other domains. The areas of overlap are more significant than the circles themselves, for within the overlapping areas "truth" can be found. While these diagrams were originally designed as models for mathematics and logic, they can also be used in the philosophy and practice of modern clinical medicine.

The "truth" in medicine represents the underlying diagnosis giving rise to a patient's symptoms and signs. In this version of the Venn diagram, the large circle represents a patient's relevant clinical history. It is the largest of the circles and where the majority of useful information can be found. Partially overlapping the patient's history is a smaller circle representing the physical examination. The exam substantiates

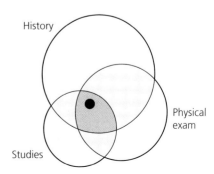

Figure 1–1. Venn diagram.

findings from the clinical history, but the non-overlapping area represents its ability to identify issues not uncovered in the patient's history. Lastly, the smallest circle represents additional clinical testing – whether laboratory, imaging, or electrophysiologic – that can further refine and confirm the true diagnosis denoted by the black dot. The true diagnosis lies within the clinical history, is supported by the physical examination, and is corroborated with other clinical studies.

In modern medicine, the bulk of clinical practice is predicated on the research question and the quality of support by which the question is answered. When critically reviewing the literature, it is paramount to understand these concepts. Indeed, an appreciation of the scientific method is necessary to fully understand the merits and pitfalls of the medical literature such that a conclusion can be properly applied to a specific clinical scenario. This chapter discusses the concepts of *validity* and *reliability*, how they give rise to sensitivity and specificity for diagnostic tests, and how the reported statistics of the various diagnostic tests should be interpreted in the clinical setting.

In contrast to observational cohort, case–control and cross-sectional studies, the evaluation of diagnostic tests is different. Most observational studies attempt to show an association between the test result (a predictor variable) and the disease. In contrast, diagnostic studies attempt to discriminate between the diseased and the non-diseased. It is insufficient to merely identify an association between the test result and the disease.[2] The concepts of specificity and sensitivity as well as positive and negative predictive value are discussed here.

Validity

Validity represents the truth, whether it be deduced, inferred, or supported by data. There are two types of validity: internal and external.[3] *Internal validity* is the degree to which the results and conclusions from a research study correctly represent the data that was measured in the study. That is, the truth in the study can be correctly explained by the results of the study. However, it is important to recognize that this may not correctly answer the clinical question at hand. While a conclusion can be properly reached based on the available study findings, if the question asked or methods used are incorrect, then meaningful interpretation of the results is suspect. Once internal validity issues are satisfied, then the greater issue is that of external validity.

External validity is the degree to which the internal validity conclusions can be generalized to situations outside of the study. This is the *sine qua non* of meaningful clinical research. That is, can the conclusion of a study that has correctly interpreted its results be used *outside* of that specific research setting? The variables designed in a study must correctly represent the phenomena of interest. A research study that is so contrived or so artificially over-simplified to a degree that does not exist in the real world clinical setting is of guarded value.

Errors in study design and measurement tools will greatly affect validity. How well a measurement represents a phenomenon is influenced by two major sources of error: sampling error and measurement error. In order for a study to be generalizable, the study population needs to parallel the target population. That is, the inclusion criteria for entrance into the study must represent the clinical characteristics and demographics of the population for which the study is intended. The sample size needs to be sufficiently large to avoid bias and increase power (see below). It is important to recognize that reporting errors can also occur, though these should be, and often are, identified in the peer review process.

Likewise, measurement errors need to be avoided so that valid conclusions can be drawn from the results. This brings up the concept of the accuracy and precision (see below) of a measurement. Accuracy is the degree to which the study measurement reflects the actual measurement. In other words, accuracy represents the validity of the study, whether internal or external. Greater accuracy increases the validity of the study.

Accuracy is influenced by systematic errors or bias. Limiting consistent distortion from the observer, subject, or instrument reduces accuracy. Observer distortion is a systematic error on the part of the observer in data gathering or reporting data. Subject bias refers to the consistent distortion of the facts as recalled or perceived by the subject. Instrument bias results from an error in the measurement device, either by malfunctioning or inappropriate usage for a study purpose for which it was not designed. Comparing the measurement to a reference standard best assesses accuracy.

Reliability

Reliability, and the related concept of precision, represents the reproducibility of a test. A test is considered reliable if repeated measurements consistently produce similar results. These results do not need to be compared to a reference standard. Precision refers to the uniformity and consistency of the repeated measurement. It is affected by random error whereby the greater the error, the lower the precision.[5]

The three primary sources of precision error are observer, subject, and instrument variability. Observer variability is dependent on the observer in gathering data points, whereas subject variability refers to innate differences within the subject population that can contribute to errors. Instrument variability is affected by environmental factors.

Research studies on diagnostic tests are inherently susceptible to random errors.[2] Patients with positive findings may not have the disease by chance alone, and vice versa. Because random errors are difficult to control, confidence intervals for sensitivity and specificity should be reported. Confidence intervals allow for the possibility of random errors given the study's sample size. The ranges of these confidence intervals are perhaps even more important than the actual sensitivity and specificity score. Standard deviations are typically used to describe precision.

The degree of concordance between paired measurements is usually expressed as a correlation coefficient (R) or as a kappa statistic (κ). The correlation coefficient is a number between −1 and +1. The absolute value indicates the strength of correlation, where 0 is poor and 1 is high; i.e., very precise. Various tests can be employed including the Pearson coefficient, where values are evaluated directly, and the Spearman rank test, where values are placed in rank order and then analyzed.

Reliability measurements need to be observed for test–retest, internal, and inter-observer and intra-observer consistency. The test–retest reliability refers to the concordance among repeated measurements on a sample of subjects. Caution must be exercised especially with physical exam maneuvers, since the test itself can create errors, by factors such as the training effect and learning curve. Internal consistency indicates that separate measures of the same variable will have internal concordance. Intra-observer consistency indicates that repeated measurements by a single observer are reproducible whereas inter-observer measurements are reproducible by separate observers of the same event.

Precision strongly influences the power of a study.[5] A more precise measurement lends greater statistical power. Power is the probability of rejecting the null hypothesis when it is in fact false. The null hypothesis suggests there is no association between the two variables in question. The power depends on the total number of end-points experienced by a population. By increasing the sample size, the power will increase.[4] This will also decrease the probability that the null hypothesis will be incorrectly accepted.

Validity and reliability are not necessarily linked nor are they mutually exclusive. Although high accuracy and precision are ideal within a given test, unfortunately this is not often the case. It is possible to have high accuracy yet low precision, and vice versa (Figure 1–2).

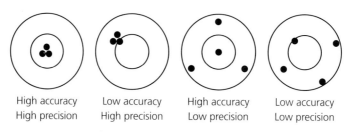

High accuracy   Low accuracy   High accuracy   Low accuracy
High precision   High precision Low precision   Low precision

Figure 1–2. Accuracy and precision.

Specificity and Sensitivity

As mentioned previously, the outcome variable of a diagnostic test is the presence or absence of disease or injury, when compared to the ideal reference standard known as the "gold standard." By convention, the gold standard is always positive in patients with the disease and negative in those without the disease. However, in the clinical setting, even the gold standard has its limitations and is not impervious to error. Generally, the quality and efficacy of a diagnostic test is obtained by calculating its sensitivity and specificity.

The outcome variable of a diagnostic test falls into one of four situations (Table 1-1):

a. A true-positive result, where the test is positive for the patient who has the disease

b. A false-positive result, where the test is positive, but the patient does not have the disease

c. A false-negative result, where the test is negative, but the patient has the disease

d. A true-negative result, where the test is negative for the patient who does not have the disease.

Ideally, the best diagnostics tests have no false-positives or false-negatives. Sensitivities and specificities are unlinked and should not affect one other. It is possible to have any combination of sensitivities and specificities – high sensitivity with high or low specificity, and vice versa. The utility of a test with both low sensitivity and specificity has dubious value.

The sensitivity of a test represents how good it is at identifying disease. Andersson et al.[1] used the mnemonic SnNout. If *Sen*sitivity is *high*, a *N*egative test result rules *out* the target diagnosis. It is calculated by the proportion of patients with the disease who have a positive test:

$$\text{Sensitivity} = \text{True positive}/[\text{True positive} + \text{False negative}]$$
$$= (a)/[(a) + (c)].$$

Table 1–1. CALCULATING SPECIFICITY AND SENSITIVITY

		Disease State	
		Present	**Absent**
Test result	Positive	(a) True positive	(b) False positive
	Negative	(c) False negative	(d) True negative
		(a) + (c) = 100%	(b) + (d) = 100%

Specificity, on the other hand, represents how good a test is at identifying those patients without disease. Using Andersson's mnemonic, SpPin, if **Sp**ecificity is *high*, a **P**ositive test result rules **in** the target diagnosis. It is calculated as the proportion of patients without the disease who have a negative test:

$$\text{Specificity} = \text{False positive}/[\text{False positive} + \text{True negative}]$$
$$= (d)/[(b) + (d)].$$

In the chapter on knee examinations (Chapter 9), various physical exam maneuvers are used to assess the integrity of the anterior cruciate ligament. Using arthroscopy as the gold standard, the Lachman test was 81.8% sensitive and 96.8% specific, the pivot shift was 81.8% sensitive and 98.4% specific, while the anterior drawer sign was only 40.9% sensitive yet 95.2% specific.[6] With the high sensitivities of the Lachman and the pivot shift test, a negative result on physical examination essentially rules out an ACL tear. Likewise, with the high specificities, a positive finding on the Lachman, pivot shift, and anterior drawer likely rules in the diagnosis. The low sensitivity of the anterior drawer test indicates that it is suboptimal at diagnosing ACL-deficient knees. Although this study was published in 1986, it is unclear why the anterior drawer test is still one of the most beloved tests of the ACL in clinical practice.

Positive and Negative Predictive Values

Once the specificity and sensitivity of a test is established, the predictive value of a positive test versus a negative test can be determined if the prevalence of the disease is known. When the prevalence of a disease increases, a patient with a positive test is more likely to have the disease. It is therefore less likely for that test to represent a false-negative. A negative result of a highly sensitive test will probably rule out a common disease. Conversely, however, if a disease is rare, the test must be much more specific for it to be clinically useful.

Predictive values are especially clinically relevant since they utilize information on both the test itself and the population being tested. This introduces the concept of prior probabilities, which is essentially the prevalence of a disease in a single test subject. Prior probability is determined based on the subject's demographics and clinical presentation. Unfortunately, delineating these values on a single subject in order to calculate the positive predictive value in a population of patients is difficult. The calculation for positive predictive value (PV), which is beyond the scope of this chapter, is provided by Bayes' theorem:

$$\text{Positive PV} = \text{Likelihood of a true-positive}/[\text{Likelihood of a true-positive} + \text{Likelihood of a false-positive}]$$

Summary

Correctly analyzing and interpreting conclusions is the cornerstone of modern medical practice. The use of the clinical history, substantiation with the clinical exam, and corroboration with clinical studies to diagnose a patient is predicated on the available scientific studies in the literature. The physical exam requires not only knowledge of how to perform a specific maneuver and its nuances, but also knowledge of how the results of a specific test support or challenge a given diagnosis. The reliability and validity of a particular diagnostic exam maneuver will establish the sensitivity and specificity statistics. Understanding the scientific method of a particular study and how its results can be applied to the community at large is critical.

REFERENCES

1. Andersson GB, Deyo RA. History and physical examination in patients with herniated lumbar discs. Spine 1996;21(suppl. 24):10–18S.
2. Browner WS, Newman TB, Cummings SR. Designing a new study. III: Diagnostic tests. In Hulley SB, Cummings SR (eds), Designing Clinical Research. Baltimore: Williams & Wilkins, 1988, pp. 87–97.
3. Hulley SB, Newman TB, Cummings SR. Getting started: the anatomy and physiology of research. In Hulley SB, Cummings SR (eds), Designing Clinical Research. Baltimore: Williams & Wilkins, 1988, pp. 1–11.
4. Hulley SB, Gove S, Browner WS, et al. Choosing the study subjects: specification and sampling. In Hulley SB, Cummings SR (eds), Designing Clinical Research. Baltimore: Williams & Wilkins, 1988, pp. 18–30.
5. Hulley SB, Cummings SR. Planning the measurements: precision and accuracy. In Hulley SB, Cummings SR (eds), Designing Clinical Research. Baltimore: Williams & Wilkins, 1988, pp. 31–41.
6. Katz JW, Fingeroth RJ. The diagnostic accuracy of ruptures of the anterior cruciate ligament comparing the Lachman test, the anterior drawer sign, and the pivot shift test in acute and chronic knee injuries. Am J Sports Med 1986;14(1):88–91.
7. Venn J. On the diagrammatic and mechanical representation of propositions and reasonings. Philosoph Magazine J Sci S 1880;9(59) July:1–18.

Chapter **2**

Sensory, Motor, and Reflex Examination

SCOTT F. NADLER, DO • LUKE RIGOLOSI, MD •
DANIEL KIM, MD • JENNIFER SOLOMON, MD

Introduction

The neurological examination is one of the most unique exercises in all of clinical medicine. Whereas the history is the most important element in defining the clinical problem, the neurological examination localizes a lesion within the central or peripheral nervous systems (CNS, PNS). Utilizing the patients' subjective complaints of sensory loss or weakness is neither sensitive nor specific for any neurologically based condition, though it may help better focus the actual examination. At the same time, clinicians must not get hung up on the textbook examples of motor, sensory, and reflex changes with nerve injury. More often than not, a patchy distribution of findings is appreciated, and the clinician is left to the art of rationale thinking in piecing together an appropriate differential diagnosis. The sensory, motor, and reflex examination will be discussed in detail to improve the overall understanding of each component and their potential pitfalls.

Sensory Testing

Evaluation of the sensory system involves an understanding of the entire peripheral and central sensory pathways from the skin to the thalamus. Light touch, deep pressure, pain, temperature, vibration, and proprioception can be assessed during the clinical evaluation. Understanding the intricate pathways that make up the sensory system allows the clinician to differentiate an injury involving a peripheral nerve from that involving the spinothalamic tracts of the spinal cord or the somatosensory cortex of the brain. In most clinical settings, sensory testing is performed through assessment of light touch and pinprick. The various sensory modalities have been elucidated over the past centuries. Cardano and Ingrassia initially described vibratory sense in the sixteenth century; this was further defined by Rinne (1864) and Rumpf (1889).[25,57,60,61] Proprioception was defined by Bell in 1826 who recognized what he termed "a sixth sense."[5,25] Brown-Sequard (1852) and Edinger (1889) in the late nineteenth century and van Gehuchten (1908) in the early twentieth century clarified the sensory pathways of pain, temperature, and position sense with the spinal cord.[9,25,27] Temperature sensation was initially utilized in the late nineteenth century. Jean-Martin Charcot (1887) used a thermometer that could be heated or cooled and placed on the patient's skin. Gowers (1888) reported that "hot and cold spoons may be employed; for ascertaining the power of differential discrimination."[25,28] Gowers noted that sensibility to cold was least on the epigastrium and sensibility to heat was least on the back, whereas heat and cold had the greatest sensitivity on the knee.[25,28]

Gowers (1888) also described the tactile sensory exam. He indicated that "in examining the tactile sensibility, it is important to ascertain, not only whether the patient can feel, but whether he is able to recognize the place touched."[25,28] The pinprick test was described by Holmes (1927), who found it useful for localization.[25,33] Weber (1846) described the two-point discrimination test in which he used a compass to determine whether patients could differentiate two simultaneously applied stimuli to the skin.[25,69] Henry Head (1900) provided the initial map of the human dermatomes using patients with herpes zoster and matching their specific spinal nerve roots.[25,32]

By 1955, the sensory examination became much like the examination used today, with tests for light touch, vibration, position sense, pinprick, temperature, and two-point discrimination.[25] A dermatome is an area of skin innervated by one spinal cord segment. On the trunk of the body, there are relatively distinct bands of skin that are sequentially innervated from the region of the shoulders down to the perineum (Figure 2–1). These bands of skin encircle the torso (both ventrally and dorsally), but within that band, all the sensory fibers still reach the same spinal cord segment via the same dorsal root. However, when it comes to the dermatome arrangement of the upper and lower extremities, the pattern is more complicated. There is still a reasonably distinct arrangement, but it is no longer a circular band on each side. There are still areas of skin innervated by one spinal cord segment, but the pattern is distorted for two main reasons: rotation of the limbs during development, and the presence of a nerve plexus between the spinal cord and the skin on the extremities.

Sherrington first delineated dermatomal sensory maps in the late 1890s in monkeys.[63] He noted an overlaying of dermatomes of more than one nerve root and individual variations.[63] Head and Campbell (1900) examined dermatomal involvement in patients with herpes zoster. They noted that the seventh cervical nerve root

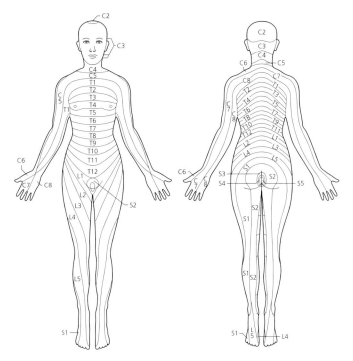

Figure 2–1. Dermatomal map.

received sensory inputs from digits I and II and the eighth cervical first thoracic nerve roots from digit V.[32] Inouye and Buchthal recorded evoked potentials from C5 to C8 just outside the intervertebral foramen after stimulation of various peripheral nerves and digits. They found dermatomal distributions that were consistent with previous research, although they noted considerable individual variability.[35] They also noted that pain testing was more sensitive and specific than light touch testing. An interesting study by Dick correlated abnormalities of cutaneous sensation with clinical and quantitative measures.[17] He found that clinical testing was better than quantitative measurement tools for thermal discrimination but nonetheless underestimated touch-pressure deficits. Quantitative testing was additionally more sensitive for pain sensation with statistically significant differences only detected for sensation of the feet. Sensory changes alone, however, are not sufficient to make any specific diagnoses. Kosteljanetz et al. demonstrated a specificity of only 18% in using reports of sensory change in individuals with lumbar disc injury[40] and in using numbness or paresthesias to predict the level of disc injury. McCombe et al. found the interobserver agreement for sensory deficit in patients with low back pain to be good with $\kappa = 0.68$.[51] Kosteljanetz et al. and Kortelainen et al. noted sensitivities of 66% and 38%, respectively, with regards to the sensory examination in lumbar disc herniation.[39,41]

Kosteljanetz et al. also noted a specificity of only 51% in the same population.[41] Overall, the area of sensory loss was a poor predictor in localizing lumbar disc herniations.[39,41] Using Semmes Weinstein pressure thresholds of more than 15 mg/mm and vibratory thresholds of more than 3.5 µm in individuals with lumbar disc herniations, Weise et al. was able to localize disc injuries in 100% of patients using the former and 88% of patients using the latter test.[70]

Two-point discrimination has been demonstrated to reliably identify those with peripheral nerve injury. Dellon et al. noted an interobserver variability to vary less than 1 mm for moving two-point discrimination in 93.3% of subjects and 86.6% for static two-point discrimination.[15] Hayes et al. evaluated reliability of sensory screening in 33 patients with incomplete spinal cord injury compared to 14 normal controls.[31] Quantitative sensory testing (QST) measures for perceptual threshold for temperature and vibration as well as the American Spinal Cord Injury Association sensory scores for light touch and pinprick were assessed. There was a low degree of association between QST and sensory scores (κ = 0.05–0.44). QST was felt to be more sensitive to detect sensory loss than standard sensory testing.[31]

Overall, the sensitivity, specificity, and reliability for the sensory examination is poorly described in the peer-reviewed literature except for mention in the diagnosis of various disease entities involving sensory loss such as in peripheral neuropathies. In this day and age, comparisons between the sensory examination and more complex diagnostic testing are more common, especially QST and nerve conduction testing.

Motor Testing

Strength is a reflection of peripheral neuromuscular function, and is generally tested by manual muscle testing. Manual muscle testing was first described by Dr Robert Lovett in 1912 as a method of following the progress of "infantile paralysis," more commonly known as poliomyelitis. This led to the utilization of muscle testing as an outcome measure in therapeutic trials. From these early days of muscle strength assessment, manual muscle testing (MMT) became the standard of force production evaluation.

Classification systems for MMT grade on some variation of the Medical Research Council 0–5 point scale.[53] This ranges from no palpable muscular contraction to full ability to resist the examiner throughout the entire range of motion.[14,38,53] Each system specifies patient testing position, examiner positioning to maximize patient stabilization and minimize substitution of agonist muscles, the force vector for examiner resistance, and a corresponding grading scheme describing the examiner's results. The grading systems for MMT all produce ordinal data with unequal rankings between grades. The near-normal range is examiner subjective, because this requires the examiner to assess the amount of force resisted as minimal, moderate, or maximum before the patient's isometric contraction is "broken." This becomes problematic in clinical trials, because conclusions are drawn based on the increase or decrease in subjective measurements. Thus, there is a need for muscle testing equipment that quantifies force production.

Quantitative muscle testing (QMT) produces interval data that describe force production. QMT is composed of isometric muscle testing (IMT), which measures maximum force production at a specific joint angle, and isokinetic muscle testing (IKT), which measures maximum torque and work across a joint as it goes through its range of motion. Isokinetic testing requires large, expensive, and specific pieces of testing equipment. For the purposes of this review, IKT testing has proven to be reliable in the majority of studies but will not be addressed further.[12,19,44,59] Isometric muscle testing uses equipment such as handheld dynamometers (HHD) and utilizes the same testing positions as those in MMT. HHD are less expensive and often portable. The interval data produced by QMT is a continuous scale with a full range of grades that describe the amount of force produced by a muscle contraction.

The primary tenet of MMT is that each muscle should be tested just proximal to the next distal joint of the muscle's insertion. This will allow for the maximal lever arm and torque, giving the examiner a biomechanical advantage.[38] For example, the biceps brachii should be tested with resistance applied to just proximal to the wrist, with the elbow at 90 degrees. The examiner must place the subject in positions that will isolate, as much as possible, the specific muscle or muscles being examined and eliminate substitution of agonist muscles.

Regardless of the type of muscle testing used, the procedure is innately subjective and depends on the subject's ability to exert a maximal contraction. Factors such as pain, motivation, cooperation, fatigue, instruction, and fear potentially magnify the subjectivity of muscle testing. Issues that may impact upon the results of muscle testing include patient comprehension of the testing procedure which makes assurance of maximum contraction questionable, and age. Escolar et al.[21] showed increased variability in the younger population, whereas Barr et al.[3] demonstrated increased variability in older patients as well as younger patients. These factors cannot be excluded from muscle testing and should be considered when reliability studies are conducted on these patient populations.

Neuromuscular diseases manifest with a decrease in muscle strength, and the importance of following muscle strength in these subjects cannot be overestimated. MMT is used as an indicator of disease progression and a measure of response to specific interventions. MMT also allows healthcare professionals to share a common language and methodology in which to evaluate and discuss patients. This is especially important when analyzing results of therapeutic trials.

Reliability of Manual Muscle Testing

Multiple studies have shown good inter-tester and intra-tester reliability with MMT and a high degree of exact consistency to within one grade using some form of the Medicine Research Council's grading sequence.[53] It is commonly acknowledged that good reliability is demonstrated by an intraclass correlation coefficient (ICC) of greater than 0.75 or consistency between examiners greater than 75%. Results outside of this range are generally considered inconsistent. The same grade or within one grade (i.e., 3+ to 4−) is generally considered reliable. Protocols for investigating neuromuscular disease have traditionally used MMT as the mechanism for studying muscle force production. Pretrial testing sessions for the examiners have been utilized by many studies, which have documented good inter-tester reliability in MMT.[3,6,8,23,24,30,42,43] This allows the examiners to have a well-defined grading scheme and established test positions for each muscle. Isolating specific individual muscles or muscle groups across a joint and minimizing substitution will allow examiners to maximize consistency. This is best performed with use of a training session prior to initiating patient testing.

Lilienfeld et al. and Iddings et al. showed MMT to be highly reliable.[34,43] Lilienfeld and colleagues used three to five examiners who graded muscle strength with a descriptive scale: normal, good, fair, poor, trace, and zero following a pretrial training period.[43] Inter-examiner reliability was found to be 70% when testing individual or groups of muscles. Inter-examiner reliability increased to 95% when including a border range (i.e., plus or minus one grade). When adding all muscles tested, the difference between examiners was found to be 3%.

Iddings did not initiate training sessions prior to testing because he felt that experienced therapists over time develop various techniques and standards of their own for grading strength.[34] In this study, nine examiners tested the same subject with post-poliomyelitis. Inter-examiner reliability was found to be 48%, but when including plus or minus one grade variability the reliability increased to 91% when individual muscle testing was analyzed. The difference in total muscle scores among all therapists was approximately 4%. Intra-tester reliability was 65%, and 97% with the addition of plus or minus one grade for individual muscle testing. The use of plus or minus grades of strength inflated inter- and intra-examiner reliability; however, it results in much less specificity and sensitivity.[34]

In 1981, Brooke investigated the reliability of MMT in subjects with Duchenne muscular dystrophy.[8] He defined a system to track disease progression by examining range of motion, functional capabilities, and MMT. Testing was continuously monitored through a central computerized system. This allowed evaluators to monitor for centers that were producing inconsistent data. Reliability ranged from 48% to 98% within one grade, and utilizing this feedback system, the reliability of the study increased over time.

Mulroy et al. investigated the maximum examiner (female and male) resistance force versus the maximum quadriceps force in subjects (female and male) with post-poliomyelitis.[54] This study utilized a handheld device to determine the maximal forces of both examiner and subject, and determined the range of knee extension forces in normal males and females. Reliability of 79% was demonstrated within one grade of MMT in subjects with post-poliomyelitis. However, examiners regardless of gender did produce enough force to detect mild to moderate decreases in strength of normal patients.[54] These results indicate that MMT is sufficient when monitoring disease states that are outside of the normal range, but, in normal subjects, mild differences were indistinguishable. This study advocated examiner self-calibration in which examiners determined their own push capability, allowing them to estimate the amount of muscle weakness they would be capable of detecting.

Florence et al. conducted a study in which 18 muscle groups were examined in subjects with Duchenne muscular dystrophy.[23] Reliability of grades for individual muscle groups using κ values ranged from 0.65 to 0.93. When individual muscles were investigated as opposed to muscle groups, a higher κ value of 0.80 to 0.99 was demonstrated in proximal muscles. Manual muscle testing is thus most reliable when performed by the same examiner on individual muscles as opposed to muscle groups. Florence et al. investigated both inter-observer and intra-observer reliability in a study of subjects with Duchenne's. A total of 34 muscles were graded on a modified MRC scale, grading strength from 0 to 10. The intra-observer ICC was 0.95 and the inter-observer ICC was 0.90. The percentage consistency (within one grade) ranged from 83% to 93% between any two of four examiners.[24]

Controversies in MMT

One of the two major criticisms of MMT is the subjectivity in the grade 4 strength measurement. Grade 4 strength encompasses the ability of a patient to go through full range of motion against gravity with no, little, or overwhelming examiner resistance. It is difficult for examiners of different strengths and sizes to exactly agree on grade 4 strength, as it requires them to assign an ordinal number to a subjective evaluation of resistance offered by the patient. Investigators have dealt with this controversy in different ways. Brooke et al. emphasized the use of a reference muscle with a strength of 4, differing in the upper and lower extremities. In the upper extremity, either the elbow flexors or shoulder abductors that are grade 4 are chosen; while in the lower extremities, the hip flexors and knee extensors are utilized. The muscles in the 4 range are then compared to that reference muscle and given a grade of "S" for stronger than that reference muscle or "W" for weaker than that reference muscle. These 4S and 4W categories are not equivalent to 4+ and 4−, but rather they are a way of defining muscle strength in the subnormal range that allows for increased consistency between examiners. This is felt to enhance the reliability of MMT in clinical trials.[8]

Florence et al.[23] suggested that the subjectivity in the 3+ range can be largely due to day-to-day variability as opposed to examiner inconsistency. Intra-tester reliability measured in a population of Duchenne's muscular dystrophy patients with a grade of 3+ had the lowest reliability coefficient. In this range, the muscle is capable of providing transient resistance but collapses suddenly. It was speculated that this range of strength exists as a transitional state and that the discrepancy in grading may be secondary to a real daily performance fluctuation.

Studies that compare the reliability of MMT and QMT often come to the conclusion that MMT may be consistent and reliable, but it is unable to detect subtle differences in strength.[6,54,67] This detracts from the ability of MMT to detect minimal asymmetry or differences in muscle strength at separate examinations. Andres et al.[2] showed a correlation coefficient of 0.77 between examiners performing MMT in a population of subjects with amyotrophic lateral sclerosis. In this study, there was considerable variation within a MMT grade when compared to grading by a strain-gauge isometric muscle testing (IMT) device. A grade of normal in MMT for shoulder flexion had a correlating IMT contraction score that varied over 55%. This supports the concept that MMT results are more consistent, whereas the variation produced by QMT will appreciate differences in strength undetectable in MMT.

The other major criticism of MMT is the overestimation of strength when a muscle is weak as identified by QMT, yet it is graded as normal by MMT. Bohannon[6] and Beasley[4] confirmed the overestimation of knee extensor strength using MMT as compared to a handheld dynamometer. A MMT grade of 5 does not necessarily correlate with a "100%" theoretical percentage as described in Kendall's definition of MMT grading.[38] A theoretical percentage score based on MMT is likely to grossly overestimate the strength of a patient. Beasley[4] showed that 50% of knee extensor strength needed to be lost before MMT was able to identify weakness. Griffin et al.[29] had similar findings when evaluating IKT and MMT in knee flexion and extension, demonstrating the value of IKT when MMT has improved to levels considered normal.

Wadsworth et al.[68] had similar conclusions in their comparison of MMT and isometric testing with a handheld dynamometer (HHD). They found test–retest reliability coefficients for MMT in the 0.63–0.98 range, whereas the HHD had reliability coefficients in the 0.69–0.90 range. MMT generated reliable results in this setting, but its accuracy must be questioned, as it did not have the ability to detect differences in strength in two muscle groups that were differentiated by HHD.

Many examiners have shown that reliability in MMT is dependent on the specific muscle being examined. Lawson et al.[42] performed a study using applied kinesiology with a grading system confined to "strong" and "weak" grades. Three clinicians tested the piriformis and the knee flexors of 32 healthy individuals, and the pectoralis and tensor fascia lata of 53 healthy individuals. They found significant agreement in strength assessment of the piriformis and pectoralis, but no agreement in that of the knee flexors or the tensor fascia lata, even with a grading scheme consisting of only two grades. Florence et al.[23] found higher reliability in the proximal muscles as opposed to the distal muscles. Barr et al.[3] found varying reliability depending on the region or group of muscles tested. The proximal muscles (ICC = 0.8) demonstrated improved reliability as compared to the distal muscles (ICC = 0.58). In addition, the upper-body muscles (ICC = 0.87) were found to be more reliably tested than the lower-body ones (ICC = 0.66). Further research is necessary to support these various claims.

In conclusion, the reliability of MMT is dependent on the muscle groups being studied. Manual muscle testing is not able to detect mild to moderate weakness, depending on the muscle group and examiner strength. The accuracy of MMT may be in question, though reliability between examiners is not affected. Quantitative muscle testing is of no added benefit over MMT in weakened states, but it will contribute accurate information in patients with undetected weakness and therefore can be a useful tool for tracking early neuromuscular disease progression and recovery. Further investigation into the accuracy and reliability of MMT needs to be conducted.

Reflex Testing

Concepts of animal automatism and reflex action were first established by Rene Descartes (1596–1650) in the early seventeenth century.[16,46] Observations of the salient physiological features of stretching muscle fibers were made by Robert Whytt in 1763 who stated that:

> whatever stretches the fibres of any muscle so far as to extend them beyond their usual length, excites them into contraction in about the same manner, as if they had been irritated by a sharp instrument, or acrid liquor.[58,71]

The concept of an anatomically and physiologically distinct sensorimotor reflex arc did not evolve until the early nineteenth century, with the work of the English physician Marshall Hall (1790–1857) in animals after removal of the brain.[30,46] The importance of the muscle stretch reflexes were noted at approximately the same time by Wilhelm Heinrich Erb (1840–1921) and Carl Friedrich Otto Westphal (1833–1890) in 1875, but only Erb correctly regarded the phenomenon as a true reflex arc.[20,46] In 1883, Erno Jendrassik reported that having the patient "hook together the flexed fingers of his right and left hands and pull them apart as strongly as possible" while the clinician taps on the tendon enhances the reflexes of a normal patient. This has been termed the *Jendrassik maneuver* and is the most common method of reinforcing reflexes, since reflexes may be difficult to elicit in normal subjects owing to global hypoexcitability of ventral horn motor neurons.[36,52,62] The Jendrassik maneuver was originally thought to enhance fusimotor drive, but it is now thought to reflect a direct excitatory effect on the alpha motor neurons, following studies by Bussel and Burke.[10,11]

Tendon reflex activity and muscle tone depend on the status of the large motor neurons of the anterior horn (the alpha motor neurons), the muscle spindles with their afferent fibers, and the small anterior horn cells (gamma neurons) whose axons terminate on the small intrafusal muscle fibers within the spindles. Beta motor neurons effect co-contraction of both spindle and non-spindle fibers, but the significance of this physiologic phenomenon is not fully understood. Some of the gamma neurons are tonically active at rest, keeping the intrafusal (nuclear chain) muscle fibers taut and sensitive to active and passive changes in muscle length. A tap on a tendon stretches the spindle and activates its nuclear bag fibers; afferent projections from these fibers synapse with alpha motor neurons in the same and adjacent spinal segments. They, in turn, send impulses to the skeletal muscle fibers, producing the familiar brief muscle contraction or monophasic (myostatic) stretch reflex (Figure 2–2). All this occurs within 25 milliseconds of stretch. The alpha neurons of antagonist muscles are simultaneously inhibited, but through disynaptic rather than monosynaptic connections.

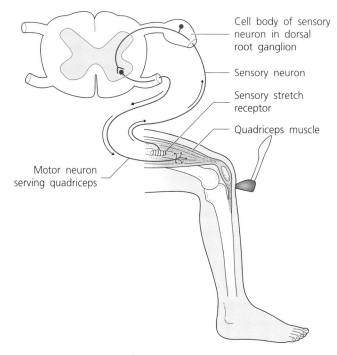

Cell body of sensory neuron in dorsal root ganglion

Sensory neuron

Sensory stretch receptor

Quadriceps muscle

Motor neuron serving quadriceps

Figure 2–2. Reflex arc.

Mainly, this is accomplished through the Renshaw cells, which are stimulated by recurrent collateral branches from alpha motor neurons. In turn, Renshaw cell axons end on inhibitory synapses of alpha motor neurons (recurrent inhibition). Thus, the setting of the spindle fibers and the state of excitability of the alpha and gamma neurons (influenced greatly by descending fiber systems) determine the level of activity of the tendon reflexes and the responsiveness of muscle to stretch.

Other mechanisms, of an inhibitory nature, involve the Golgi tendon organs, for which the stimulus is tension produced by active contraction of muscle. These encapsulated receptors, which lie in the tendinous and aponeurotic insertions of muscle, activate afferent fibers that end on internuncial cells, which, in turn, project to alpha motor neurons, thus forming a disynaptic reflex arc. They are silent in relaxed muscle and during passive stretch, serving with muscle spindles to monitor or calibrate the length and force of contraction under different conditions.

The large neurons of the anterior horns of the spinal cord contain high concentrations of choline acetyltransferase and utilize acetylcholine as their transmitter. Glycine is the neurotransmitter released by Renshaw cells, which are responsible for recurrent inhibition, and by interneurons that mediate reciprocal inhibition during reflex action. There are also descending cholinergic, adrenergic, and dopaminergic axons, which play a less well defined role in reflex functions, but both alpha and gamma motor neurons are influenced by descending fiber systems from supraspinal levels.[1]

Although muscle stretch reflexes are often called "deep tendon reflexes," this name is a misnomer because tendons have little to do with the response other than being responsible for mechanically transmitting the sudden stretch from the reflex hammer to the muscle spindle. In addition, some muscles with stretch reflexes have no tendons (e.g., "jaw jerk" of the masseter muscle).[52]

Common muscle stretch reflexes that are tested are the brachioradialis and biceps (C5–C6), triceps (C7–C8), quadriceps or patellar (L3–L4), and Achilles or ankle (S1).[17] The medial hamstring reflex has been shown to be mainly innervated by the L5 and S1 roots; and, in the presence of symmetrically active gastrocsoleus reflexes, asymmetry of the medial hamstring reflexes indicates an L5 root lesion.[22] Jensen evaluated the medial hamstring reflex in 52 hospitalized patients with a suspected lumbar nerve root compression syndrome.[37] The patient was placed in the supine position with the knee semiflexed and supported with one of the examiner's hands. The ipsilateral hip was also slightly flexed, externally rotated, and abducted. The medial hamstring reflex was then elicited by using a reflex hammer to strike the index finger of the supporting hand placed on the tendons of the medial hamstrings. An abnormal medial hamstring reflex as a sign of L4/L5 disc herniation affecting the L5 nerve root was found to have a positive predictive value of 85–89% and a negative predictive value of 51–61%, and it is therefore recommended to include the medial hamstring reflex in the neurological examination of patients with a suspected lumbar disc protrusion.[37] In a study by Malanga and Campagnolo,[48] a Teca reflex hammer was used to produce the pronator muscle stretch reflex, and standard bar surface recording EMG electrodes were placed over the muscle belly of the pronator quadratus and pronator teres in 10 healthy subjects. Because the location of the pronator teres and pronator quadratus is relatively superficial, surface EMG electrodes effectively demonstrated the muscle activation in this reflex. Subjects were tested with their arms resting comfortably on a table in the seated position. After placing the elbow in approximately 90 degrees of flexion with the forearm in a neutral position, the reflex was elicited by a gentle tapping on the medial aspect of the distal radius. A reproducible response was found in all patients when recordings were made over the pronator teres, and no response was found in any of the subjects when recordings were made over the pronator quadratus. Therefore, it was concluded that the pronator reflex represents a muscle stretch reflex of the pronator teres (and not the pronator quadratus), which would make it helpful in evaluating C6 and C7 root lesions.

Muscle stretch reflexes are elicited by a short, sharp blow with a tendon hammer delivered to the tendon of a gently extended muscle, and they are difficult to elicit from a contracting muscle (in an anxious patient) or from a flaccid muscle (limb in the wrong position). Furthermore, whereas the presence of pathologically brisk or completely absent deep tendon reflexes has clear significance, absent or exaggerated reflexes by themselves may not signify neurological disease. Up to 50% of elderly persons without neurological disease lack the ankle jerk bilaterally, and a small percentage of normal individuals have generalized hyperreflexia, even with a few beats of clonus, especially in anxious individuals.[17,52] Instead, the absent or exaggerated reflex is significant only when it is associated with one of the following clinical settings. The absent reflex should be associated with other findings of lower motor neuron disease such as weakness, atrophy, or fasciculations. The exaggerated reflex should be associated with other findings of upper motor neuron disease such as weakness, spasticity, Babinski's sign, or Hoffman's sign.[52]

Several types of reflex hammers are popular today. The Taylor hammer is a tomahawk-shaped soft rubber hammer; the original handle ended in an open loop, but the pointed end was added in about 1920 for use in eliciting cutaneous reflexes. The Babinski hammer has a handle that can be removed and attached either perpendicular or parallel to the disc-shaped head, and some models have built-in pins. The Queen Square hammer has a rubber-lined disc attached to the end of a long rod, like a wheel on an axle.[52] In one study by Marshall and Little,[50] peak tap force for eliciting reflexes was similar in the hyperreflexic and normoreflexic ranges for all three hammers, but in the hyporeflexic range, peak tap forces with the Taylor hammer were lower and had a ceiling effect. Otherwise, no study has demonstrated any hammer to be superior to another.

The most important observation during reflex examination is the reflex's amplitude. If the reflex amplitude is asymmetric, this suggests either lower motor neuron disease of the side with diminished reflex or upper motor neuron disease of the side with the exaggerated reflex. Unlike examination of motor strength, examination of reflexes lacks a single universally accepted grading system.[52] Two popular muscle stretch reflex scales are the Mayo Clinic scale (Table 2–1) and the National Institute of Neurological Disorders and Stroke (NINDS) scale. The Mayo Clinic scale has 9 points, where −4 is absent, −3 is just elicitable, −2 is low, −1 is moderately low, 0 is normal, +1 is brisk, +2 is very brisk, +3 is exhaustible clonus, and +4 is continuous clonus.[49,50] The NINDS scale has 5 points grading reflexes from 0 to 4, where 0 is absent, 1 is slight and less than normal (includes a trace response or a response brought out only by reinforcement), 2 is in lower half of normal range, 3 is in the upper half of normal range, and 4 is enhanced and more than normal (includes clonus if present, which optionally can be noted in an added verbal description of the reflex).[45,49] Litvan et al.[45] performed a study on the NINDS reflex scale in which moderate to substantial inter-observer reliability was reported with a κ correlation coefficient ranging from 0.50 to 0.64, but all examinations were performed by four clinical neurologists with similar backgrounds (also three of the authors were from NINDS and another author was from NIH).

Manschot et al.[49] set out to establish inter-observer reliability of the NINDS as well as that of the older Mayo Clinic scale. They had expected the NINDS scale to show higher inter-observer agreement, because fewer options for grading are available and

Table 2–1. MAYO CLINIC SCALE FOR TENDON REFLEX ASSESSMENT

Description	Score
Absent	−4
Just elicitable	−3
Low	−2
Moderately low	−1
Normal	0
Brisk	+1
Very brisk	+2
Exhaustible clonus	+3
Continuous clonus	+4

Reproduced with permission from Manschot S, van Passel L, Buskens E, et al. Mayo and NINDS scales for assessment of tendon reflexes: between observer agreement and implications for communication. J Neurol Neurosurg Psychiat 1998;64:253–255.

accordingly there is less margin for disagreement. However, the agreement among doctors was never better than "fair" for both scales with a κ correlation coefficient of 0.35, and they concluded that neither the use of the NINDS nor the Mayo Clinic scale yielded acceptable reliability in the performance of different observers. The NINDS scale does not have one separate category for "normal," and thus it is necessary to choose between low-normal or high-normal, which often proves difficult. Varying clinical background and experience may have also been an underlying cause for lack of agreement, although only neurologists and trainees in neurology were involved. Some reflexes were recorded as absent by one physician whereas another had no problem eliciting them. In day-to-day practice, many physicians of different specialties and training use various techniques and reflex hammers with different amounts of force applied, different sites of the tendon tapped, and different positioning of the patient. These may all contribute to variations in the excitation of muscle spindles and consequently of the reflex responses. Numeric codes have been assigned to the steps in both scales and imply a degree of precision, which Manschot and associates believe is unrealistic. Instead, they believe a plain verbal description of the observed tendon reflexes using terms that are understood and used by everyone (absent, low, average, brisk, a few beats of clonus, and permanent clonus) may be most satisfactory. However, a formal classification using words instead of numbers would again require assessment of its reliability.[49]

Vogel[67] designed a study to determine how additional information (referring to the patient's history and the results of other parts of the physical examination) influences results of the neurological examination. This study measured the reliability of attainment of reflexes, with reliability declining considerably in re-examinations under conditions deviating from the normal situation (if only parts of the examination were performed or the history was not known). Only with the availability of historical information did more experienced examiners score better, not because they performed the physical examination itself more reliably, but because they used the patient's history more reliably and probably more adequately. Part of the disagreement among experienced examiners may be explained by personality-specific differences in "style," such as the readiness to make extreme judgments, or to give more optimistic or more pessimistic evaluations in equivocal situations.

Marshall and Little[50] suggested a possible systematic method for delivering tendon taps and testing patellar reflexes. If a weak tap as judged by a clinician results in large knee excursion, the patient is hyperreflexic; i.e., a muscle stretch reflex (MSR) of 4 out of 4. If there is a small response, the patient is normoreflexic (an MSR of 3 out of 4). If there is no response, a medium tap is delivered; if there is a large response, the patient is normoreflexic (an MSR of 2 out of 4), but if there is a small response, the patient is hyporeflexic (an MSR of 1 out of 4). If there is no response, then a strong tap is delivered; if there is a reflex response, then the patient is hyporeflexic (an MSR of 1 out of 4). If there is no response, then a strong tap in conjunction with reinforcement is repeated; if there is an observable response, then the patient is hyporeflexic (an MSR of 1 out of 4 with reinforcement). If there is no response, the patient is areflexic (an MSR of 0 out of 4).

O'Keeffe et al.[56] compared two techniques for ankle jerk assessment in elderly subjects, and the aim of the study was to assess the intra-observer and inter-observer agreement in the detection of ankle jerks in elderly people by both techniques. In the conventional tendon strike method, the leg to be tested lies flexed and everted, and the Achilles tendon is struck with a tendon hammer. The Achilles reflex can also be elicited by the alternative plantar strike method, in which the reflex hammer strikes the clinician's hand, which is resting on the ball of the foot. Their results showed that there is substantial intra-observer and inter-observer disagreement about the presence of the ankle jerk with the tendon strike method, possibly due to paratonic rigidity induced by the need to put the limb into a certain posture, causing resistance to passive movement.

Bowditch et al.[7] assessed the prevalence of ankle reflexes in normal adult patients without known pathologic causes of reflex loss. All patients aged under 30 years had both reflexes. Few had absent reflexes at between 30 and 40 years, but in those over 40 the proportion with both reflexes absent increased rapidly from 5% (40–50 years) to 80% (90–100 years). However, unilateral absence did not show the same pattern of increase, with 3–5% at 40–60 years and 7–10% at over 60 years. They concluded that a small number of "normal" adults have unilateral absence of an ankle reflex, but this finding is rare enough to be a definite clinical sign, irrespective of age.

Stam and van Crevel[65] measured tendon reflexes by surface EMG in normal subjects using an ordinary clinical reflex hammer attached to a piezoelectric transducer. It is common knowledge that a large variation in the amplitude of reflexes can be observed in healthy persons, and in their study, the maximal amplitude of the Achilles reflex was about 50 times as large as the smallest, with other reflexes showing comparable ranges. Over 40% of the reflex pairs showed some degree of asymmetry on clinical examination, and many of these left-to-right differences were very small and would be rightly glossed over in a routine clinical examination. Some differences, however, were not negligible and measurement occasionally showed that the maximum reflex on one side of a subject was twice as large as on the other side.

Stam et al.[64] also performed a study to determine the effect of voluntary mental influences on the patellar tendon reflexes in healthy subjects with reflexes recorded by surface electrodes. Ten subjects were instructed to increase the right patellar reflex and decrease the left by mental effort, and measurement showed reflex asymmetry in seven subjects consistent with the instruction. The experiment was repeated in another 20 subjects with symmetric reflexes at rest. Ten of these subjects were, after random assignment, instructed to increase either the right or the left knee jerk and then were examined by a neurologist without knowledge of the instruction. Three of the ten instructed subjects were correctly judged to be asymmetric, which seemed to imply that mental influence on reflexes can sometimes be clinically relevant. However, two of the ten symmetric subjects who were not instructed were judged to be asymmetric incorrectly, and the concordance between mental instruction and clinical neurologic judgment showed a trend but was not statistically significant ($p = 0.09$).

The muscle stretch reflexes are important physical signs, and they are one of the main components of the clinical examination of the nervous system. Reflexes can aid anatomical diagnosis, such as when reflex asymmetry is present, and give an important indicator to whether a patient's disorder arises from the central or peripheral nervous system. Taken in conjunction with the overall history and neurological examination, muscle stretch reflexes can be quite useful. However, even though muscle stretch reflexes have long been assumed to be "hard" objective signs, the grading of muscle stretch reflexes between different observers for the same subject is quite variable and subjective due to both patient and physician factors. Therefore, muscle stretch reflexes may be misleading if used in isolation.

Conclusion

The sensory, motor, and reflex examination is a valuable component of the neuromusculoskeletal evaluation. Proper performance will enable the clinician to readily differentiate central from peripheral involvement and may be useful in monitoring response to treatment. Reliability issues are important to understand when multiple examiners are involved in care, as well as the fact that small differences may not be detectable in healthy, normal individuals. The neurological examination cannot be replaced by simple subjective reporting and is invaluable in the context of the overall physical examination.

REFERENCES

1. Adams RD, Victor M, Ropper AH. Principles of Neurology, 6th edn. New York: McGraw-Hill, 1997, pp. 46–47.
2. Andres PL, Skerry LM, Thornell B, et al. A comparison of three measures of disease progression in ALS. J Neurol Sci 1996;139:64–70.
3. Barr AE, et al. Reliability of testing measures in Duchenne or Becker muscular dystrophy. Arch Phys Med Rehabil 1991;72:315–319.
4. Beasley WC. Quantitative muscle testing: principle and applications to research and clinical services. Arch Phys Med Rehabil 1961;42:398–425.
5. Bell C. On the nervous circle which connects the voluntary muscles with the brain. Phil Trans (pt 2) 1826:116.
6. Bohannon RW. Manual muscle test scores and dynamometer test scores of knee extension strength. Arch Phys Med Rehabil 1986;67:390–392.

7. Bowditch MC, Sanderson P, Livesey JP. The significance of an absent ankle reflex. J Bone Joint Surg 1996;78B:276–279.
8. Brooke MH, Griggs RC, et al. Clinical trial in Duchenne dystrophy. Muscle Nerve 1981;4:186–197.
9. Brown-Sequard C. Experimental researches applied to physiology and pathology. In Medical Examiner, Vol. 8. Philadelphia: Baillière, 1852, pp. 481–504.
10. Burke D, McKeon B, Skuse NF. Dependence of the Achilles tendon reflex on the excitability of spinal reflex pathways. Ann Neurol 1981;10:551–556.
11. Bussel B, Morin C, Pierrot-Deseilligny E. Mechanism of monosynaptic reflex reinforcement during Jendrassik manoeuvre in man. J Neurol Neurosurg Psychiat 1978;41:40–44.
12. Callaghan MJ, et al. The reproducibility of multi-joint isokinetic and isometric assessments in a healthy and patient population. Clin Biomech 2000;15:678–683.
13. Charcot JRP. Les Demoniaques dans l'art. Paris: A. Delhaye & E. Lecrosnier, 1887.
14. Daniels L, Worthingham C. Muscle Testing: Techniques of Manual Examination, 4th edn. Philadelphia: WB Saunders, 1980.
15. Dellon AL, Mackinnon SE, Crosby PM. Reliability of two-point discrimination measurements. J Hand Surg 1987;12A:693–696.
16. Haldane ES, Ross GRT (trans.). Philosophical Works of Descartes. Cambridge: Cambridge University Press, 1911.
17. Dick JP. The deep tendon and the abdominal reflexes. J Neurol Neurosurg Psychiat 2003;74(2):150–153.
18. Edinger L. Anatomie des centres nerveux. Paris: JB Baillière et Fils, 1889.
19. Emery CA, et al. Test–retest reliability of isokinetic hip adductor and flexor muscle strength. Clin J Sport Med 1999;9:79–85.
20. Erb WH. Über Sehnenreflexe bei Gesunden und Rückenmarkskranken. Arch Psychiatr Nervenkrankh 1875;5:792–802.
21. Escolar DM, et al. Clinical evaluator reliability for quantitative and manual muscle testing measures of strength in children. Muscle Nerve 2001;24:787–793.
22. Felsenthal G, Reischer MA. Asymmetric hamstring reflexes indicative of L5 radicular lesion. Arch Phys Med Rehabil 1982;63(8):377–378.
23. Florence JM, et al. Intrarater reliability of manual muscle test (Medical Research Council Scale) grades in Duchenne's muscular dystrophy. Phys Ther 1992;72(2):115–122.
24. Florence JM, et al. Clinical trials in Duchenne dystrophy: standardization and reliability of evaluation procedures. Phys Ther 1984;64(1):41–45.
25. Freeman C, Okun MS. Origins of the sensory examination in neurology. Semin Neurol 2002;22:399–408.
26. Frese E, Brown M, Norton BJ. Clinical reliability of manual muscle testing. Phys Ther 1987;7:1072–1076.
27. Gehuchten AV. Les centres nerveux cerebrospinaux. Louvain: Uyastpruyst-Dieudonne, 1908.
28. Gowers WR. A Manual of Disease of the Nervous System, Vol. 1. London: Churchill, 1888, pp. 6–10.
29. Griffin JW, McClure MH, Bertorini TE. Sequential isokinetic and manual muscle testing in patients with neuromuscular disease. Phys Ther 1986;66(1):32–35.
30. Hall M. Synopsis of the Diastatic Nervous System. London: Joseph Mallett, 1850.
31. Hayes KC, Wolfe DL, Hsieh JT, et al. Clinical and electrophysiological correlates of quantitative sensory testing in patients with incomplete spinal cord injury. Arch Phys Med Rehabil 2002;83:1612–1619.
32. Head H, Campbell AW. The pathology of herpes zoster and its bearing on sensory localization. Brain 1900;23:353–523.
33. Holmes G. Disorders of sensation produced by cortical lesions. Brain 1927;50:413–427.
34. Iddings DM, et al, Muscle testing. 2: Reliability in clinical use. Phys Ther Rev 1961;41:249–256.
35. Inouye Y, Buchthal F. Segmental sensory innervation determined by potentials recorded from cervical spinal nerves. Brain 1977;100:731–748.
36. Jendrassik E. Beitrage zur Lehre von den Sehnenreflexen. Deutsch Arch Klin Med 1883;33:177–199.
37. Jensen OH. The medial hamstring reflex in the level-diagnosis of a lumbar disc herniation. Clin Rheumatol 1987;6:570–574.
38. Kendall FP, McCreary EK. Muscle Testing and Function, 3rd edn. Baltimore: Williams & Wilkins, 1983.
39. Kortelainen P, Puranen J, Kovisto E, Lahde S. Symptoms and signs of sciatica and their relation to the localization of the lumbar disc herniation. Spine 1985;10:88–92.
40. Kosteljanetz M, Bang F, Schmidt-Olsen S. The clinical significance of straight leg raising (Lasegue's sign) in the diagnosis of prolapsed lumbar disc. Spine 1988;13:393–395.
41. Kosteljanetz M, Espersen JO, Halaburt H, Miletic T. Predictive value of clinical and surgical findings in patients with lumbago–sciatica: a prospective study (pt 1). Acta Neurochir 1984;73:67–76.

42. Lawson A, Calderon L. Interexaminer agreement for applied kinesiology manual muscle testing. Percept Motor Skills 1997;84:539–546.

43. Lilienfeld AM, et al. A study of the reproducibility of muscle testing and certain other aspects of muscle scoring. Phys Ther Rev 1954;34:279–289.

44. Li RC, et al. Eccentric and concentric isokinetic knee flexion and extension: a reliability study using the Cybex 6000 dynamometer. Br J Sports Med 1996;30:156–160.

45. Litvan I, Mangone CA, Werden W, et al. Reliability of the NINDS myotatic reflex scale. Neurology 1996;47:969–972.

46. Louis ED, Kaufmann P. Erb's explanation for the tendon reflexes. Arch Neurol 1996;53:1187–1189.

47. Lunsford BR, Perry J. The standing heel-rise test for ankle plantar flexion: criterion for normal. Phys Ther 1995;75:694–698.

48. Malanga GA, Campagnolo DI. Clarification of the pronator reflex. Am J Phys Med Rehabil 1994;73:338–340.

49. Manschot S, van Passel L, Buskens E, et al. Mayo and NINDS scales for assessment of tendon reflexes: between observer agreement and implications for communication. J Neurol Neurosurg Psychiat 1998;64:253–255.

50. Marshall GL, Little JW. Deep tendon reflexes: a study of quantitative methods. J Spinal Cord Med 2002;25(2):94–99.

51. McCombe PF, Fairbank JCT, Cockersole BC, Pynsent PB. Reproducibility of physical signs in low back pain. Spine 1989;14:908–918.

52. McGee S. Evidence-based Physical Diagnosis. Philadelphia: WB Saunders, 2001, pp. 772–777.

53. Medical Research Council. Aids to the Investigation of the Peripheral Nervous System. London: HMSO, 1975.

54. Mulroy SJ, Lassen KD, Chambers SH, Perry J. The ability of male and female clinicians to effectively test knee extension strength using manual muscle testing. J Orthop Sports Phys Ther 1997;26(4):192–199.

55. Nadler SF, DePrince M, Hauesien N, et al. Portable dynamometer anchoring station for measuring strength of the hip extensors and abductors. Arch Phys Med Rehabil 2000;81:1072–1076.

56. O'Keeffe ST, Smith T, Valacio R, et al. A comparison of two techniques for ankle jerk assessment in elderly subjects. Lancet 1994;344:1619–1620.

57. Pearce JM. Early days of the tuning fork tests. Am J Otol 1993;14:100–105.

58. Pearce JM. Robert Whytt and the stretch reflex. J Neurol Neurosurg Psychiat 1997;62:484.

59. Pincivero DM, et al. Reliability and precision of isokinetic strength and muscular endurance for the quadriceps and hamstrings. Int J Sports Med 1997;18:113–117.

60. Rinne RF, Heinrich F. Beitrage zur Physiologie des menschlichen Ohres. Leipzig: Zeitschrift fur rationelle Medicin, 1864, p. 12.

61. Rumpf H. Ueber einen Fall von Syringomyelie nebst Beitrag zur Untersuchung der Sensibilitat. Neurologisches Zentralblatt, 1889.

62. Schiller F. The reflex hammer: in memoriam Robert Wartenberg (1887–1956). Med Hist 1967;11:75–85.

63. Sherrington C. Experiments in the examination of the peripheral distribution of the fibres of the posterior roots of some spinal nerves. Phil Trans B 1898;190:45–186.

64. Stam J, Speelman HD, van Crevel H. Tendon reflex asymmetry by voluntary mental effort in healthy subjects. Arch Neurol 1989;46:70–73.

65. Stam J, van Crevel H. Measurement of tendon reflexes by surface electromyography in normal subjects. J Neurol 1989;236:231–237.

66. van der Ploeg RJO, Oosterhuis HJ, Reuvekamp J. Measuring muscle strength. J Neurol 1984;231:200–203.

67. Vogel HP. Influence of additional information on interrater reliability in the neurologic examination. Neurology 1992;42:2076–2081.

68. Wadsworth CT, et al. Intrarater reliability of manual muscle testing and hand-held dynametric muscle testing. Phys Ther 1987;67:1342–1347.

69. Weber E. Ueber die Gestalt des Gehirns der Schleie, Cyprinus tinca, im Aler von einem Jahr und bei dem erswachsnen Thiere. Berlin: Arch Anat Physiol wissen Med., 1846, p. 478.

70. Weise MD, Garfin SR, Gelberman RH, Katz MM, Thorne RP. Lower-extremity sensibility testing in patients with herniated lumbar intervertebral discs. J Bone Joint Surg Am 1985;67:1219–1224.

71. Whytt R. On the vital and involuntary movements of animals. Edinburgh, 1763. Cited by G. Jefferson in Selected Papers of Sir Geoffrey Jefferson. London: Pitman, 1960, pp. 73–93.

72. Ziter FA, Allsop KG, Tyler FH. Assessment of muscle strength in Duchenne muscular dystrophy. Neurology 1977;27:981–984.

Chapter 3

Physical Examination of the Cervical Spine

PHILLIP LANDES, MD • GERARD A. MALANGA, MD •
SCOTT F. NADLER, DO • JAMES FARMER, MD

Introduction

Neck pain is common in the general population. Its causes include whiplash injury from motor vehicle crashes and sports-related activities. Many specialized provocative tests have been described for physical examination of the neck and cervical spine. The majority of these relate to identification of plexus, nerve root, or spinal cord pathology. These tests are routinely performed by clinicians with varying experience and skill. This may lead to error in both the technique and the interpretation of findings.

This chapter provides a comprehensive overview of the physical examination of the cervical spine. For each test, the original description, currently performed technique, reliability, validity, and clinical significance are discussed, based on a comprehensive search of the existing literature. The goal is not necessarily to learn every examination maneuver performed for neck pain, but rather to understand the limitations, reliability, and scientifically proven validity of some of the commonly used tests.

Inspection

Inspection should begin by noting the position of the head in relation to the line of gravity, which passes through the external auditory meatus, odontoid process, cervical, thoracic, thoracolumbar, and lumbosacral spine and the sacral promontory. One should carefully assess not only the upper cervical region but also the relative curvature of the thoracolumbar and lumbosacral spines, as the relative positioning of the cervical spine may be influenced by the curvature below. The forward-head position can also be the direct cause of the loss of cervical motion. Caillet[10] reported a 25–50% loss of head rotation with a forwardly protruded head and a significant increase in the gravity-induced weight of the head brought on by this postural abnormality. The forward-head posture thus increases the work requirements of the capital and cervical musculature

Palpation

A segmental evaluation can be incorporated for those skilled in manual treatment, realizing that at C1/C2 almost pure rotation is present while coupled side-bending and rotation is the general rule for the C2–C7 region. This may be performed by translating segments from right to left and left to right in flexed, extended, and neutral positions of the neck to identify segments with limited mobility. Segmental evaluation of the various facet joints determining translatory motion of the individual segments can be helpful in diagnosing headache related to the C2/C3 facet joint. In 1995, Sandmark and Nisell[41] reported that palpation over the facet joints was the most appropriate screening to corroborate self-reported neck dysfunction. Range of motion assessment had poor overall sensitivity.

Palpation is a key component of the evaluation for cervical myofascial pain. For the purpose of this section, palpation discussion will be limited to the trapezius, sternocleidomastoid, scalenes, and posterior cervical and capital musculature. The trapezius is a large muscle group with upper, middle, and lower fibers. The large area of this muscle makes it susceptible to the effects of whiplash injury. The upper trapezius is greatly affected by postural insufficiency and has been noted in dentists, secretaries, and sewing machine operators.[3,27,33] The sternocleidomastoid should always be palpated along both sternal and clavicular heads (Figure 3–1). Evaluation of the

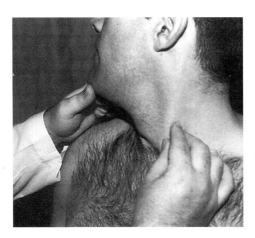

Figure 3–1. Palpation of the sternocleidomastoid. Reproduced with permission from Nadler SF, Cooke P: Myofascial pain in whiplash injuries: diagnosis and treatment. In Spine: State of the Art Reviews 12, Philadelphia: Hanley & Belfus, 1998, p. 366.

Figure 3–2. Scalene cramp test. Reproduced with permission from Nadler SF, Cooke P: Myofascial pain in whiplash injuries: diagnosis and treatment. In Spine: State of the Art Reviews 12, Philadelphia: Hanley & Belfus, 1998, p. 366.

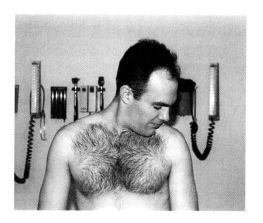

posterior musculature including the splenius, semispinalis, multifidi, and suboccipital muscles should be included. All of these muscle groups can cause radiation of pain in or about the head.

The scalenes can be evaluated during physical exam by the *scalene cramp test,* which is performed by having the patient turn the head toward the painful side and pulling the chin down into the supraclavicular fossa (Figure 3–2). This position causes contraction of the scalenes and should reproduce distal radiation of pain. The individual scalene muscles can be evaluated by stretching the head to the opposite side (Figure 3–3), looking straight forward (middle scalene), looking away (anterior scalene), and looking towards the elbow (posterior scalene). Stretching of the various portions of the scalenes may also reproduce symptoms. The *scalene relief test* attempts to relax the scalenes by increasing the space between the clavicle and the scalenes. The clinician evaluating these various structures must have a thorough understanding of both structural and functional anatomy.

Range of Motion

The amount of motion that occurs between contiguous vertebrae in the cervical spine is dictated mainly by the anatomic orientation of the facet joints. Paired superior and inferior articular processes project from each pedicle–lamina junction. The superior articular processes of each vertebra articulate with the inferior articular processes of the next higher vertebra to form hyaline cartilage-covered synovial facet joints. These joints are true synovial joints with hyaline cartilage, synovial lining, and a joint capsule that encloses the joint space. Mechanoreceptors and nociceptors richly innervate each cervical zygapophyseal joint. The facet joint capsule for the subatlantoaxial zygapophyseal joints are generally sufficiently lax to permit gliding movements of the

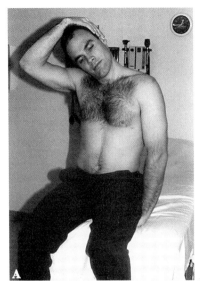

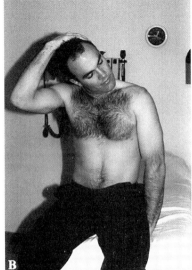

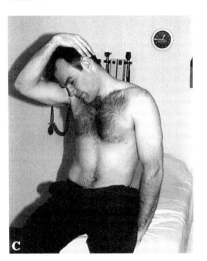

Figure 3–3. Provocative scalene stretching. Reproduced with permission from Nadler SF, Cooke P: Myofascial pain in whiplash injuries: diagnosis and treatment. In Spine: State of the Art Reviews 12, Philadelphia: Hanley & Belfus, 1998, p. 371.

facet joints in planes compatible with their facing direction.[56] The atlanto-occipital (AO) and atlantoaxial (AA) joints are not true facet joints. True joints extend from C2/C3 to the C7–T1 level. Biomechanical studies have identified flexion and extension motion of the AO joint to be approximately 13 degrees. Lateral bending motion at the AO joint averages 8 degrees with negligible rotation. The AA joint articulates at three locations creating a medial atlantodental and two lateral AA joints.[56] Rotation is the key movement of the AA joint, which averages 47 degrees and is limited by the lateral atlantoaxial facet joint capsule and the opposite alar ligament. The AA joint accounts for 50% of the total rotation of the cervical spine.[4] There is 10 degrees of total flexion and extension at the AA joint with a negligible amount of lateral bending. Distal to C2, the superior articular processes of the facet joints are oriented in a posterior and superior direction, at a 45-degree angle from the horizontal plane. Flexion and extension are greatest at the C5/C6 and C6/C7 interspaces, where they amount to 17 degrees and 16 degrees, respectively.[34] Lateral bending and rotation of the five lower cervical facet joints tend to be most extensive at the C3/C4 and C4/C5 levels, averaging 11–12 degrees.[41]

Range of motion ideally should be assessed actively using a goniometer placed at the external auditory meatus for flexion and extension, at the top of the head for rotation, and at the nares for side-bending (Figure 3–4). Cervical flexion has been identified to range between 54 and 69 degrees with extension ranging between 73 and 93 degrees.[8,14,25] Youdas et al.[59] identified extension to range between 20 and 74 degrees with a mean of 52 degrees in patients older than 90 years and a range of 61 to 106 degrees with a mean of 86 degrees in patients between 11 and 19 years. Lateral bending ranged between 11 and 38 degrees, while rotation ranged between 26 and 74 degrees in those older than 90 years. In patients between 11 and 19 years, lateral bending ranged between 30 and 66 degrees, whereas rotation ranged between 50 and 94 degrees. Intra-class correlation coefficients range from 0.84 to 0.95 for intra-tester reliability of goniometric assessment, and the inter-tester reliability ranged between 0.73 and 0.92.[58]

Neuromuscular Evaluation

The neuromuscular screen should be performed on any individual being evaluated with radicular symptoms or signs. The comprehensive neuromuscular examination should include a detailed sensory examination (Table 3–1), motor examination (Table 3–2), and assessment of reflexes (Table 3–3). The results of these tests should be considered in the context of the patient's complaints and in conjunction with other provocative maneuvers such as Spurling's test. This evaluation is described in greater detail below.

Non-organic Physical Examination Findings

Clinicians evaluating patients with neck pain with or without radicular symptoms may also want to evaluate them for non-organic findings consistent with abnormal illness behavior. Sobel et al.[45] reported on the use of cervical non-organic signs to assess abnormal illness behavior in 26 patients with chronic neck pain. In this study, a standardized assessment was developed to determine agreement between examiners

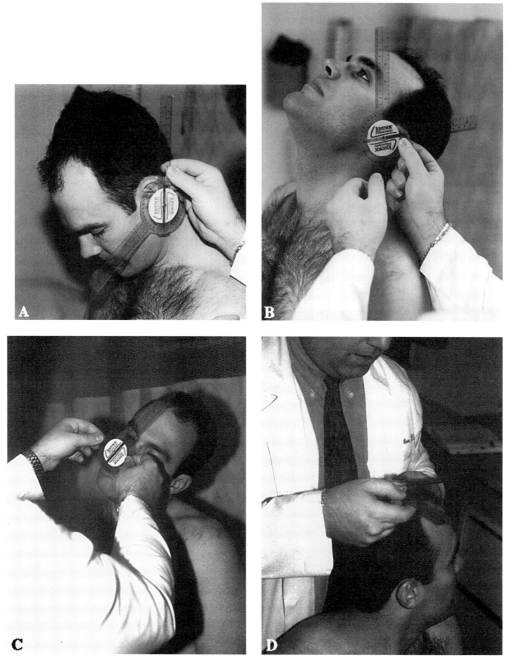

Figure 3–4. Assessment of active cervical range of motion using goniometer. Reproduced with permission from Nadler SF, Cooke P: Myofascial pain in whiplash injuries: diagnosis and treatment. In Spine: State of the Art Reviews 12, Philadelphia: Hanley & Belfus, 1998, p. 364.

Table 3–1. SENSORY EXAMINATION

Spine Level	Sensation
C3	Supraclavicular fossa
C4	Tip of acromion
C5	Lateral epicondyle
C6	Thumb
C7	Middle digit
C8	Fifth digit

Table 3–2. MOTOR EXAMINATION

Spine Level	Nerve	Muscle	Testing
C5/C6	Axillary	Deltoid	Arm abducted to the side
C5/C6	Musculocutaneous	Biceps	Elbow flexion
C5–C7	Radial	Triceps	Elbow extension
C6/C7	Median	Pronator teres	Pronation of extended forearm
C6/C7	Radial	Extensor carpi radialis	Wrist extension
C8/T1	Ulnar	Abductor digiti minimi	Abduction of the fifth digit

Table 3–3. REFLEX EXAMINATION

Spine Level	Reflexes
C5/C6	Biceps
C5/C6	Brachioradialis
C6/C7	Pronator teres
C7/C8	Triceps

using a standardized set of physical examination signs. Non-anatomic findings included complaints of pain with light touch or pinching of the skin over the cervical region or complaints of widespread tenderness with local palpation in the cervical or upper thoracic region. Reports were of neck pain with rotation of the head, trunk, and pelvis in unison while standing, and limited neck rotation – less than 50% of normal in each direction. Additionally, patient reports of diminished sensation in a pattern not corresponding to a specific dermatome of a nerve root or peripheral nerve, giveaway weakness on motor testing, and signs of overreaction were utilized. Regional sensory or motor loss were found to be signs demonstrating high agreement among examiners in order to detect abnormal illness behavior in neck pain patients.

Cervical Spine Tests that Provoke or Relieve Pain

Spurling's Neck Compression Test

Spurling and Scoville first described Spurling's neck compression test, also known as the *foraminal compression test*, *neck compression test*, or *quadrant test*, in 1944 as "the most important diagnostic test and one that is almost pathognomonic of a cervical intraspinal lesion."[46] Their observations were based on the presentation of 12 patients with "ruptured cervical discs" verified during surgery in 1943 at Walter Reed Army Hospital. The authors state that during the same period many more of these cases were diagnosed but not verified surgically. They described "the neck compression test" as follows.

> Tilting the head and neck toward the painful side may be sufficient to reproduce the characteristic pain and radicular features of the lesion. Pressure on the top of the head in this position may greatly intensify the symptoms. Tilting the head away from the lesion usually gives relief.

Currently, the test is performed by extending the neck and rotating the head and then applying downward pressure on the head (Figure 3–5). The test is considered positive if pain radiates into the limb ipsilateral to the side at which the head is rotated.[30] Some authors advocate performing the components of the test in a staged manner and halting with the onset of radicular symptoms, preferably reproducing the

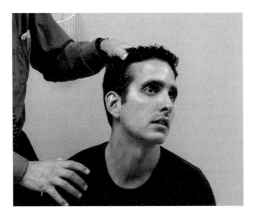

Figure 3–5. Spurling's maneuver.

patient's presenting symptoms.[9,17,29] Radicular symptoms are described as pain or paresthesias occurring distant from the neck, in the distribution of a cervical spinal nerve root.

Viikari-Juntura[53] performed a prospective study assessing the inter-examiner reliability of common tests performed in the clinical examination of patients with neck and radicular pain. Two blinded expert examiners, who were trained together in the identical performance of the clinical tests, independently examined 52 patients referred for cervical myelography. The neck compression test was performed with each patient in both supine and sitting positions. The patient's neck was passively flexed laterally and slightly rotated ipsilaterally, and the head was then compressed with approximately 7 kg of pressure. A positive test was considered to be the appearance or aggravation of pain, numbness, or paresthesias in the shoulder or upper extremity. For the sitting position, κ values ranged from 0.40 to 0.77, which was considered to be "fair to excellent," and the proportion of specific agreement was found to be 0.47 to 0.80, which was also considered to be "fair to excellent." For the supine position, κ values ranged from 0.28 to 0.63, which was considered to be "poor to good," and the proportion of specific agreement was found to be 0.36 to 0.67, which was also considered to be "poor to good." The author concluded that this test has good reliability when performed in the sitting position. This is one of the only studies in the literature assessing inter-examiner reliability for Spurling's neck compression test and other provocative test maneuvers of the cervical spine. However, the results are analyzed according to the area of symptom radiation (e.g., "right shoulder or upper arm," "right forearm or hand," "left shoulder or upper arm," "left forearm or hand"), instead of classifying the test as positive or negative. This fragments statistical analysis and makes interpretation difficult.

In 1989, Viikari-Juntura et al.[52] published a prospective study assessing the validity of Spurling's neck compression test in diagnosing cervical radiculopathy, along with the axial manual traction and shoulder abduction tests. Forty-three patients who presented for myelography were interviewed and examined prior to performing the procedure. Spurling's neck compression test was performed with the patient sitting as previously described.[53] The criterion standard used was myelography combined with neurological exam findings. Based on the study population's myelographic and clinical findings, statistical analysis was performed only for cervical roots C6–C8. Sensitivity ranged from 40% to 60% and specificity was 92–100%. The authors concluded that the test has high specificity but low sensitivity.[53] The results are presented in a manner making interpretation difficult.[52,53]

Tong and Haig[49] reported a sensitivity of 30% and specificity of 93% utilizing electrodiagnostic studies as a criterion standard in 224 patients. Sandmark and Nisell[41] reported a specificity of 92%, sensitivity of 77%, positive predictive value of 80%, and negative predictive value of 91%. However, their study used neck pain symptoms as the criterion standard, and Spurling's neck compression test was considered to be positive if neck pain, not radicular symptoms, was produced. This interpretation is inconsistent with the original and commonly accepted descriptions of Spurling's sign. Due to these methodological issues the results should be viewed cautiously. Uchihara et al.[51] reported a sensitivity of 28% and a specificity of 100%. However, the criterion standard used was spinal cord deformity on MRI in 65 patients.

In summary, there are few methodologically sound studies that assess the inter-examiner reliability, sensitivity, and specificity of Spurling's neck compression test. The literature appears to indicate high specificity and low sensitivity. More research is needed to better explore the utility of this commonly used clinical test.

Shoulder Abduction Test

Spurling[13] was reported to have first described the shoulder abduction test, also described as the *shoulder abduction relief sign*, in 1956. In a review on the examination maneuver, Davidson et al.[13] described Spurling's initial description as follows: "raising the arm above the head sometimes brings relief of radicular symptoms caused by cervical intervertebral disc pathology."

Davidson et al.[13] described 22 patients who presented with severe cervical radicular pain, sensory and motor symptoms, initially unresponsive to outpatient measures. All were found to have large lateral extradural lesions on myelography. Fifteen (68%) of these patients experienced relief of their radicular symptoms with ipsilateral shoulder abduction. The authors hypothesized that reduced nerve root tension is the most likely cause for symptom relief with shoulder abduction. They concluded that the shoulder abduction relief sign is indicative of nerve root compression and predictive of excellent response to surgical treatment.

The shoulder abduction relief test is currently described as:

active or passive abduction of the ipsilateral shoulder so that the hand rests on top of the head, with the patient either sitting or supine [Figure 3–6]. Relief or reduction of ipsilateral cervical radicular symptoms is indicative of a positive test.[29]

Beatty et al.[6] described this sign to be indicative of radiculopathy secondary to cervical disc pathology but not from cervical spondylosis. Ellenberg and Honet[17] described the shoulder abduction relief sign as helpful in distinguishing cervical radiculopathy from shoulder pathology, when present. In their experience the sign is "frequently not present" with cervical radiculopathy.

Viikari-Juntura[53] prospectively studied the inter-examiner reliability of the shoulder abduction relief test in 31 patients with radicular pain, paresthesias, or numbness. It was performed in the seated position with the patient instructed to "lift" his hand above the head. The decrease or disappearance of radicular symptoms indicated a

Figure 3–6. Hyperabduction test.

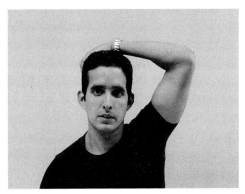

positive test. Kappa scores were poor to fair and ranged from 0.21 to 0.40. The proportion of specific agreement was fair to good, ranging from 0.57 to 0.67. Overall, the test's reliability was described as "fair." Viikari-Juntura et al.[52] later investigated the validity of the shoulder abduction relief test on 22 patients. Sensitivity ranged from 43% to 50% and specificity ranged from 80% to 100%. The authors concluded that the test is highly specific for cervical radiculopathy with low sensitivity.

The literature seems to indicate high specificity with low sensitivity for the shoulder abduction relief test. However, the only available prospective study examined a small number of subjects for this test. The only investigation of inter-examiner reliability concluded the test to be "fair." Interestingly, incorporation of the abduction maneuver into a non-surgical treatment program is reported as beneficial for patients with a positive test.[20]

Neck Distraction Test

The neck distraction test is also described as the *axial manual traction test*. The origin of this maneuver is uncertain although it is well described in the current literature.

> To perform the distraction test, the examiner places one hand under the patient's chin and the other hand around the occiput, then slowly lifts the patient's head. The test is classified as positive if the pain is relieved or decreased when the head is lifted or distracted, indicating pressure on nerve roots that has been relieved.[29]

This test is commonly performed in the supine position in the presence of radicular symptoms (Figure 3–7). A positive test is indicated by relief or lessening of the radicular symptoms and is thought to indicate cervical radiculopathy caused by discogenic pathology.[18,52,53] Viikari-Juntura[53] concluded that the inter-examiner reliability of the neck distraction test is "good." In his prospective study, a traction force of 10–15 kg was applied to 29 subjects. Kappa values ranged from 0.50 to 0.71. Using the same

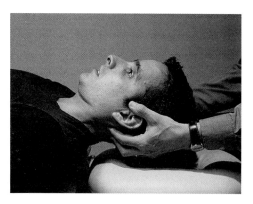

Figure 3–7. Neck distraction test.

examination technique in a 1989 study, Viikari-Juntura et al.[52] reported a specificity of 100% and a sensitivity of 40–43%. The authors concluded that the axial manual traction test has low sensitivity but is highly specific for radicular pain, neurologic, and radiologic signs of radiculopathy from cervical disc disease. No other studies of inter-examiner reliability or validity are reported in the literature.

Lhermitte's Sign

What is now referred to as Lhermitte's sign was first described by Marie and Chatelin in 1917, at a meeting of the Centres of Military Neurology in Paris.[23] They described "transient 'pins and needles' sensations traveling the spine and limbs on flexion of the head" in some patients with head injuries. It was believed that these symptoms were caused by positional pressure on cervical nerve roots.[31]

In 1918, Babinski and Dubois[5] described a patient with a Brown–Sequard syndrome who reported sensations of "electric discharge" upon flexing the head, sneezing, or coughing. They attributed the symptom to the presence of an intramedullary lesion. Lhermitte first wrote on this topic in 1920 when he further elaborated on the symptom's origin in patients with "concussion of the spinal cord."[26] He attributed these symptoms to posterior and lateral column pathology in the cervical spinal cord.[23,26] Lhermitte attributed the "electric discharge" symptoms to demyelination of cervical spinal cord segments and believed this to be an early finding in multiple sclerosis.[26]

Lhermitte's test is currently described as being performed in a variety of ways. It is most commonly described as passive cervical flexion to end range with the patient seated (Figure 3–8). A positive test is indicated by the presence of an "electric-like" sensation down the spine or in the extremities. This is described to occur with cervical spinal cord pathology from a wide variety of conditions, including multiple sclerosis, spinal cord tumor, cervical spondylosis, and radiation myelitis.[17,18,30] The test is also currently described as performed in the following manner, although different from the descriptions above.

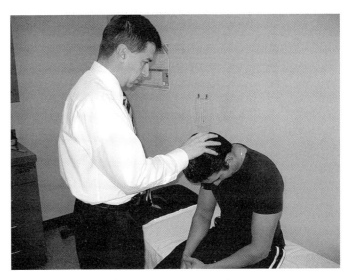

Figure 3–8. Lhermitte's sign.

The patient is in the long leg sitting position on the examining table. The examiner passively flexes the patient's head and one hip simultaneously, with the leg kept straight. A positive test occurs if there is a sharp pain down the spine and into the upper or lower limbs; it indicates dural or meningeal irritation in the spine or possible cervical myelopathy.[29]

No reports investigating the inter-examiner reliability of Lhermitte's sign could be found in the literature. There are two studies describing the validity of Lhermitte's sign, although both have methodological flaws. Sandmark and Nissell[41] reported a sensitivity of 27%, specificity of 90%, positive predictive value of 55%, and negative predictive value of 75% for the *active flexion and extension test*, which partly resembles Lhermitte's test. Uchihara et al.[51] reported a high sensitivity and less than 28% specificity, although exact percentages are difficult to discern.

Lhermitte's sign was originally described anecdotally, and experience with this test continues to be primarily based on anecdotal observation.

Hoffmann's Sign

The origin of what is now described as Hoffmann's sign remained controversial through the late 1930s until a medical student named Otto Bendheim found a reference to the reflex in a paper written by Hans Curschmann on uremia in 1911.[7] In 1916, Keyser published a paper suggesting the name "Hoffmann's sign" be dropped for "digital reflex" after an extensive search failed to identify the origin of the reflex.[7,24] The sign is attributed to Johann Hoffmann, professor of neurology at Heidelberg,

Germany, in the late nineteenth and early twentieth centuries, a pupil of Erb. Hoffmann was reported to demonstrate the sign routinely in lectures and clinics, although he did not discuss it through publication.[7,12] Hoffmann's assistant, Hans Curschmann, who became professor of medicine at the University of Rostock, Germany, described the reflex in the literature in 1911 and named it Hoffmann's sign.[12,16] In 1908, Jakobson described a similar sign, independently and after Hoffmann. Jakobson tapped the distal radius instead of snapping the nail.[7] In 1913, Tromner described the reflex as well.[11,50] In response to an inquiry, Dr Curschmann later wrote:

> The finger phenomenon mentioned by me originates from Johann Hoffmann, Professor of Neurology at Heidelberg (died 1919). I learned it while his pupil and assistant from 1901 to 1904. He demonstrated it in his classes and clinics as a sign of hyperreflexia of the upper extremity. So far as I know he never published it.[12,16]

Hoffmann's sign was originally described as follows (Figure 3–9):

> The test is performed by supporting the patient's hand so that it is completely relaxed and the fingers partially flexed. The middle finger is firmly grasped, partially extended, and the nail snapped by the examiner's thumb nail. The snapping should be done with considerable force, even to the point of causing pain. The sign is present if quick flexion of both the thumb and index finger results. Finger nails other than the middle one are sometimes selected for the snapping. The sign is said to be incomplete if only the thumb or only the fingers move.[16]

There continues to be disagreement as to whether the sign is present if only the thumb flexes.[28,44] Keyser described the test to be positive "if definite flexion of either the thumb or one or more fingers results."[24]

The clinical significance of Hoffmann's sign has been long disputed.[16,28,36] There are three general views of the meaning of this reflex. One theory is that Hoffmann's sign is a "pathologic sign, indicating pyramidal tract involvement."[28] A second, popular

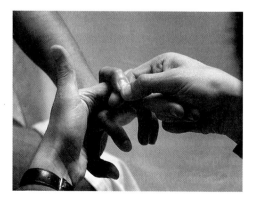

Figure 3–9. Hoffmann's sign.

view is that it "indicates pyramidal-tract involvement" but that, owing to its frequent presence in other conditions, "its clinical value is doubtful."[28] Finally, many "do not consider the Hoffmann sign as pathologic or of any clinical value."[28] In 1929, Pitfield observed the sign to be inconsistent in individual patients and to be frequently present in patients with cardiovascular disease.[36] He devised a scale classifying the degree in which the response follows the nail snapping into four groups, "plus 1" to "plus 4." Pitfield also described a maneuver to reinforce or negate if absent as follows:

> The upper arm is encircled by the cuff of a blood pressure apparatus; this is blown to 300 mm; if then the prone hand is examined by snapping the nail an apparently absent reflex will become positive and faint ones will be exalted to a plus three or four. After releasing the pressure and removing the cuff, it sometimes can be noted that a condition of exultation will persist for some minutes, the reflex being more active than it was before compression.[36]

Denno and Meadows[15] described "the dynamic Hoffman's sign" as a modification to assist in the diagnosis of early spondylotic cervical myelopathy. This is performed by "multiple active full flexion to extension of the neck" prior to performing the Hoffmann's sign maneuver as originally described. Echols[16] examined 2017 students at the University of Michigan and observed a Hoffmann's sign in 159 using the lenient criteria of any suggested flexion of the index finger, the thumb, or both. After 4 months, 153 were re-examined and 32 patients no longer demonstrated the sign, 68 had an "incomplete Hoffmann's sign" with flexion of only one or more fingers, and 53 had a "true Hoffmann's sign" with flexion of both the thumb and index fingers in response to snapping the middle finger, the ring finger, or both. Of the 53 students with "true Hoffmann's signs," only 33 had no history of prior head injury or other central nervous system pathology. The incidence of a "true Hoffmann's sign" was 2.62%, the incidence of an "incomplete Hoffmann's sign" was 3.37%, and the incidence of an unexplained "true Hoffmann's sign" was 1.63%. Echols concluded that "the (true) Hoffmann sign almost always indicates a disturbance of the pyramidal pathway" and "the significance of an incomplete Hoffmann's sign is still unsettled." It should be noted that 62% of the patients with true Hoffman's signs in Echols' study (33/53) were unexplained.

In 1946, Schneck published a preliminary report of a 2.5–3% incidence of Hoffmann's sign in more than 2500 subjects in the military.[44] No history or physical examination findings consistent with neurologic disease were elicited in the majority of subjects tested. Madonick[28] noted the overall incidence of Hoffmann's sign to be 2.08% in a study of 2500 patients without neurologic disease, and the sign was more frequent with advancing age. The incidence was 0.7% in those aged 0 to 19 years, 1.2% in those 20 to 39 years, 3.4% in those 40 to 59 years, and 4% in those older than 60 years. The question remained as to whether the Hoffmann sign was due to a functional disturbance of the pyramidal tract or indicated a state of increased muscle tone.

Sung and Wang[47] prospectively evaluated 16 asymptomatic patients with a positive Hoffmann's reflex using cervical radiographs and magnetic resonance imaging (MRI). Fourteen of 16 (87.5%) cervical spine x-rays were abnormal with spondylosis, and all 16 MRIs were interpreted as abnormal with spondylosis and cord compression in 15. The authors concluded that "the presence of a positive Hoffman's reflex was found to be highly associated with the presence of a cervical spine lesion causing neural compression." Imaging studies or further evaluation is not recommended, as the cohort studied remained asymptomatic, with continued yearly follow-up. The small number of subjects and lack of a control group makes strong conclusions pertaining to this study difficult.

There are no known studies assessing the inter-examiner reliability of the Hoffman's sign. Glaser et al.[22] reported a sensitivity of 58%, specificity of 78%, positive predictive value of 62%, and negative predictive value of 75% in a study of 124 patients presenting with cervical complaints. Imaging of the cervical spinal canal for evidence of cord compression with CT or MRI was used as the criterion standard. When only results of the patients with cervical spine MRIs were evaluated using blinded neuroradiologists, the sensitivity was 33%, specificity 59%, positive predictive value 26%, and negative predictive value 67%. The authors concluded that the Hoffman's sign "without other clinical findings" is not a reliable test to screen for cervical spinal cord compression. This retrospective study is useful despite its methodological flaws.

In summary, the significance of the Hoffman's sign remains disputed in the literature. The validity has not been well studied although poor to fair sensitivity and fair to good specificity are reported. Inter-examiner reliability has not been reported. Further studies exploring the validity and inter-examiner reliability of Hoffmann's sign are indicated.

Thoracic Outlet Syndrome

The thoracic outlet syndrome (TOS) is ascribed to a constellation of symptoms into the upper extremities including pain, weakness, numbness, or paresthesias. Symptoms are caused by compression of the subclavian artery and vein, axillary artery and vein, lower trunk or cords of the brachial plexus. Anatomically, the outlet can be defined by its bony borders including the first rib, first thoracic vertebra, clavicle, and manubrium of the sternum or within the muscular space between the anterior and middle scalenes. The four main sites of compression described are (Figure 3–10):

- within the scalene musculature (scalenus anticus syndrome)
- under a congenital band or bony extension of the 7th cervical transverse process (cervical rib)

Figure 3–10. Thoracic outlet anatomy. Reproduced with permission from Bennett JB, Mehlhoff TL: Thoracic outlet syndrome. In Delee JC, Drez D (eds), Orthopedic Sports Medicine: Principles and Practices. Philadelphia: WB Saunders, 1994, p. 795.

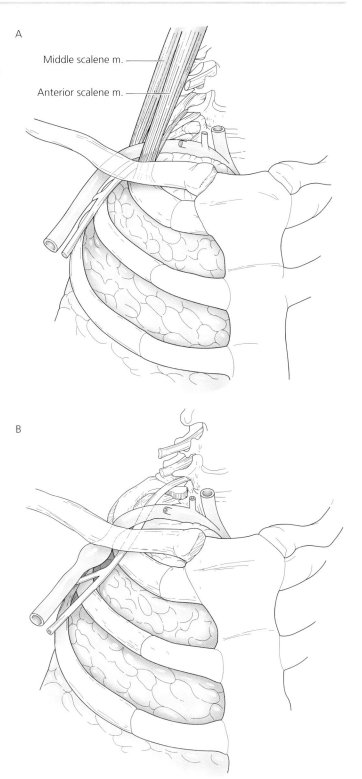

A

Middle scalene m.

Anterior scalene m.

B

- between the clavicle and the 1st rib (costoclavicular syndrome)
- under the pectoralis minor (pectoralis minor syndrome).

The syndrome is controversial, and the diagnostic tests used to assess this condition are of questionable value. Warrens and Heaton[55] found that 58% of 64 randomly chosen individuals had at least one diagnostic test positive including the Adson's, costoclavicular, and hyperabduction tests. Only 2% had more than one test positive, bringing into question the specificity of the various tests. Rayan and Jensen[39] found that 91% of normal individuals developed symptoms from at least one of the tests for TOS.

Adson's Test

In 1927, Adson and Coffey[1] described a physical exam maneuver that could be used to assess compression of the subclavian artery between a cervical rib and the scalenus anticus muscle; this maneuver later became known as Adson's maneuver (Figure 3–11). Simply stated:

> sitting upright, with arms resting on knees [the patient] takes a deep breath, extends the neck, and turns the head toward the affected side. An alteration of the radial pulse or blood pressure in the affected arm was considered "a pathognomonic sign of the presence of a cervical rib or scalenus anticus syndrome."

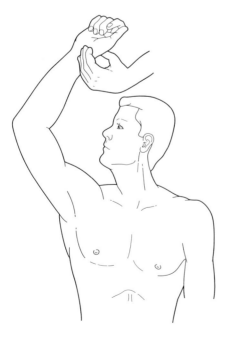

Figure 3–11. Adson's test. Reproduced with permission from Bennett JB, Mehlhoff TL: Thoracic outlet syndrome. In Delee JC, Drez D (eds), Orthopedic Sports Medicine: Principles and Practices. Philadelphia: WB Saunders, 1994, p. 796.

However, the efficacy of this test remains controversial. Based on the biomechanics of the Adson test, one would expect that the scalene angle should increase, not decrease, thus causing the aforementioned compression. Instead, the scalene angle actually increases and, in fact, this would allow more room for the brachial plexus to exit the neck and reduce the likelihood of compression.[2,35,48,54] Moreover, to date, no studies have been performed to document the reliability of this test. The specificity has been noted to range from 18% to 87%, but the sensitivity has been documented to approach 94%.[32]

Wright's Hyperabduction Test

In 1945, Wright[57] originally described the obliteration of the radial pulse in at least one upper extremity in 93% of 150 asymptomatic subjects with the arm held overhead at a 90-degree angle with the elbow flexed. He attributed the neurovascular symptom to entrapment by pectoralis minor tendon (Figure 3–12). Gilroy and Meyer[21] and Raaf[38] found that arm elevation induced radial pulse obliteration or bruit in the former, in 60% to 69% of normal subjects. The existing research clearly demonstrates that pulse diminution is a normal phenomena in the general population with overhead activity. According to Roos, "these studies clearly indicate that pulse

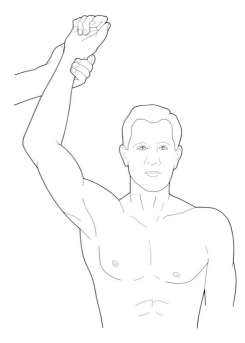

Figure 3–12. Wright's hyperabduction test. Reproduced with permission from Bennett JB, Mehlhoff TL: Thoracic outlet syndrome. In Delee JC, Drez D (eds), *Orthopedic Sports Medicine: Principles and Practices.* Philadelphia: WB Saunders, 1994, p. 797.

obliteration with the arms and head in various positions is a normal finding in the majority of asymptomatic people and therefore has no relation to the etiology or presence of symptoms."[40] Rayan and Jensen[39] suggested modification of the hyperabduction test with the elbow maintained in extension to avoid inducing ulnar nerve symptoms with elbow flexion. No studies have described the reliability, sensitivity, or specificity of this test.

Roos Test

In 1976, Roos described this elevated arm stress test as follows:

> [The patient holds the] brachium at right angles to the thorax and the forearm flexed to 90 degrees. The patient is instructed to open and close his fist at moderate speed for 3 minutes, with the elbows braced somewhat posteriorly. It reproduces the patient's usual symptoms within 3 minutes [Figure 3–13].[40]

Symptoms produced with this test include early fatigue and heaviness of the involved arm, gradual onset of numbness and tingling of the hand, increasing vocal complaints, sudden dropping of the limb into the lap, involved limb slow to recover to normal, and totally abnormal response commonly seen while radial pulses are strong.[40] Roos indicated that his elevated arm test was perhaps the most reliable of all and will delineate TOS from other problems with similar symptoms. Unfortunately, no specific data are presented to support these claims.

Plewa and Delinger[37] demonstrated in a study of four of the common tests for TOS in normal subjects that the elevated arm stress test resulted in diminution of pulse in 62% compared to 11% for Adson's or costoclavicular tests. This points to the

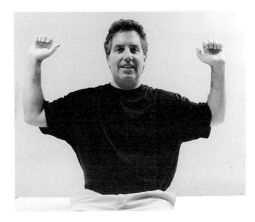

Figure 3–13. Roos test.

high false-positive rate among these tests and brings into question the sensitivity and specificity of this maneuver.

Costoclavicular Test

The original description of the costoclavicular maneuver may be ascribed to Falconer and Wedell who, in 1943, reported in a case series of three subjects with subclavian artery and vein compression that:

> costoclavicular compression of the subclavian vessels can be recognized by observing the effect of postural maneuvers of the shoulder girdle on the arterial pulse of the limb. Backward and downward bracing of the shoulders is the movement which obliterates the pulses most readily.[19]

The test is performed with the patient asked to retract and then depress the shoulders. This is followed by protrusion of the chest and a request to hold the position for 1 minute (Figure 3–14). The examiner identifying the radial pulse on the involved extremity monitors the pulse for reduction. Telford and Modershead[48] found an alteration of the radial pulse in 64% of normal individuals with shoulder depression and 68% after shoulder retraction. No studies are available that identify the sensitivity or specificity of this maneuver.

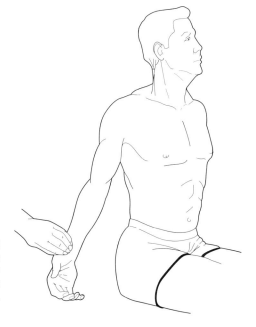

Figure 3–14. Costoclavicular test. Reproduced with permission from Bennett JB, Mehlhoff TL: Thoracic outlet syndrome. In Delee JC, Drez D (eds), Orthopedic Sports Medicine: Principles and Practices. Philadelphia: WB Saunders, 1994, p. 797.

Conclusion

The majority of the specialized provocative tests commonly used in examination of the cervical spine and related neck structures are purported to assist in identification of radiculopathy, spinal cord pathology, or brachial plexus pathology. Each of the tests described originated from the anecdotal observations of experienced, well-respected clinicians. They are summarized in Table 3–4.

Table 3–4. CERVICAL SPINE AND THORACIC OUTLET TESTS

Test	Original Description	Reliablity Studies	Validity Studies
Spurling's/neck compression test	Passive lateral flexion and compression of head. Positive test is reproduction of radicular symptoms distant from neck.	Viikari-Juntura 1987[53] Seated position. Kappa = 0.40–0.77 Proportion specific agreement = 0.47–0.80	Viikari-Juntura 1989[52] Seated position. Sensitivity: 40–60% Specificity: 92–100%
Shoulder abduction (relief) sign	Active abduction of symptomatic arm, placing patient's hand on head. Positive test is relief or reduction of ipsilateral cervical radicular symptoms.	Viikari-Juntura 1987[53] Seated position. Kappa = 0.21–0.40 Proportion specific agreement = 0.57–0.67	Viikari-Juntura 1989[52] Seated position. Sensitivity: 43–50% Specificity: 80–100%
Neck distraction test	Examiner grasps patient's head under occiput and chin and applies axial traction force. Positive test is relief or reduction of cervical radicular symptoms.	Viikari-Juntura 1987[53] Supine position. 10–15 kg traction force applied. Kappa = 0.50 Proportion specific agreement = 0.71	Viikari-Juntura 1989[52] Supine position. 10–15 kg traction force applied. Sensitivity: 40–43% Specificity: 100%
Lhermitte's sign	Passive anterior cervical flexion. Positive test is presence of "electric-like" sensations down spine or extremities.	Not reported.	Uchihara 1994[51] Sensitivity: < 28% Specificity: "high"
Hoffmann's sign	Passive snapping flexion of middle finger distal phalanx. Positive test is flexion-adduction of ipsilateral thumb and index finger.	Not reported	Glaser 2000[22] Sensitivity: 58% Specificity: 78% Positive predictive value: 62% Negative predictive value: 75%
Adson's test	Inspiration, chin elevation, and head rotation to affected side. Positive test is alteration or obliteration of radial pulse.	Not reported	Marx 1999[32] Specificity: 18–87% Sensitivity: 94%

Table 3–4. CERVICAL SPINE AND THORACIC OUTLET TESTS—*cont'd*

Test	Original Description	Reliablity Studies	Validity Studies
Wright's hyperabduction test	Arms elevated to 90 degrees, pulse palpated at wrist. Positive test is obliteration of radial pulse.	Not reported	Not reported
Roos test	Arms and elbows flexed to 90 degrees. The patient is instructed to open and close his fist at moderate speed for 3 minutes. Positive test reproduces the patient's usual symptoms within 3 minutes.	Not reported	Not reported
Costoclavicular test	Patient asked to retract and then the depress the shoulders, followed by protrusion of the chest. Positive test indicated by reduction in radial pulse.	Not reported	Not reported

Few studies have been performed addressing the inter-examiner reliability or validity of these tests. Of the studies performed, most were not methodologically sound or had other limitations. The existing literature appears to indicate high specificity, low sensitivity, and good to fair inter-examiner reliability for Spurling's neck compression test, the neck distraction test, and the shoulder abduction (relief) test when performed as described. For Hoffmann's sign, the existing literature does not address inter-examiner reliability but appears to indicate fair sensitivity and fair to good specificity. For Lhermitte's sign and Adson's test, not even tentative statements can be made with regard to inter-examiner reliability, sensitivity, and specificity, based on the existing literature. It should be emphasized that more research is indicated to understand the clinical utility of all these tests.

REFERENCES

1. Adson AW, Coffey JR. Cervical rib: a method of anterior approach for relief of symptoms by division of the scalenus anticus. Ann Surg 1927;85:839–857.
2. Adson AW. Cervical ribs: symptoms, differential diagnosis, and indications for section of the insertion of the scalenus anticus muscle. J Int Coll Surg 1951;16:546–559.
3. Anderson JH, Gaardbol O. Musculoskeletal disorders of the neck and upper limb in serving machine operators: a clinical investigation. Am J Industr Med 1993;24:689–700.
4. Aprill C, Bogduk N. The prevalence of cervical zygapophysial joint pain: a first approximation. Spine 1992;17:744–747.

5. Babinski J, Dubois R. Douleurs a forme de decharge electrique, consecutives aux traumatismes de la nuque. Presse Med 1918;26:64.

6. Beatty RM, et al. The abducted arm as a sign of ruptured cervical disc. Neurosurgery 1987;21:731–732.

7. Bendheim OL. On the history of Hoffmann's sign. Bull Inst Hist Med 1937;5:684–685.

8. Bennett JG, Bergmanis LE, Carpenter JK, Skowlund HV. Range of motion of the neck. J Am Phys Ther Assoc 1963;43:45–47.

9. Bradley JP, Tibone JE, Watkins RG. History, physical examination, and diagnostic tests for neck and upper-extremity problems. In Watkins RG (ed.), The Spine in Sports. St Louis: Mosby–Year Book, 1996.

10. Caillet R. Neck and Arm Pain. Philadelphia: FA Davis, 1991, pp. 81–123.

11. Cooper MJ. Mechanical factors governing the Tromner reflex. Arch Neurol Psychiat 1933;30:166–169.

12. Curschmann H. Uber die diagnostiche bedeutung des Babinskischen phanomens im prauramischen zustand. Munch Med Wchnschr 1911;58:2054–2057.

13. Davidson RI, et al. The shoulder abduction relief test in the diagnosis of radicular pain in cervical extradural compressive monoradiculopathies. Spine 1981;6:441–446.

14. Defibaugh JJ. Measurement of head motion. II: An experimental study of head motion in adult males. Phys Ther 1964;44:163–168.

15. Denno JJ, Meadows GR. Early diagnosis of cervical spondylotic myelopathy: a useful clinical sign. Spine 1991;16:1353–1355.

16. Echols DH. The Hoffmann sign: its incidence in university students. J Nerv Ment Dis 1936;84:427–431.

17. Ellenberg M, Honet JC. Clinical pearls in cervical radiculopathy. Phys Med Rehabil Clin N Am 1996;7:487–508.

18. Ellenberg MR, Honet JC, Treanor WJ. Cervical radiculopathy. Arch Phys Med Rehabil 1994;75:342–352.

19. Falconer MA, Weddell G. Costoclavicular compression of the subclavian artery and vein. Lancet 1943;2:539–543.

20. Fast A, Parikh S, Marin EL. The shoulder abduction relief sign in cervical radiculopathy. Arch Phys Med Rehabil 1989;70:402–403.

21. Gilroy J, Meyer JS. Compression of the subclavian artery, a cause of ischemic brachial neuropathy. Brain 1963;86:733–746.

22. Glaser JA, et al. Cervical cord compression and the Hoffman's sign. Presented at the 14th Annual Meeting of the North American Spine Society, 21 October 1999.

23. Gutrecht JA. Lhermitte's sign: from observation to eponym. Arch Neurol 1989;46:557–558.

24. Keyser TS. Hoffmann's sign or the "digital reflex." J Nerv Ment Dis 1916;44:51–62.

25. Kottke FJ, Blanchard RS. A study of degenerative changes of the cervical spine in relation to age. Bull Univ Minn Hosp 1953;24:470–479.

26. L'hermitte J. Les formes douloureuses de commotion de la moelle epiniere. Rev Neurol 1920;36:257–262.

27. Lundervold AL. Electromyographic investigation during sedentary work, especially typewriting. Br J Phys Med 1951;14:32–36.

28. Madonick MJ. Statistical control studies in neurology. III: The Hoffmann sign. Arch Neurol Psychiat 1952;68:109–115.

29. Magee DJ. Cervical spine. In Orthopedic Physical Assessment, 3rd edn. Philadelphia: WB Saunders, 1997.

30. Malanga GA. The diagnosis and treatment of cervical radiculopathy. Med Sci Sports Exerc 1997;29(7)(Suppl.):S236–S245.

31. Marie P, Chatelin C. Sur certains symtomes vraisemblablement d'orogine radiculaire chez les blesses du crane. Rev Neurol 1917;31:336.

32. Marx RG, Bombardier C, Wright JG. What we know about the reliability and validity of physical examination tests used to examine the upper extremity. J Hand Surg 1999;24A(1):185–192.

33. Milerad E, Ericson MO, Nisell R, Kilbom A. An electromyographic study of dental work. Ergonomics 1991;34:953–962.

34. Mooney V, Robertson J. Facet joint syndrome. Clin Orthop 1976;115:149–156.

35. Nachlus IW. Scalenus anticus syndrome or cervical foraminal compression? South Med J 1942;35:663–667.

36. Pitfield RL. The Hoffmann reflex: a simple way of reinforcing it and other reflexes. J Nerv Ment Dis 1929;69:252–258.

37. Plewa MC, Delinger M. The false positive rate of thoracic outlet syndrome shoulder maneuvers in healthy subjects. Acad Emerg Med 1998;5:337–342.

38. Raaf J. Surgery for cervical rib and scalenus anticus syndrome J Am Med Assoc 1965;157:219.

39. Rayan GM, Jensen C. Thoracic outlet syndrome: provocative examination maneuvers in a typical population. J Shoulder Elbow Surg 1995;4:113–117.

40. Roos DB. Congenital anomalies associated with thoracic outlet syndrome: anatomy, symptoms, diagnosis, and treatment. Am J Surg 1976;132:771–778.

41. Sandmark H, Nisell R. Validity of five common manual neck pain provoking tests. Scand J Rehab Med 1995;27:131–136.

42. Savitsky N, Madonick MJ. Statistical control studies in neurology. I: The Babinski sign. Arch Neurol Psychiat 1943;49:272–276.

43. Schneck CD. Functional and clinical anatomy of the spine. In Spine: State of the Art Reviews 9. Philadelphia: Hanley & Belfus, 1995, pp. 525–558.

44. Schneck JM. The unilateral Hoffmann reflex. J Nerv Ment Dis 1946;104:597–598.

45. Sobel JB, Sollenberger P, Robinson R, Polatin PB, Gatchel RJ. Cervical nonorganic signs: a new clinical tool to assess abnormal illlness behavior in neck pain patients: a pilot study. Arch Phys Med Rehabil 2000;81:170–175.

46. Spurling RG, Scoville WB. Lateral rupture of the cervical intervertebral discs: a common cause of shoulder and arm pain. Surg Gynecol Obstet 1944;78:350–358.

47. Sung RD, Wang JC. Correlation between a positive Hoffman's reflex and cervical pathology in asymptomatic individuals. Spine 2001;26:67–70.

48. Telford E, Modershead S. Pressure of the cervical brachial junction: an operative and anatomical study. J Bone Joint Surg (B) 1948;308:249–265.

49. Tong HC, Haig AJ. Spurling's test and cervical radiculopathy. Presented at the American Academy of Physical Medicine and Rehabilitation Annual Assembly, San Francisco, 2000.

50. Tromner E. Ueber sehnen-respective muskelreflexe und die merkmale ihrer schwachung und steigerung. Berl Klin Wchnschr 1913;50:1712–1715.

51. Uchihara T, Furukawa T, Tsukagoshi H. Compression of brachial plexus as a diagnostic test of cervical cord lesion. Spine 1994;19:2170–2173.

52. Viikari-Juntura E, Porras M, Laasonen EM. Validity of clinical tests in the diagnosis of root compression in cervical disease. Spine 1989;14:253–257.

53. Viikari-Juntura E. Interexaminer reliability of observations in physical examinations of the neck. Phys Ther 1987;67:1526–1532.

54. Walshe FMR, Jackson H, Wyburn-Mason R. On some pressure effects associated with rudimentary and "normal" first ribs, and the factors entering into their causation. Brain 1944;67:141–177.

55. Warren AN, Heaton JM. Thoracic outlet compression syndrome: the lack of reliability of its clinical assessment. Ann R Coll Surg Engl 1987;69(5):203–204.

56. White AA, Panjabi MM. Clinical Biomechanics of the Cervical Spine. Philadelphia: JB Lippincott, 1978.

57. Wright IS. The neurovascular syndrome produced by abduction of the arms: the immediate changes produced in 150 normal controls and the effects on some persons of prolonged hyperabduction of the arms as in sleeping and some occupations. Am Heart J 1945;29:1–19.

58. Youdas JW, Carey JR, Garrett TR. Reliability of measurements of cervical range of motion comparison of three methods. Phys Ther 1991;71:98–104.

59. Youdas JW, Garrett TR, Suman VJ, et al. Normal range of motion of the cervical spine: an initial goniometric study. Phys Ther 1992;72:770–780.

Chapter 4

Physical Examination of the Shoulder

JAY E. BOWEN, DO • GERARD A. MALANGA, MD •
TUTANKHAMEN PAPPOE, MD •
EDWARD MCFARLAND, MD

Introduction

The shoulder girdle allows for a large degree of motion in multiple planes, with the glenohumeral joint being the most mobile joint in the body. The tradeoff for this freedom of motion is a relative lack of stability, which makes the shoulder girdle susceptible to an array of injuries. A number of physical exam maneuvers have been developed to assist the examiner in diagnosing shoulder problems. Performing these maneuvers accurately and understanding their reliability and validity are paramount to a proper shoulder exam. In this chapter, we review common shoulder examination maneuvers, identifying the original descriptions and presenting research examining the sensitivity, specificity, positive predictive value (PPV) and negative predictive value (NPV) of the various tests.

Examination of the Shoulder

A thorough examination of shoulder complaints should include the cervical spine, contra-lateral shoulder, elbow, trunk and upper-limb neurovascular structures. We will limit our focus to the shoulder girdle which includes the sternoclavicular (SC), acromioclavicular (AC), glenohumeral (GH), and scapulothoracic (ST) joints.

Inspection

The patient should be examined in various positions when possible, especially from behind where elements such as muscle bulk and scapular positioning can be easily observed. Posture should be observed in both the seated and standing positions and from different angles. Inspection for scars, atrophy, swelling, ecchymosis, erythema, rashes, deformities, shoulder heights, and scapular positioning should be evaluated. Posture in the standing and seated position should be observed for a forward set, protracted head and/or rounded shoulders (humeral internal rotation and scapular protraction) which both will cause functional narrowing of the subacromial space. Scapular winging may be seen and can be accentuated by muscle activation (Figure 4–1). Observing the shoulder girdle from the back of the patient during arm flexion and abduction may demonstrate altered movement of the scapula secondary to muscle weakness or imbalances in flexibilities.

Palpation

The sternal notch, SC joint, clavicle, acromioclavicular joint, long head of the biceps tendon, subacromial bursae, greater and lesser tuberosities of the humerus, coracoid process, supraclavicular fossa, and the spine of the scapula with its borders are the superficial structures which should be evaluated (Figure 4–2). The acromioclavicular

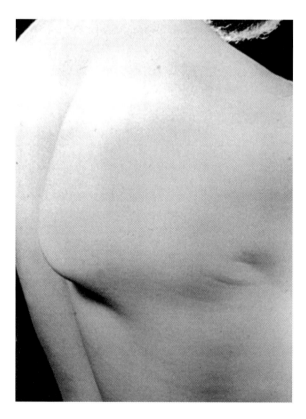

Figure 4–1. Winging of the scapula. Reproduced with permission from Hawkins RJ, Bokor DJ: Clinical evaluation of shoulder problems. In Rockwood CA, Matsen FA (eds), The Shoulder, 2nd edn. Philadelphia: WB Saunders, 1998, p. 172.

Figure 4–2. The subacromial bursa region. Adapted from Jobe CM: Gross anatomy of the shoulder. In Rockwood CA, Matsen FA (eds), The Shoulder, 2nd edn. Philadelphia: WB Saunders, 1998, p. 88.

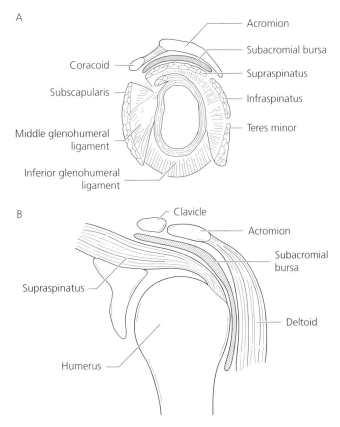

joint is superficial and is identified with palpation of the clavicle and spine of the scapula until they meet laterally. The long head of the biceps is anterior between the lesser and greater humeral tuberosities and more easily palpated with some external rotation of the arm (Figure 4–3). The coracoid process lies medial to the long head of the biceps inferior to the clavicle. The scapula should be examined as the patient resists forward flexion or does a push-up against the wall to evaluate for weakness of the serratus anterior secondary to injury of the long thoracic nerve or disuse atrophy (Figure 4–1). This results in the scapula being situated more medially secondary to the unopposed action of the middle trapezius. In addition, the examiner may look for weakness of the upper trapezius secondary to injury of the spinal accessory nerve by monitoring the scapula during active as well as resisted arm abduction. This will result in a more laterally situated scapula, secondary to the unopposed action of the serratus anterior. The examiner can place hands over both scapulae while the patient abducts his or her arms to monitor for dysrhythmia. Kibler has described measurement from the spinous processes to the medial border of the scapula with side-to-side comparison to note a lateral displaced (protracted) scapula. This can be done with the arms at the sides and at various degrees of abduction. The superior angle of the

A

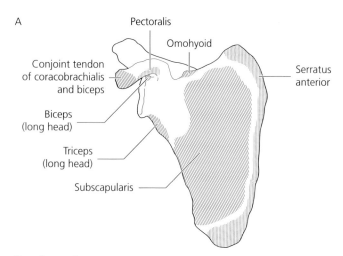

Pectoralis

Omohyoid

Conjoint tendon
of coracobrachialis
and biceps

Biceps
(long head)

Triceps
(long head)

Subscapularis

Serratus
anterior

Figure 4–3. Muscular anatomy about the
scapula. **A:** Anterior view. **B:** Posterior view.
Adapted from Jobe CM: Gross anatomy of the
shoulder. In Rockwood CA, Matsen FA (eds), The
Shoulder, 2nd edn. Philadelphia: WB Saunders,
1998, p. 44.

B

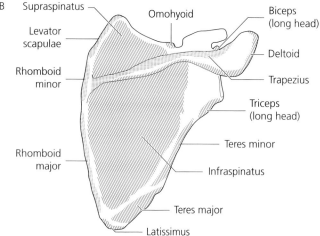

Supraspinatus

Levator
scapulae

Rhomboid
minor

Rhomboid
major

Omohyoid

Biceps
(long head)

Deltoid

Trapezius

Triceps
(long head)

Teres minor

Infraspinatus

Teres major

Latissimus

scapula corresponds to the second rib, the spine of the scapula to the level of third
thoracic vertebra (T3), and the inferior border to T7.

The axilla should be evaluated for masses, lymph nodes, and palpation of the
muscles. The pectoralis lies anterior and the minor portion is commonly tight leading
to an internally rotated position of the humerus. The latissimus dorsi forms the
posterior border.

Range of Motion Testing

Active range of motion is usually performed first to allow the patient to feel comfortable and avoid painful positions. Passive motion can then be performed to isolate
motions for accurate evaluation. The planes of shoulder girdle motion include forward
flexion, extension, internal/external rotation, abduction/adduction, and a combination

called *circumduction*. Range of motion is noted by degrees from a reference position; usually the anatomic position is used without scapular fixation unless otherwise specified.

Forward flexion is from 0 to 180 degrees and extension to 60 degrees. Internal rotation cannot be accurately measured in the anatomic position since the trunk impedes the motion. Functional internal rotation can be assessed by using the Apley scratch test (Figure 4–4). To isolate glenohumeral motion, the arm should be abducted to 90 degrees and the scapula manually fixed. The neutral position is with the arm and forearm in the horizontal plane (Figure 4–5). Internal/external rotation from this position can vary greatly, particularly in overhead athletes. Generally, external rotation is 90 degrees or more, and internal rotation is 60–70 degrees. Adduction is also limited secondary to the trunk position. With the arm crossing in front of the trunk, 30 degrees is normal (Figure 4–6). Normal abduction range of motion is from 0 to 180 degrees (Table 4–1).[21]

Apley Scratch Test

In the 1940s, A. G. Apley described the Apley scratch test in courses he taught to assess range of motion of the shoulder (see Figure 4–4). The test is commonly performed by having the patient reach behind the back in internal rotation and behind the neck in adduction and external rotation.[48,68] The degree of rotation can be quantified by documenting the level of the spinous process that can be reached.

Despite being widely utilized for testing shoulder range of motion, our search of the literature was unable to locate any studies that discuss the sensitivity, specificity, positive predictive value, or negative predictive value of this maneuver.

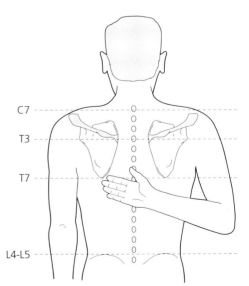

Figure 4–4. Functional internal rotation using the "Apley scratch test." Adapted from Matsen FA, Lippitt SB, Sidles JA, Harryman DT: Practical Evaluation and Management of the Shoulder. Philadelphia: WB Saunders, 1994, p. 782.

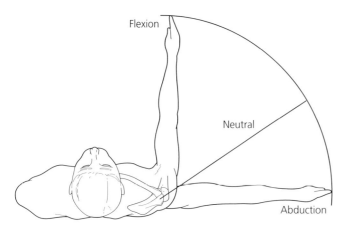

Figure 4–5. Neutral plane of the shoulder. Adapted from Perry J: Anatomy and biomechanics of the shoulder in throwing, swimming, gymnastics, and tennis. Clin Sports Med 1983;2(2):255.

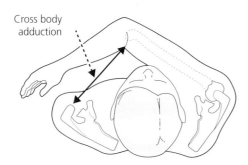

Figure 4–6. Cross-body adduction. Adapted from Matsen FA, Lippitt SB, Sidles JA, Harryman DT: Practical Evaluation and Management of the Shoulder. Philadelphia: WB Saunders, 1994.

Table 4–1. RANGE OF MOTION

Position	Degrees
Forward flexion/elevation[a]	0–180
Extension[a]	0–60
Abduction[a]	0–180
Adduction (humerus passes in front of trunk)[a]	0–30
Glenohumeral internal rotation[b]	0–70
Glenohumeral external rotation[b]	0–90

[a]Zero begins at the anatomic position.
[b]Zero begins with the humerus abducted to 90 degrees.
Reproduced with permission from Moore KL: The upper limb. In Clinically Oriented Anatomy, 2nd edn. Baltimore: Williams & Wilkins, 1985.

Muscles, Innervations, and Biomechanics

The muscles of the shoulder consist of the stabilizing rotator cuff (supraspinatus, infraspinatus, teres minor, and subscapularis; Figure 4–7), trapezius, serratus anterior, rhomboids, and the prime movers (pectoralis major/minor, latissimus dorsi, teres major, triceps, biceps, and deltoid; Figure 4–8). Most of the shoulder girdle is supplied by the fifth and sixth cervical roots through the upper trunk of the brachial plexus.

The suprascapular nerve (C5–C6) innervates the supraspinatus and infraspinatus, which originate from the supraspinatus and infraspinatus fossa, respectively. The supraspinatus inserts onto the superior facet of the greater tuberosity while the infraspinatus inserts on the middle facet. The axillary nerve (C5–C6) innervates the deltoid and teres minor. The deltoid originates from the lateral third of the clavicle and scapular spine and includes the acromioclavicular joint; it inserts onto the deltoid tuberosity of the humerus. The teres minor originates from the superior lateral portion of the scapula and inserts onto the inferior aspect of the greater tuberosity. The subscapularis is innervated by the nerve to the subscapularis (upper and lower) composed of the cervical 5, 6, and 7 roots. It originates from the anterior portion of the scapula (subscapularis fossa) and inserts onto the lesser tuberosity of the humerus.

The trapezius contains three portions, upper, middle, and lower. It is innervated by the spinal accessory, eleventh cranial nerve (C3–C4). It has a vast origin from the occipital protuberance and superior nuchal line superiorly to the twelfth thoracic vertebra inferiorly. It inserts onto the lateral third of the clavicle, acromion and spine of the scapula. The long thoracic nerve (C5–C7) innervates the serratus anterior. It originates from the lateral portions of the first eight ribs and inserts on to the anterior surface of the medial border of the scapula. The rhomboids include the major and minor divisions and are innervated by the dorsal scapular nerve (C5). They originate from the ligamentum nuchae and spinous processes from C7 to T5 and insert on to the medial border of the scapula from the scapular spine to the inferior angle.

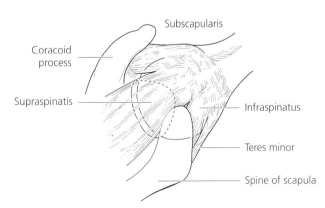

Figure 4–7. The stabilizing effect of the rotator cuff muscles on the humeral head. Adapted from Perry J: Anatomy and biomechanics of the shoulder in throwing, swimming, gymnastics, and tennis. Clin Sports Med 1983;2(2):252.

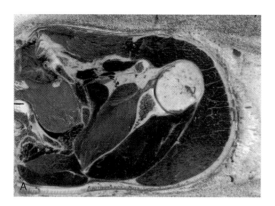

Figure 4–8. Prime movers about the shoulder girdle: **1,** pectoralis major; **2,** pectoralis minor; **3,** first rib; **4,** serratus anterior; **5,** second rib; **6,** third rib; **7,** rhomboid; **8,** trapezius; **9,** subscapularis; **10,** infraspinatus; **11,** deltoid. Adapted from Jobe CM: Gross anatomy of the shoulder. In Rockwood CA, Matsen FA (eds), The Shoulder, 2nd edn. Philadelphia: WB Saunders, 1998, p. 43.

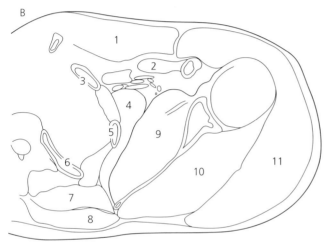

The pectoralis major has two components, the clavicular and sternocostal divisions, which are innervated by the lateral and medial pectoral nerves (clavicular, C5–C6 and sternocostal, C7–T1). The pectoralis minor is also innervated by these nerves (C6–C8). The major originates from the medial portion of the clavicle, sternum, and second to sixth ribs and inserts on to the humeral lateral lip of the intertubercular groove. The minor originates from ribs 3–5 and inserts onto the medial coracoid. The latissimus dorsi is supplied by the thoracodorsal nerve (C6–C8) and has a large origin of the spinous processes of T6 to the sacrum, the thoracolumbar fascia, iliac crest, and the caudal three ribs while inserting onto the floor of the intertubercular groove. The teres major is supplied by the lower subscapular nerve (C6–C7). It originates on the dorsal surface of the inferior angle of the scapula and inserts on to the medial lip of the intertubercular groove. The triceps has three heads, the long, lateral, and medial, which are supplied by the radial nerve (C6–C8). The long head originates from the infraglenoid tubercle of the scapula and the lateral and medial heads from the posterior surface of the humerus superior and inferior to the spiral groove, respectively.

They insert on to the proximal ulna (olecranon). The biceps is comprised of the long and short heads innervated by the musculocutaneous nerve (C5–C6). The long head originates from the supraglenoid tubercle of the scapula and the short head from the coracoid process of the scapula and both insert on to the radial tuberosity and flow into the bicipital aponeurosis.

Scapular Biomechanics

Saha[71] has discussed three layers of muscles, which stabilize the scapula and assist in force production from the musculature. The rotator cuff muscles (supraspinatus, infraspinatus, subscapularis, and teres minor) are the inner layer. The middle layer compromises the teres major, pectoralis major, latissimus dorsi, and the short fibers of the anterior and posterior deltoid. The superficial layer is the triceps, long head of the biceps, coracobrachialis, and the superficial fibers of the anterior and posterior deltoid. The trapezius, rhomboids, and serratus anterior provide stabilizing forces since the scapula lacks rigid, bony fixation.

The upper trapezius, levator scapula, and superior serratus anterior elevate the scapula; the pectoralis minor and major and latissimus dorsi depress the scapula; the serratus anterior, pectoralis minor, and levator scapula protract the scapula; the trapezius, rhomboids, and latissimus dorsi retract the scapula; the superior and inferior portions of the trapezius and inferior portion of the serratus anterior cause lateral scapula rotation; and the levator scapula, rhomboids, pectoralis minor, and major and latissimus dorsi cause medial scapular rotation. These muscles fire in a coordinated fashion to perform the resultant actions in a smooth and effective manner, which are known as *force couples*.

Proper positioning of the scapula throughout motion allows for the muscles associated with the scapula to have the appropriate length tension relations for the greatest efficiency of limb positioning. With the scapula stabilized, the glenoid can be maintained for humeral motion upon it. As the humerus is abducted, the glenohumeral to scapulothoracic range of motion occurs at approximately a 2:1 ratio. This ratio changes through the arc of motion; that is, the 2:1 ratio is not constant throughout the entire range of motion. In the initial portion of abduction, glenohumeral motion predominates and the ratio has been found to be 4.4 of glenohumeral for every degree of scapulothoracic motion. As the shoulder moves above 90 degrees of abduction, this ratio becomes 1.1 degrees of GH to 1 degree of ST motion. This scapular rotation during abduction also elevates the acromion to prevent impingement.[34,66]

As the muscles are the dynamic stabilizers, the static stabilizers of the ligaments and joint capsule cannot be forgotten (Figure 4–9). The primary stabilizer of anterior translation with the arm abducted to 90 degrees is the anterior band of the inferior glenohumeral ligament complex (IGHLC). With the arm in lesser degrees of abduction,

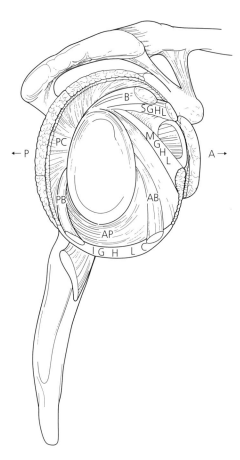

Figure 4–9. Anatomy of the glenohumeral liga-ments. A, anterior; P, posterior; B, long head of biceps; PC, posterior capsule; PB, posterior band; AB, anterior band; SGHL, superior glenohumeral ligament; MGHL, middle glenohumeral ligament; IGHLC, inferior glenohumeral ligament complex. Reproduced with permission from Bowen MK, Warren RF: Ligamentous control of shoulder stability based on selective cutting and static translation experiments. Clin Sports Med 1991;10:763.

the middle glenohumeral ligament restricts motion. Limitation of posterior translation is the posterior band of the IGHLC while inferior translation is limited by superior glenohumeral ligament (Figure 4–10).[76] Recently it has been noted that the inferior glenohumeral ligament also affords limitation of inferior motion with the arm abducted.[15]

Tests of Rotator Cuff Strength and Integrity

See Table 4–2.

Dynamic stability of the glenohumeral joint is provided by contraction of the rotator cuff and the long head of the biceps, which increases compression across the glenohumeral joint and dynamically maintains co-optation of the humeral head within the glenoid.[1,3,8,11,13]

Jenp et al.[27] used electromyography to detect the most specific positions for activating particular rotator cuff muscles. The supraspinatus could not be effectively isolated. The subscapularis' greatest activation was with the arm in the scapular plane at 90 degrees of elevation and neutral humeral rotation. The infraspinatus-teres minor

Figure 4–10. The superior glenohumeral ligament (SGHL): the primary restraint to inferior translation. AB, anterior band; MGHL, middle glenohumeral ligament; PB, posterior band. Reproduced with permission from Bowen MK, Warren RF: Ligamentous control of shoulder stability based on selective cutting and static translation experiments. Clin Sports Med 1991;10:769.

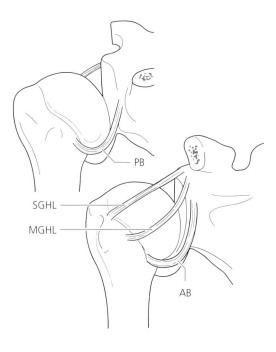

Table 4–2. ROTATOR CUFF PATHOLOGY

Test	Description	Reliability/Validity Tests
Empty can test	The supraspinatus test is first performed by assessing the deltoid with the arm at 90 degrees of abduction and neutral rotation. The shoulder is then internally rotated and angled forward 30 degrees: the thumb should be pointing toward the floor. Muscle testing against resistance is then performed.	Malanga et al.[49] Sensitivity and specificity not reported. Noted supraspinatus activated but not isolated with empty can maneuvers Naredo et al.[57] For detecting supraspinatus lesion: Sensitivity 79.3% Specificity: 50% For detecting supraspinatus tendonitis: Sensitivity: 77.2% Specificity: 38.4% For detecting supraspinatus tears: Sensitivity: 18.7% Specificity: 100%
Drop arm test	The examiner abducts the patient's shoulder to 90 degrees and then asks the patient to slowly lower the arm to the side in the same arc of movement. A positive test is indicated if the patient is unable to return the arm to the side slowly or has severe pain when attempting to do so.	Bryant et al.[7] For detecting RTC tear PPV: 100% Sensitivity: 10%

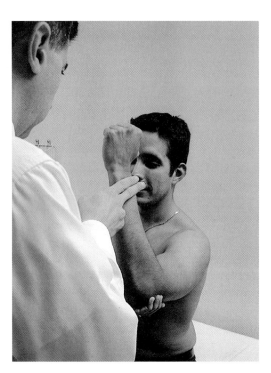

Figure 4–11. Hornblower's position for testing the infraspinatus and teres minor.

muscles were isolated with the arm in the sagittal plane and the humerus elevated to 90 degrees in mid-range of external rotation. This is also referred as the "hornblower's position" (Figure 4–11).

Kelly et al.[31,33] performed a similar study and noted isolation was greatest at the following positions: supraspinatus, arm elevation to 90 degrees in the scapular plane, and 45 degrees of humeral external rotation; infraspinatus, 0 degrees of arm elevation, 45 degrees of humeral internal rotation and resisted external rotation; and the subscapularis, with the Gerber lift-off test.

Empty Can Test

Jobe[29] described the "empty can test" – also known as the supraspinatus test – to help in evaluating the strength of the supraspinatus muscle. It was originally described as follows (Figure 4–12):

> The supraspinatus test is first performed by assessing the deltoid with the arm at 90 degrees of abduction and neutral rotation. The shoulder is then internally rotated and angled forward 30 degrees: the thumb should be pointing toward the floor. Muscle testing against resistance is then performed.

Blackburn and colleagues[6,54] have noted that strengthening of the posterior rotator cuff is greatest with the humerus abducted to 90 degrees, full humeral internal

Figure 4–12. The empty can test.

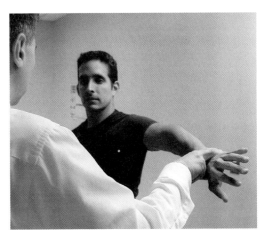

rotation, and horizontal adduction to 30 degrees. With the patient in the prone position and the arm abducted with humeral external rotation, the supraspinatus and other posterior cuff musculature is maximally exercised.

Malanga et al.[49] examined the rotator cuff muscles via electromyography utilizing two different testing positions based on Jobe and Blackburn's recommendations. They noted the supraspinatus was sufficiently activated in both positions. However, isolation of the supraspinatus was not achieved in either position as surrounding muscle activity was always noted.

In a comparison of Jobe's test to findings on ultrasound, Naredo et al.[57] found that the test had a sensitivity of 79.3%, specificity of 50%, positive predictive value of 95.8, and negative predictive value of 14.2 for detecting supraspinatus lesions; a sensitivity of 77.2%, specificity of 38.4%, positive predictive value of 61.9%, and negative predictive value of 50% for detecting supraspinatus tendonitis; and a sensitivity of 18.7%, specificity of 100%, positive predictive value of 100%, and negative predictive value of 53.7% for detecting supraspinatus tears. The "lesions" were not specifically defined, but appear to represent a tendinopathy. They examined the Jobe position to assess rotator cuff pathology, not strength.

Drop Arm Test

The drop arm test has been used to assess for rotator cuff tear, particularly of the supraspinatus. Although the original description of the drop arm test remains obscure, it has been ascribed to Codman and described by Magee as follows:

> The examiner abducts the patient's shoulder to 90 degrees and then asks the patient to slowly lower the arm to the side in the same arc of movement. A positive test is indicated if the patient is unable to return the arm to the side slowly or has severe pain when attempting to do so.[48]

Bryant et al.[7] studied 53 patients with a suspicion for rotator cuff (RTC) tear and compared physical examination tests to the results of MRI and ultrasonography of the shoulder. They found the drop arm test to have a 100% PPV (i.e., if present the patient has a tear) and 10% sensitivity (if negative the patient could still have a tear). Other authors have looked at the drop arm test as a part of other physical tests without reporting the reliability of the drop test itself.[14]

Tests of Infraspinatus and Teres Minor Integrity

See Table 4–3.

As noted above, previous electromyographic data have failed to differentiate the function of the infraspinatus and teres minor.[27,31] Jenp et al. found the infraspinatus and teres minor muscles were best isolated with the arm in the sagittal plane and the humerus elevated to 90 degrees in mid-range of external rotation. The "hornblower's sign" was first described in an obstretic plexus palsy and referred to weakness of external rotation of the shoulder as manifested by difficulty raising the hand to the mouth with external rotation of the shoulder.[82] This weakness would be manifested by the affected elbow falling inferiorly.

Table 4–3. TESTS OF INFRASPINATUS AND TERES MINOR INTEGRITY

Test	Description	Reliability/Validity Tests
Patte's test	The examiner supports the patient's elbow in 90 degrees of forward elevation in the plane of the scapula while the patient is asked to rotate the arm laterally in order to compare the strength of lateral rotation. Jobe's and Patte's maneuvers can produce three types of responses: (a) absence of pain, indicating that the tested tendon is normal; (b) the ability to resist despite pain, denoting tendonitis; or (c) the inability to resist with gradual lowering of the arm or forearm, indicating tendon rupture.	Naredo et al.[57] For detecting infraspinatus lesions: Sensitivity: 70.5% Specificity: 90% For detecting infraspinatus tendonitis: Sensitivity: 57.1% Specificity: 70.8% For detecting infraspinatus tears: Sensitivity: 36.3% Specificity: 95%
Lift-off test	This test is performed with the patient standing or seated with the arm internally rotated behind their back. They are then asked to lift the forearm off of their back against examiner resistance. A patient with a subscapularis rupture is unable to lift the dorsum of his hand off his back, a finding that we call a "pathological lift-off test."	Greis and Kuhn[19] Statistically significant difference in muscle activity when test performed from midback and buttocks regions Naredo et al.[57] For detecting subscapularis lesions: Sensitivity: 50% Specificity: 84.2% For detecting subscapularis tears: Sensitivity: 50% Specificity: 95.4%

Patte's "Dropping" Test

Naredo et al. reported a test described by Patte in 1995 for assessing tears of the infraspinatus and teres minor (Figure 4–13). They write:

> The examiner supports the patient's elbow in 90 degrees of forward elevation in the plane of the scapula while the patient is asked to rotate the arm laterally in order to compare the strength of lateral rotation. Jobe's and Patte's maneuvers can produce three types of responses: (a) absence of pain, indicating that the tested tendon is normal; (b) the ability to resist despite pain, denoting tendonitis; or (c) the inability to resist with gradual lowering of the arm or forearm, indicating tendon rupture.[57]

Naredo and colleagues compared Patte's test to findings on ultrasound and showed the test to have a sensitivity of 70.5%, specificity of 90%, positive predictive value of 85.7%, and negative predictive value of 70.5% for detecting infraspinatus lesions; a sensitivity of 57.1%, specificity of 70.8%, positive predictive value of 36.2%, and negative predictive value of 85% for detecting infraspinatus tendonitis; and a sensitivity of 36.3%, specificity of 95%, positive predictive value of 80%, and negative predictive value of 73% for detecting infraspinatus tears.

Tests of Subscapularis Strength

Lift-off Test

Muscle strength of the subscapularis can be tested with the lift-off maneuver. The test was first described by Gerber and Krushell in 1991 and was originally described as follows (Figure 4–14):

> This test is performed with the patient standing or seated with the arm internally rotated behind their back. They are then asked to lift the forearm off of their back against examiner resistance. A patient with a subscapularis rupture is unable to lift the dorsum of his hand off his back, a finding that we call a "pathological lift-off test".[17]

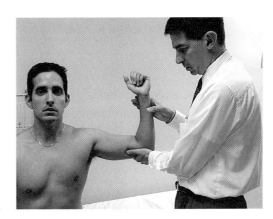

Figure 4–13. The Patte test.

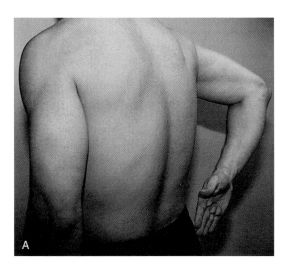
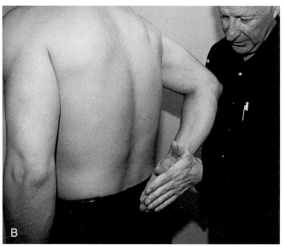

Figure 4–14. The lift-off test. Reproduced with permission from Hawkins RJ, Bokor DJ: Clinical evaluation of shoulder problems. In Rockwood CA, Matsen FA (eds), The Shoulder, 2nd edn. Philadelphia: WB Saunders, 1998, p. 192.

Greis and Khun[19] showed a statistically significant difference in muscle activity between the subscapularis muscle and the other muscles tested when the test was performed both from the midback and buttocks regions.

Naredo et al.[57] compared findings of the lift-off test to findings on ultrasound and showed the test to have a sensitivity of 50%, specificity of 84.2%, positive predictive value of 66.6, and negative predictive value of 72.7 for detecting subscapularis lesions; a sensitivity of 50%, specificity of 88%, positive predictive value of 56%, and negative predictive value of 88% for detecting subscapularis tendonitis: and a sensitivity of 50%, specificity of 95.4%, positive predictive value of 75%, and negative predictive value of 87.5% for detecting subscapularis tears.

Tests of the Scapula

See Table 4–4.

The dynamic scapulothoracic stabilizers, including the serratus anterior, trapezius, and rhomboids, allow for proper positioning of the glenoid for articulation and subsequent movement of the humeral head. Dysfunction of any of the dynamic stabilizers can lead to subsequent instability. Without dynamically fixing the scapula functionally throughout motion by the use of the stabilizing muscles, the base on which the humerus moves will be compromised and result in dysfunction. This impaired glenohumeral motion may result in rotator cuff impingement as improper clearance of the humeral head under the coraco-acromial arch occurs.[1,3,8,11,13]

Table 4–4. SCAPULAR PATHOLOGY

Test	Description	Reliability/Validity Tests
Lateral slide test	The first position of the test is with the arm relaxed at the side. The second is with the hands on the hips with the fingers anterior and the thumb posterior with about 10 degrees of shoulder extension. The third position is with the arms at or below 90 degrees of arm elevation with maximal internal rotation at the glenohumeral joint. These positions offer a graded challenge to the functioning of the shoulder muscles to stabilize the scapula. The final position presents a challenge to the muscles in the position of most common function at 90 degrees of shoulder elevation.	Odom et al.[64] With 1.5 cm difference as positive: In first position: Sensitivity: 28% Specificity: 53% In second position: Sensitivity: 50% Specificity: 58% In third position: Sensitivity: 34% Specificity: 52% With 1 cm difference: In first position: Sensitivity: 35% Specificity: 48% In second position: Sensitivity: 41% Specificity: 54% In third positin: Sensitivity: 43% Specificity: 56%
Isometric pinch test	A good provocative maneuver to evaluate scapular muscle strength is to do an isometric pinch of the scapulae in retraction. Scapular muscle weakness can be noted as a burning pain in less than 15 seconds. Normally, the scapula can be held in this position for 15–20 seconds with the patient having no burning pain or muscle weakness.	Unable to find any tests of sensitivity or specificity
Scapular assistance test	The scapular assistance test involves assisting the lower trapezius by manually stabilizing the upper medial border [of the scapula] and rotating the inferomedial border as the arm is abducted or adducted. The test is positive, indicating lower trapezius weakness as part of the injury, when it gives relief of symptoms of impingement, clicking, or rotator cuff weakness.	We have found no tests assessing the sensitivity, specificity, positive predictive value, or negative predictive value, of this test.
Scapular retraction test	The test involves manually positioning and stabilizing the entire medial border of the scapula. This test is helpful in two groups of patients. The first group has decreased retraction and apparent muscle weakness. The test is positive when retesting reveals increased muscle strength with the scapula in the stabilized position. The second group has a positive Jobe relocation test. The test is positive when scapular retraction decreases the pain or impingement associated with the Jobe relocation test. This indicates that decreased scapular retraction is a component of the overall injury and must be addressed in rehabilitation. A positive scapular retraction test indicates trapezius and rhomboid weakness.	We have found no tests assessing the sensitivity, specificity, positive predictive value, or negative predictive value, of this test.

Lateral Scapular Slide Test

Kibler[36] described the lateral scapular slide test (LSST) in identification of subtle scapulothoracic motion abnormalities. The test is described by Kibler as follows (Figure 4–15):

> The first position of the test is with the arm relaxed at the side. The second is with the hands on the hips with the fingers anterior and the thumb posterior with about 10 degrees of shoulder extension. The third position is with the arms at or below 90 degrees of arm elevation with maximal internal rotation at the glenohumeral joint.

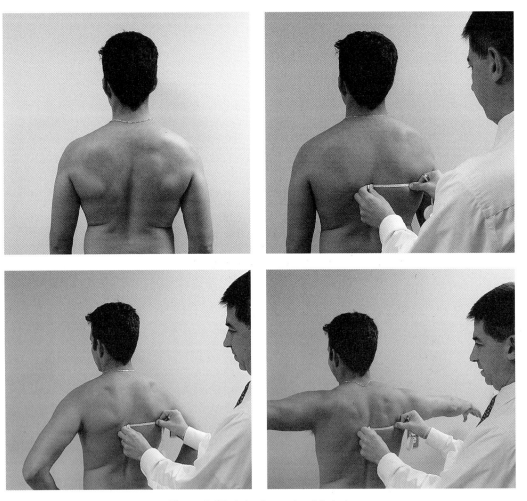

Figure 4–15. Lateral scapular slide test.

These positions offer a graded challenge to the functioning of the shoulder muscles to stabilize the scapula. The final position presents a challenge to the muscles in the position of most common function at 90 degrees of shoulder elevation.

The reference point on the spine is the nearest spinous process, which is then marked with an X. The measurements from the reference point on the spine to the inferomedial border of the scapula are measured on both sides. In the second position, the new position of the inferomedial border of the scapula is marked, and the reference point on the spine is maintained. The distances once again are calculated on both sides. The same protocol is done for the third position.[34]

Odom et al.[64] reported 1 cm of asymmetry as being positive for a pathologic scapulothoracic motion abnormality. Kibler[36] defined 1.5 cm of asymmetry as positive for a scapulothoracic motion abnormality. Odom et al.[64] found the LSST to have a sensitivity of 28% and specificity of 53% in the first position, a sensitivity of 50% and specificity of 58% in the second position, and a sensitivity of 34% and 52% for the third position when a positive result was considered a difference of 1.5 cm. The authors also conducted the test using a positive result as a 1 cm difference. Under these conditions, the test had a sensitivity 35% and specificity of 48% in the first position, a sensitivity of 41% and specificity of 54% in the second position, and a sensitivity of 43% and 56% for the third position. The authors felt that "the LSST should not be used to identify people with [or] without shoulder dysfunction."

Isometric Pinch Test

In Kibler's 1998 paper, "the role of the scapula in athletic shoulder function" is described by a provocative maneuver for evaluating scapular muscular strength.[36] Kibler writes:

A good provocative maneuver to evaluate scapular muscle strength it to do an isometric pinch of the scapulae in retraction. Scapular muscle weakness can be noted as a burning pain in less than 15 seconds. Normally, the scapula can be held in this position for 15 to 20 seconds with the patient having no burning pain or muscle weakness.[34]

We have been unable to find any tests assessing the sensitivity, specificity, positive predictive value, or negative predictive value of this maneuver.

Scapular Assistance Test

Another test for the strength of the scapular stabilizers is the scapular assistance test described by Kibler et al. in 2000. The test is described as follows:

The scapular assistance test involves assisting the lower trapezius by manually stabilizing the upper medial border [of the scapula] and rotating the inferiomedial border as the arm is abducted or adducted. The test is positive, indicating lower trapezius weakness as part of the injury, when it gives relief of symptoms of impingement, clicking, or rotator cuff weakness.[37]

We have found no tests assessing the sensitivity, specificity, positive predictive value, or negative predictive value of this test.

Scapular Retraction Test

In 2000, Kibler et al. described his scapular retraction test as follows:

> The scapular retraction test involves manually positioning and stabilizing the entire medial border of the scapula. This test is helpful in two groups of patients. The first group has decreased retraction and apparent muscle weakness. The test is positive when retesting reveals increased muscle strength with the scapula in the stabilized position. The second group has a positive Jobe relocation test. The test is positive when scapular retraction decreases the pain or impingement associated with the Jobe relocation test. This indicates that decreased scapular retraction is a component of the overall injury and must be addressed in rehabilitation. A positive scapular retraction test indicates trapezius and rhomboid weakness.[37]

We have found no tests assessing the sensitivity, specificity, positive predictive value, or negative predictive value of this test.

Tests of the Biceps Tendon

See Table 4–5.

As mentioned in the previous section, dynamic stability can be assisted by contraction of the rotator cuff and by the long head of the biceps (particularly when there is a loss of rotator cuff force), which increases compression across the glenohumeral joint. Along with being a possible source of instability, inflammation at the biceps tendon can be a significant source of pain.

Ludington Test

In 1923, Nelson Ludington described a test for diagnosing rupture of the long head of the biceps[46] (Figure 4–16). Ludington writes:

> The patient is directed to rest his folded hands, palms down, on the top of his head and allow the interlocked fingers to support the weight of the arms. In this position there is maximum relaxation of the long head [of the biceps tendon]. The examiner then places two fingers on the tendon of the long head of the biceps in each arm, and directs the patient to simultaneously contract and relax his biceps muscles. The contraction of the long head tendon on the sound side is plainly felt while it is absent on the affected side if the tendon is ruptured.[46]

Table 4–5. BICEPS TENDON TESTS

Test	Description	Reliability/Validity Tests
Ludington test	The patient is directed to rest his folded hands, palms down, on the top of his head and allow the interlocked fingers to support the weight of the arms. In this position there is maximum relaxation of the long head [of the biceps tendon]. The examiner then places two fingers on the tendon of the long head of the biceps in each arm, and directs the patient to simultaneously contract and relax his biceps muscles. The contraction of the long head tendon on the sound side is plainly felt while it is absent on the affected side if the tendon is ruptured.	There are no reported studies assessing the sensitivity, specificity, positive predictive value, or negative predictive value of this maneuver.
Yergason's test	If the elbow is flexed to ninety degrees, the forearm being pronated and the examining surgeon holds the patient's wrist so as to resist supination, and then directs that active supination be made against his resistance; pain, very definitely localized in the bicipital groove, indicates a condition of wear and tear of the long head of the biceps, or synovitis of the tendon sheath. In fractures of the lesser tuberosity of the humerus, even without displacement, the supination sign will be positive. The sign will be negative in cases of partial or complete rupture of the supraspinatus tendon, which are very common.	Calis et al.[9] For diagnosis of subacromial impingement (not evaluating the biceps tendon) using MRI and Neer's injection test as the gold standards: Sensitivity: 37% Specificity: 86.1%
Speed's test	Have the patient flex his shoulder [elevate it anteriorly] against resistance while the elbow is extended and the forearm supinated. The test is considered positive when pain is localized to the bicipital groove.	Bennett[4] Sensitivity: 90% Specificity: 13.8% Calis et al.[9] For subacromial impingement: Sensitivity: 68.5% Specificity: 55.5%

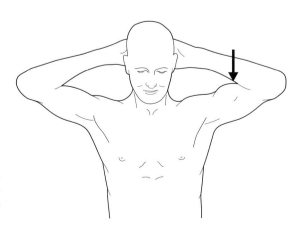

Figure 4–16. Ludington's test. Adapted from Burkhead WZ, et al.: The biceps tendon. In Rockwood CA, Matsen FA (eds), The Shoulder, 2nd edn. Philadelphia: WB Saunders, 1998, p. 1037.

There are no reported studies assessing the sensitivity, specificity, positive predictive value, or negative predictive value of this maneuver.

Yergason's Test

Robert M. Yergason originally described his "supination sign" for evaluating tendonitis of the biceps tendon in 1931. He described the test as follows (Figure 4–17):

> If the elbow is flexed to 90 degrees, the forearm being pronated and the examining surgeon holds the patient's wrist so as to resist supination, and then directs that active supination be made against his resistance; pain, very definitely localized in the bicipital groove, indicates a condition of wear and tear of the long head of the biceps, or synovitis of it tendon sheath ... In fractures of the lesser tuberosity of the humerus, even without displacement, the supination sign will be positive. ... The sign will be negative in cases of partial or complete rupture of the supraspinatus tendon, which are very common.[85]

To validate the exam, Yergason presented a case report of a patient complaining of shoulder and arm pain for a year. The supination test was positive in this patient. When reviewing the patient's history it was found that a large amount of her daily

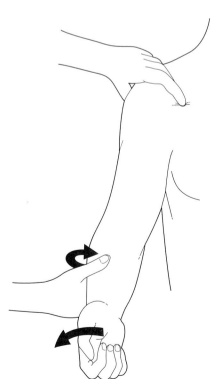

Figure 4–17. Yergason's sign. Adapted from Burkhead WZ, et al: The biceps tendon. In Rockwood CA, Matsen FA (eds), The Shoulder, 2nd edn. Philadelphia: WB Saunders, 1998, p. 1036.

activities involved washing clothes by hand and it was extrapolated that these actions would be enough to produce wear and tear of the biceps tendon in its groove. Buying a washing machine and reducing the patient's level of activity brought about complete recovery in less than a month.

Calis et al.[9] found the Yergason's test to have a sensitivity of 37%, specificity of 86.1%, positive predictive value of 86.8%, and negative predictive value of 35.6% for diagnosis of subacromial impingement using MRI and Neer's injection test as the gold standards. The authors described the test for a disorder of the long head of the biceps tendon, but did not specify how this related to the diagnosis of impingement.

Speed's Test

The earliest reference of this study in the literature was by Crenshaw and Kilgore on "the surgical treatment of bicipital tenosynovitis" in 1996.[12] They cite a personal communication with Speed in 1952. They describe the test as follows (Figure 4–18):

> [Have] the patient flex his shoulder [elevate it anteriorly] against resistance while the elbow is extended and the forearm supinated. The test is considered positive when pain is localized to the bicipital groove.

Bennett[4] found Speed's test to have a specificity of 13.8%, sensitivity of 90%, positive predictive value of 23%, and negative predictive value of 83%.

Calis et al.[9] noted the Speed's test to have a sensitivity of 68.5%, specificity of 55.5%, positive predictive value of 79.2%, and negative predictive value 41.6% for subacromial impingement. Again, these authors do not specify how this test assists in the diagnosis of impingement syndrome.

Burkhart et al.[8] evaluated Speed's test for labral pathology.

Impingement Tests

See Table 4–6.

Impingement syndrome is a clinical entity involving compression of the structures that course through the subacromial space (i.e., the supraspinatus tendon and the overlying subdeltoid bursae). This space can be compromised primarily by arthritic or

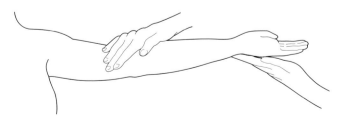

Figure 4–18. Speed's test. Adapted from Burkhead WZ, et al: The biceps tendon. In Rockwood CA, Matsen FA (eds), The Shoulder, 2nd edn. Philadelphia: WB Saunders, 1998, p. 1035.

Table 4–6. IMPINGEMENT TESTS

Test	Description	Reliability/Validity Tests
Neer's sign test	Elevation of the arm in internal rotation or in the anatomical position of external rotation causes the critical area to pass under the coracoacromial ligament or the anterior process of the acromion. The critical area does not touch the posterior two-thirds of the acromion. With scapular rotation the acromion is tilted backwards, leaving the anterior process as the leading edge. At about 80 degrees of abduction, the critical area of the supraspinatus tendon passes beneath the acromioclavicular joint and this joint tilts with overhead elevation of the arm. With the joint in this position, it is logical to assume that excrescences on the undersurface if the anterior margin of the acromion may impinge on the cuff.	Calis et al.[9] Sensitivity: 88.7% Specificity: 30.5% MacDonald et al.[47] For assessing subacromial bursitis: Sensitivity: 75% Specificity: 47.5% For detecting rotator cuff pathology: Sensitivity: 83.3% Specificity: 50.8%
Neer's test (subacromial injection test)	Hemorrhage is often present and blood may be aspirated from the bursa. Pain may be temporarily stopped by instilling 1% Xylocaine into the bursa.	There are no studies which validate Neer's test.
Hawkin's test	This involves forward flexing the humerus to 90 degrees and forcibly internally rotating the shoulder. This maneuver drives the greater tuberosity farther under the coracoacromial ligament, similarly reproducing the impingement pain.	MacDonald et al.[47] For assessing subacromial bursitis: Sensitivity: 91.7% Specificity: 44.3% For rotator cuff pathology: Sensitivity: 87.5% Specificity: 42.6% Calis et al.[9] Sensitivity: 92.1% Specificity: 25% MacDonald et al.[47] When Neer's and Hawkin's were both positive for detecting bursitis: Sensitivity 70.8% Specificity: 50.8% For detecting rotator cuff pathology: Sensitivity: 83.3% Specificity: 55.7% If only one of the two tests was positive: For detecting bursitis: Sensitivity: 95.8% Specificity: 41% For detecting rotator cuff pathology: Sensitivity: 87.5% Specificity: 37.7%
Yocum's test	The patient is asked to place the hand on his or her other shoulder and to raise the elbow without elevating the shoulder. This test is positive when it elicits the pain usually experienced by the patient.	Naredo et al.[57] Yocum's test in combination with Hawkin's and Neer's test: Sensitivity: 65% Specificity: 72.7% There are no studies evaluating the Yocum test in isolation.

hypertrophic changes to the acromion or secondarily from instability of the shoulder joint causing the humeral head to migrate superiorly. Chronic compression of these structures can cause inflammation, rotator cuff wear, and resultant tears.

Neer's Sign

In 1972, Neer hypothesized impingement of the rotator cuff with forward flexion of the arm, and a physical exam maneuver has become synonymous with his name[58] (Figure 4–19).

> Thus, elevation of the arm in internal rotation or in the anatomical position of external rotation causes the critical area to pass under the coracoacromial ligament or the anterior process of the acromion. The critical area does not touch the posterior two-thirds of the acromion. With scapular rotation the acromion is tilted backwards, leaving the anterior process as the leading edge. At about 80 degrees of abduction, the critical area of the supraspinatus tendon passes beneath the acromioclavicular joint and this joint tilts with overhead elevation of the arm. With the joint in this position, it is logical to assume that excrescences on the undersurface of the anterior margin of the acromion may impinge on the cuff.[55]

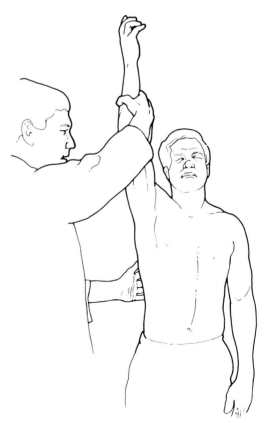

Figure 4–19. Neer's impingement test. Reproduced with permission from Jobe FW, Bradley JP: Diagnosis of shoulder injuries. Clin Sports Med 1989; 8:425.

The Calis et al. study[9] of 125 painful shoulders demonstrated Neer's sign to have a sensitivity of 88.7%, specificity of 30.5%, positive predictive value of 75.9%, and negative predictive value 52.3% when compared to MRI findings.

MacDonald et al.[47] noted the Neer's sign to have a sensitivity of 75%, specificity of 47.5%, positive predictive value 36%, and a negative predictive value 82.9% for assessing subacromial bursitis; and a sensitivity of 83.3%, specificity of 50.8%, positive predictive value 40.0%, and a negative predictive value 88.6% for detecting rotator cuff pathology in 85 patients.

Neer's Subacromial Injection Test

In 1977, Neer developed a test to evaluate possible impingement of the rotator cuff tendon.[58] Neer states in reference to acute traumatic subacromial bursitis that "hemorrhage is often present and blood may be aspirated from the bursa. Pain may be temporarily stopped by instilling 1% Xylocaine into the bursa."

In 1980, Hawkins referenced Neer's above article for stage I impingement, noting "relief of pain by injecting 10 mL of 1% lidocaine beneath the anterior acromion helps confirm the diagnosis [of impingement]."[23] This is also generically referred to as the subacromial injection test (SIT).

There are no studies that validate Neer's test. However, Calis et al.[9] did use a positive SIT (relief of pain and restoration of passive and/or active motion 30 minutes after the injection) to separate pathology of impingement from other causes to identify the sensitivity, specificity, positive predictive value, and negative predictive value of the physical examination maneuvers. They noted the most sensitive to be Hawkins' test at 92.1%, Neer's test at 88.7%, and the horizontal adduction test at 82%; while the most specific tests were the arm drop test at 97.2%, Yergason test at 86.1%, and painful arc test at 80.5%.

In 1998, Bergman and Fredericson noted that the fluid remains for less than 3 days, and MRI should be deferred during this time period;[5] whereas Wright et al. found that testing could be completed after 24 hours.[84]

Kirkley et al.[40] used the test unsuccessfully to predict outcomes from subacromial decompression for rotator cuff tendinosis. There was no correlation in the Western Ontario Rotator Cuff Index scores and the classic impingement test.

Hawkins' Test

Hawkins and Schutte[25] described this impingement physical exam test as follows (Figure 4–20):

> Another less reliable method of demonstrating this impingement involves forward flexing the humerus to 90 degrees and forcibly internally rotating the shoulder. This maneuver drives the greater tuberosity farther under the coracoacromial ligament, similarly reproducing the impingement pain.

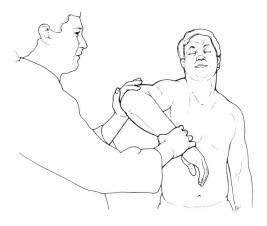

Figure 4–20. Hawkin's impingement test. Reproduced with permission from Jobe FW, Bradley JP: Diagnosis of shoulder injuries. Clin Sports Med 1989; 8:426.

MacDonald et al.[47] found in 85 patients that, when compared to the findings at time of arthroscopy, the Hawkins test had a sensitivity of 91.7%, specificity of 44.3%, positive predictive value 39.3%, and negative predictive value 93.1% for assessing subacromial bursitis; and a sensitivity of 87.5%, specificity of 42.6%, positive predictive value 37.5%, and negative predictive value 89.7% for detecting rotator cuff pathology.

Calis et al.[9] found the test to have a sensitivity of 92.1%, specificity of 25%, positive predictive value of 75.2%, and negative predictive value of 56.2% when compared with MRI.

MacDonald and Clark[47] evaluated the ability of different combinations of Neer's test and Hawkins' test to detect subacromial bursitis and rotator cuff pathology when compared to the findings at time of arthroscopy. The authors found that when they were both positive the combined tests had a sensitivity of 70.8%, specificity of 50.8%, positive predictive value of 36.2%, and negative predictive value of 81.6% for detecting bursitis; and a sensitivity of 83.3%, specificity of 55.7%, positive predictive value of 42.6%, and negative predictive value of 55.7% for detecting rotator cuff pathology. If only one of the two tests was positive, the combination had a sensitivity of 95.8%, specificity of 41%, positive predictive value of 39%, and negative predictive value 96% for detecting bursitis; and a sensitivity of 87.5%, specificity of 37.7%, positive predictive value of 35.6%, and negative predictive value of 88.5% for detecting rotator cuff pathology. This means there was an improved sensitivity and negative predictive value for detecting bursitis and rotator cuff pathology with lower specificity and positive predictive value.

Yocum's Test

Naredo describes a test developed by Lewis Yocum for assessing impingement (Figure 4–21).[57,86] The test is described as follows:

> The patient is asked to place the hand on his or her other shoulder and to raise the elbow without elevating the shoulder. This test is positive when it elicits the pain usually experienced by the patient.

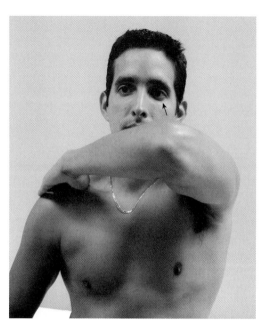

Figure 4–21. Yocum's test (elbow elevated).

Naredo[57] showed that Yocum's test in combination with Hawkins' and Neer's test had a sensitivity of 65%, specificity of 72.7%, positive predictive value of 81.2%, and negative predictive value of 53% when compared to findings on ultrasound. There are no studies evaluating the Yocum test in isolation.

See also the description of the posterior apprehension test below; this maneuver also assists in assessment of impingement.

Testing Shoulder Stability: Basics

As mentioned in the introduction, the tradeoff for the shoulder complex's significant degree of motion is a relative lack of stability. Static stability is achieved through the interaction of the glenoid, humeral head, labrum, capsule, and glenohumeral and coracohumeral ligaments.[73,74] Dynamic stability is maintained by the rotator cuff musculature, long head of the biceps, and scapular stabilizers. Contraction of the muscles around the shoulder and proprioceptive feedback also play a role by protecting the relatively weak ligamentous structures from being overwhelmed by excessive tension. A lax shoulder from a damaged labrum, capsule, or ligaments can be a significant source of pain if the dynamic musculature cannot control the excess motion and resultant impingement of tissues. Instability exists when laxity causes clinical symptoms.

Tests for Shoulder Anterior Stability

See Table 4–7.

Table 4–7. STABILITY TESTS

Test	Description	Reliability/Validity Tests	Comments
Apprehension test	This test can be carried out with the patient in either a standing or supine position. As the shoulder is moved passively into maximal external rotation in abduction and forward pressure is applied to the posterior aspect of the humeral head, the patient suddenly becomes apprehensive and complains of pain in the shoulder.	Holovacs et al.[26] For diagnosing labral pathology: Sensitivity: 69% Specificity: 50% Liu and Henry[44] For predicting labral tears in combination with the relocation, load and shift, inferior sulcus sign and crank tests: Sensitivity: 90% Specificity: 85%	
Fowler's sign (relocation test)	The examiner first performs the apprehension test and at the point where the patient feels pain or apprehension the examiner applies a posteriorly directed force to the humeral head. If the pain is related to primary impingement, it will persist despite the posteriorly applied force. If the pain and discomfort is from instability and secondary impingement, this action should "relocate" the humeral head and allow full pain-free external range.	Speer et al.[77] Without the provocative maneuver in regard to pain Sensitivity: 30% Specificity: 58% In regard to apprehension without the provocative maneuver: Sensitivity: 57% Specificity: 100% With the provocative maneuver for pain: Sensitivity: 54% Specificity 44% With the provocative maneuver for apprehension: Sensitivity: 68% Specificity 100% Burkhart et al.[8] For diagnosing anterior labral lesions: Sensitivity: 4% Specificity: 27% For assessing posterior labral lesions: Sensitivity: 85% Specificity: 68% For assessing combined labral lesions: Sensitivity: 59% Specificity: 54%	Without the provocative maneuver, accuracy of 80% in regard to apprehension With the provocative maneuver, accuracy of 85% for apprehension This study of SLAP lesions did not include patients with traditional anterior, inferior instability.

Continued

Table 4–7. STABILITY TESTS—*cont'd*

Test	Description	Reliability/Validity Tests	Comments
		Liu and Henry[44] In predicting labral tears when testing in combination with the apprehension, load and shift, inferior sulcus sign and crank test: Sensitivity: 90% Specificity: 85%	
Anterior release test	This test is performed with the patient in the supine position, with the affected shoulder over the edge of the examining table. The patient's arm is abducted 90 degrees while the examiner places a posteriorly directed force on the patient's humeral head with his hand. The posterior force is maintained while the patient's arm is brought into the extreme of external rotation. The humeral head is then released. The test result is considered positive when the patient experiences a sudden pain, a distinct increase in pain, or when the patient states that his or her symptoms have been reproduced.	Gross and Distefano[20] Sensitivity: 91.9% Specificity: 88.9%	
Fulcrum test	The patient lies supine at the edge of the examination table with the arm abducted to 90 degrees. The examiner places one hand on the table under the glenohumeral joint to act as a fulcrum. The arm is gently and progressively extended and externally rotated over this fulcrum. Maintenance of gentle passive external rotation for a minute fatigues the subscapularis, challenging the capsular contribution to the anterior stability of the shoulder. The patient with anterior instability will usually become apprehensive as this maneuver is carried out.	There are no studies on the sensitivity or specificity for the fulcrum test for assessing stability.	Holovacs and Osbahr[26] reported the fulcrum test to have sensitivity of 69% and specificity of 50% for detecting labral pathology when compared to findings on arthroscopy.
Anterior drawer test	The affected shoulder is held in 80–120 degrees of abduction, 0–20 degrees of forward flexion, and 0–30 degrees of lateral rotation; this position should be quite comfortable. The examiner holds the patient's scapula with his left hand,	No studies have been conducted on sensitivity or specificity.	

Table 4–7. STABILITY TESTS—*cont'd*

Test	Description	Reliability/Validity Tests	Comments
	pressing the scapular spine forward with his index and middle fingers; his thumb exerts counter-pressure on the coracoid process. The scapula is now held firmly in the examiner's left hand. With his right hand, he grasps the patient's relaxed upper arm in its resting position and draws anteriorly with a force comparable to that used in the knee Lachman's test.		
Protzman's test	The anterior aspect of the humeral head is palpated with the fingers of one hand deep in the axilla, while the fingers of the other hand are placed over the posterior aspect of the humeral head. The humeral head is then forced anteriorly and inferiorly with the posterior fingers. If the glenohumeral joint subluxates, pain will accompany anterior–inferior displacement. The examiner will often sense excessive anterior–posterior glenohumeral excursion of the symptomatic side when compared to the normal shoulder. Examination of the asymptomatic side is an integral part of a complete shoulder examination.	There are no studies assessing sensitivity or specificity.	
Load and shift test	With the patient sitting or supine, the scapula is stabilized by securing the coracoid and the spine process with one hand. The humeral head is then grasped with the other hand to glide it anteriorly and posteriorly. The degree of glide is graded mild, moderate, or severe.	Neer [61] In diagnosing Bankart lesions: Sensitivity: 90.9% Specificity: 93.3%	Liu and Henry [44] In predicting labral tears when the load and shift test was combined with apprehension, relocation, inferior sulcus sign, and crank tests: Sensitivity: 90% Specificity: 85%
Posterior drawer test	Assuming the left shoulder is being tested, the examiner grasps the patient's proximal forearm with left hand, flexes the elbow to about 120 degrees, and positions the shoulder into 80–120 degrees of abduction and 20–30 degrees of forward flexion. The examiner holds the scapula with his right hand, with his index and middle	There are no studies on the sensitivity or specificity of this test.	

Table 4–7. STABILITY TESTS—*cont'd*

Test	Description	Reliability/Validity Tests	Comments
	fingers on the scapular spine; his thumb lies immediately lateral to the coracoid process, so that its ulnar aspect remains in constant contact with the coracoid while performing the test. With his left hand, the examiner slightly rotates the upper arm medially and flexes it to about 60 or 80 degrees. During this maneuver, the thumb of the examiner's right hand subluxates the humeral head posteriorly.		
Posterior apprehension sign	This tests posterior instability and subacromial impingement by flexing the humerus to 90 degrees and internally rotating it fully reproduced symptoms of instability.	There are no studies on the sensitivity or specificity of this test.	
Jerk test	The patient sits with the arm internally rotated and flexed forward to 90 degrees. The examiner grasps the elbow andaxially loads the humerus in a proximal direction. While axial loading of the humerus is maintained, the arm is moved horizontally across the body. A positive result is indicated by a sudden jerk as the humeral head slides off the back of the glenoid. When the arm is returned to the original position of 90 degree abduction a second jerk may be observed, that of the humeral head returning to the glenoid.		Holovacs and Osbahr[26] reported the test to have sensitivity of 19% and specificity of 95% for *labral* injury when compared to the findings at arthroscopy.
Sulcus sign	The test is performed with the patient upright and the shoulder in the neutral position and relaxed. Stress is applied to the upper arm and not the forearm; this eliminates the effect of the biceps and the triceps brachii. A positive result invariably points to a more complex (multidirectional) instability.	There are no studies that have examined the sensitivity or specificity of the sulcus sign for inferior instability.	Liu and Henry[44] In predicting labral tears in combination with the relocation, load and shift, apprehension and crank tests: Sensitivity: 90% Specificity: 85%
Hyperabduction test	To measure the range of passive abduction, the physician stands behind the patient with his forearm pushed down firmly on the shoulder girdle in its lowest position, while lifting the relaxed upper limb in abduction with the other hand. During the test, the elbow is flexed at 90 degrees and the forearm horizontal. Under these conditions, the shoulder girdle should not move and any movement is measured by a goniometer.	The sensitivity and specificity have not been established in any studies.	

The anterior band of the inferior glenohumeral ligament complex is considered to be the primary restraint for anterior translation at 90 degrees of shoulder abduction. At lesser degrees of shoulder abduction, the middle glenohumeral ligament and superior glenohumeral ligament are believed to assist in resisting continued translation. The labrum, which is the major site of attachment for these ligaments, plays an important role as well.[1,3,8,11,13]

Apprehension Test

The apprehension test was first described by Rowe and Zarins in 1981 (Figure 4–22).[71] The test is classically described as follows:

> This test can be carried out when the patient is either in a standing or in a supine position. As the shoulder is moved passively into maximal external rotation in abduction and forward pressure is applied to the posterior aspect of the humeral head, the patient suddenly becomes apprehensive and the patient complains of pain in the shoulder.

> In a study presented at the American Academy of Orthopedic Surgery's 67th annual meeting, Holovacs and Osbahr reported the apprehension test to have a sensitivity of 69% and specificity of 50% for diagnosing labral pathology when compared to findings at the time of arthroscopy.[26]

> Liu and Henry[44,45] evaluated the apprehension test in combination with the relocation, load and shift, inferior sulcus sign, and crank tests. The authors found that the combination of these physical exam maneuvers had a sensitivity of 90% and specificity of 85% in predicting labral tears when comparing findings at the time of arthroscopy.

Relocation Test (Fowler's Test)

The relocation test initially described by Jobe (1989), with credit also given to Fowler (1982), is complementary to the apprehension test.[28,77] The test is used to help

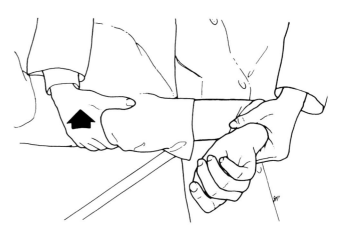

Figure 4–22. Apprehension test. Reproduced with permission from Jobe FW, Bradley JP: Diagnosis of shoulder injuries. Clin Sports Med 1989; 8:427.

discern whether the pain or discomfort from the apprehension test is attributed to anterior instability or primary impingement (Figure 4–23).

The examiner first performs the apprehension test and at the point where the patient feels pain or apprehension the examiner applies a posteriorly directed force to the humeral head. If the pain is related to primary impingement, it will persist despite the posteriorly applied force. If the pain and discomfort is from instability and secondary impingement, this action should 'relocate' the humeral head and allow full pain free external range.[28]

Speer et al.[77] evaluated the relocation test with and without the application of an anterior force to the proximal humerus. The authors found that when compared to operative findings of anterior instability, the test without the relocation maneuver had a sensitivity of 30%, specificity of 58%, positive predictive value of 38%, and negative predictive value of 49%. With relocation, the test had a sensitivity of 54%, specificity of 44%, positive predictive value of 45%, and negative predictive value of 53%. They noted that only patients with anterior instability reported apprehension; however, it was also noted that many patients do not innately understand what is happening in their shoulders so they report that they only feel "pain."

Burkhart et al.[8] showed that, when compared to the findings at time of arthroscopy or open surgery, the relocation test had a sensitivity of 4% and specificity of 27% for diagnosing anterior labral lesions, a sensitivity of 85% and specificity of 68% for assessing posterior labral lesions, and a sensitivity of 59% and specificity of 54% for assessing combined labral lesions. However, this study of SLAP lesions did not include patients with traditional anterior, inferior instability.

Liu and Henry[44] found that combining the relocation test with the apprehension, load and shift, inferior sulcus sign, and crank tests produced a sensitivity of 90% and specificity of 85% in predicting labral tears when comparing findings at the time of

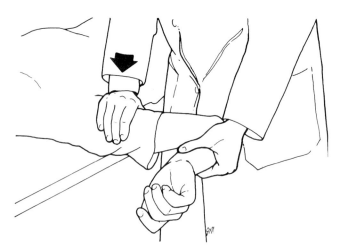

Figure 4–23. Relocation test. Reproduced with permission from Jobe FW, Bradley JP: Diagnosis of shoulder injuries. Clin Sports Med 1989; 8:427.

arthroscopy. Further comment cannot be made since these patients were not evaluated separately.

Anterior Release Test

Gross and Distefano describe the anterior release test as a test for assessing anterior glenohumeral instability (Figure 4–24).[20] They write:

> The anterior release test is performed with the patient in the supine position, with the affected shoulder over the edge of the examining table. The patient's arm is abducted 90 degrees while the examiner places a posteriorly directed force on the patient's humeral head with his hand. The posterior force is maintained while the patient's arm is brought into the extreme of external rotation. The humeral head is then released. The test result is considered positive when the patient experiences a sudden pain, a distinct increase in pain, or when the patient states that his or her symptoms have been reproduced.

This test differs from the apprehension test in that a positive test is indicated by pain on release of the posterior force on the humeral head. With the apprehension test, a positive test is pain or apprehension in the abducted and externally rotated position without a posteriorly directed force. It should also be performed with caution to avoid subluxation.

The authors found the anterior release test to have a sensitivity of 91.9%, specificity of 88.9%, positive predictive value of 87.1%, and negative predictive value of 93%, when compared to the findings at time of surgery. The patients were considered to have anterior instability if one or more of the following was present: (1) subluxation or gross dislocation on examination under anesthesia, (2) abnormal glenohumeral excursion during arthroscopic examination, (3) a Hill Sach's lesion, or (4) a Bankart lesion.

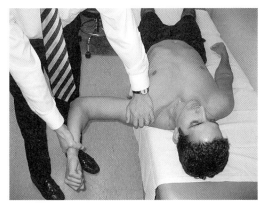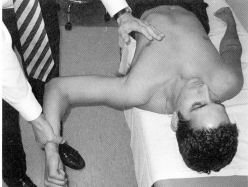

Figure 4–24. Anterior release test.

Fulcrum Test

We were unable to find the original description of the fulcrum test. It is classically described as follows (Figure 4–25):

> The patient lies supine at the edge of the examination table with the arm abducted to 90 degrees. The examiner places one hand on the table under the glenohumeral joint to act as a fulcrum. The arm is gently and progressively extended and externally rotated over this fulcrum. Maintenance of gentle passive external rotation for a minute fatigues the subscapularis, challenging the capsular contribution to the anterior stability of the shoulder. The patient with anterior instability will usually become apprehensive as this maneuver is carried out (watch the eyebrows for a clue that the shoulder is getting ready to dislocate). In this test, normally no translation occurs because it is performed in a position where the anterior ligaments are placed under tension.[51]

Holovacs and Osbahr[26] reported the fulcrum test to have sensitivity of 69% and specificity of 50% for detecting labral pathology when compared to findings on arthroscopy. In their study, the authors did not specify the type of labral pathology.

Anterior Shoulder Drawer Test

This test was described by Gerber and Ganz[16] to assess anterior instability of the shoulder. They describe the test as follows (Figure 4–26):

> The test is performed with the patient supine. The examiner stands facing the affected shoulder. Assuming the left shoulder is being tested, the examiner fixes the patient's left hand in his own right axilla by adducting his own humerus. The patient should lightly hold the examiner's upper arm and remain relaxed.

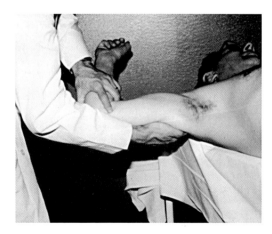

Figure 4–25. Fulcrum test. Reproduced with permission from Matsen FA, et al: Glenohumeral instability. In Rockwood CA, Matsen FA (eds), The Shoulder, 2nd edn. Philadelphia: WB Saunders, 1998, p. 680.

Figure 4–26. Anterior shoulder drawer test.

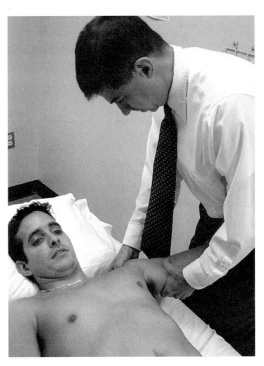

The affected shoulder is held in 80 to 120 degrees of abduction, 0 to 20 degrees of forward flexion, and 0 to 30 degrees of lateral rotation; this position should be quite comfortable. The examiner holds the patient's scapula with his left hand, pressing the scapular spine forward with his index and middle fingers; his thumb exerts counter-pressure on the coracoid process. The scapula is now held firmly in the examiner's left hand. With his right hand, he grasps the patient's relaxed upper arm in its resting position and draws anteriorly with a force comparable to that used in the knee Lachman's test.

The relative movement between the fixed scapula and the moveable humerus can easily be appreciated and can be graded as with knee instability. An occasional audible click on forward movement of the humeral head, probably due to labral pathology, is usually associated with apprehension. Its presence should be noted in addition to recording the degree of anterior displacement of the humeral head.

Levy et al.[42] evaluated the inter- and intra-observer reproducibility of gleno-humeral laxity on examination. They evaluated anterior, posterior and inferior humeral head translation using a 0–4 grading of laxity. When grade 0 and 1 laxity were grouped together, inter-observer reproducibility was 78% and intra-observer 74%. When groups were separated, the scores were 47% and 46%, respectively, and the κ values noted were no better than chance.

Protzman's Test

In 1980, Protzman described his test for anterior instability as follows (Figure 4–27):

> The patient is examined while seated, with the elbow supported on the examiner's hip, or while lying supine with the elbow supported on a pillow. The shoulder muscles must be completely relaxed to avoid intrinsic stabilization of the joint. The anterior aspect of the humeral head is palpated with the fingers of one hand deep in the axilla, while the fingers of the other hand are placed over the posterior aspect of the humeral head. The humeral head is then forced anteriorly and inferiorly with the posterior fingers. If the glenohumeral joint subluxates, pain will accompany anterior–inferior displacement. The pain is often felt posteriorly, strongly suggesting that it originates in those tightened posterior structures that are preventing further anterior displacement of the humerus. The examiner will often sense excessive anterior–posterior glenohumeral excursion of the symptomatic side when compared to the normal shoulder. Examination of the asymptomatic side is an integral part of a complete shoulder examination. Infrequently there will be a palpable click in the involved shoulder, resembling a positive McMurray sign in the knee, as the humeral head glides over an abnormal glenoid rim or loose body.[67]

No studies assess the sensitivity, specificity, positive predictive value, or negative predictive value of this exam maneuver.

Load and Shift Test

The load and shift test is used to test stability of the shoulder in the anterior and posterior directions. Credit is given to Hawkins, Abrams, and Schutte for developing this exam maneuver. The only documentation we could find of this study was an

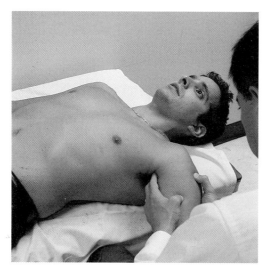

Figure 4–27. Protzman's test.

abstract published in 1987, which contains no specific description of the test.[22] The test is classically described as follows (Figure 4–28):

> With the patient sitting or supine, the scapula is stabilized by securing the coracoid and the spine process with one hand. The humeral head is then grasped with the other hand to glide it anteriorly and posteriorly. The degree of glide is graded mild, moderate or severe.[28]

The grading system mentioned in the description was devised by Hawkins and Schutte in a later study assessing their exam maneuver[25]:

- Grade I: 0–25% movement (minimal movement)
- Grade II: 25–50% movement (feeling the humeral head ride up on the glenoid rim)
- Grade III: greater than 50% movement (feeling the humeral head ride up and over the glenoid rim).

Neer and Foster's[61] findings using the load and shift test were a positive predictive value of 93.8%, sensitivity of 90.9%, and specificity of 93.3% in diagnosing Bankart lesions when compared to findings at the time of arthroscopy or open surgery.

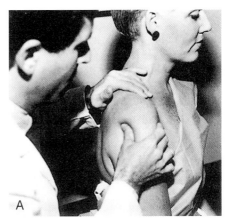

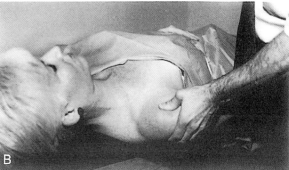

Figure 4–28. Load and shift test. Reproduced with permission from Abrams J: Special shoulder problems in the throwing athlete: pathology, diagnosis, and non-operative management. Clin Sports Med 1991;10:855.

Liu et al.[45] found that combining the load and shift with the apprehension, relocation, inferior sulcus sign, and crank tests produced a sensitivity of 90% and specificity of 85% in predicting *labral tears* when comparing findings at the time of arthroscopy.

Tests for Shoulder Posterior Stability

See Table 4–7.

The posterior band of the inferior glenohumeral ligament complex is the primary restraint to posterior translation of the humeral head. The superior glenohumeral ligament, coracohumeral ligament, and the rotator interval (anterior–superior portion of the capsule) play a role as well. As will be discussed later, the labrum assists in all aspects of stability.[1,3,8,11,13]

Posterior Drawer Test

Gerber and Ganz[16] described the posterior drawer test to evaluate posterior translation of the shoulder (Figure 4–29). This test can also be used to evaluate posterior instability. They describe the test as follows:

> The patient lies supine and the examiner stands level with the affected shoulder. Assuming the left shoulder is being tested; he/she grasps the patient's proximal forearm with his/her left hand, flexes the elbow to about 120 degrees, and positions the shoulder into 80 to 120 degrees of abduction and 20 degrees to 30 degrees of forward flexion. The examiner holds the scapula with his/her right hand, with his/her index and middle fingers on the scapular spine; his thumb lies immediately lateral to the coracoid process, so that its ulnar aspect remains in constant contact with the coracoid while performing the test. With his/her left hand, the examiner slightly rotates the upper arm medially and flexes it to about 60 or 80 degrees. During this maneuver, the thumb of the examiner's right hand subluxates the humeral head posteriorly. This posterior displacement can be appreciated as the thumb slides along the lateral

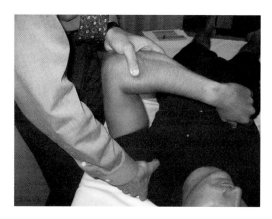

Figure 4–29. Posterior drawer test.

aspect of the coracoid process towards the glenoid, and the humeral head abuts against the ring finger of the examiner's right hand. This maneuver is pain free, but often associated with a slight to moderate degree of apprehension enabling the patient to identify the position of instability with certainty.

There are no studies assessing the sensitivity, specificity, positive predictive value, and negative predictive value of this exam maneuver.

Posterior Apprehension Sign

O'Driscoll[63] was the first to describe the test that is now referred to as the posterior apprehension sign (Figure 4–30). This tests posterior instability and "subacromial impingement by flexing the humerus to 90 degrees and internally rotating it fully reproduced symptoms of instability."

At the same time, O'Driscoll reported a prospective study of two groups, one with posterior instability and the other subacromial impingement. Both groups had reproduction of their symptoms on exam testing. The two groups had been separated by radiographs and subacromial lidocaine injections. The instability group had continued pain with this physical exam maneuver after injection while the impingement group did not. An intra-articular lidocaine injection eliminated the pain in the instability group.

Beyond O'Driscoll's description, there are no studies assessing the sensitivity, specificity, positive predictive value, and negative predictive value.

Jerk Test

We were unable to find the original description of the jerk test. The test for glenohumeral instability is described as follows (Figure 4–31):

The patient sits with the arm internally rotated and flexed forward to 90 degrees. The examiner grasps the elbow and axially loads the humerus in a proximal direction.

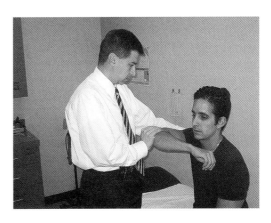

Figure 4–30. Posterior apprehension sign.

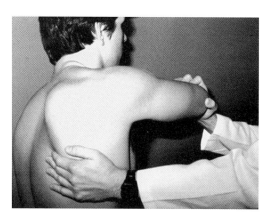

Figure 4–31. Jerk test. Reproduced with permission from Matsen FA, et al: Glenohumeral instability. In Rockwood CA, Matsen FA (eds), The Shoulder, 2nd edn. Philadelphia: WB Saunders, 1998, p. 681.

While axial loading of the humerus is maintained, the arm is moved horizontally across the body. A positive result is indicated by a sudden jerk as the humeral head slides off the back of the glenoid. When the arm is returned to the original position of 90-degree abduction a second jerk may be observed, that of the humeral head returning to the glenoid.[43,51]

Holovacs and Osbahr,[26] in a study presented at the AAOS 67th annual meeting, reported the test to have a sensitivity of 19% and specificity of 95% for *labral* injury when compared to the findings at arthroscopy.

Tests for Shoulder Inferior Stability

See Table 4–7.

The superior glenohumeral ligament and coracohumeral ligaments are the primary restraints to translation of the humeral head in the adducted position. At 45 degrees of abduction and beyond, the inferior glenohumeral ligament assists in stability. The rotator interval and labrum also play roles.[1,3,8,11,13]

Sulcus Sign

Credit is given to Neer and Foster[61] for development of the sulcus sign, which is used to test for inferior stability of the shoulder (Figure 4–32). There is no exact description of this test by Neer and Foster and the earliest written description of the test comes from Gerber and Ganz:

> The test is performed with the patient upright and the shoulder in the neutral position. It is important that the shoulder muscles are relaxed and that the stress is applied to the upper arm and not the forearm; this eliminates the effect of the biceps and the triceps brachii. A positive result invariably points to a more complex (multidirectional) instability.[16]

Figure 4–32. Sulcus sign. Reproduced with permission from Yamaguchi K, Flatow EL: Management of multidirectional instability. Clin Sports Med 1995;14:899.

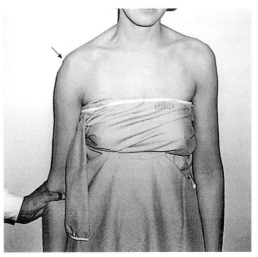

There are no studies that have examined the scientific validity of the sulcus sign for inferior instability. Liu et al.[45] found that combining the sulcus sign with the apprehension, relocation, and crank tests produced a sensitivity of 90% and specificity of 85% in predicting *labral tears* when comparing findings at the time of arthroscopy. With regard to the validity of the sulcus sign, no studies have assessed the sensitivity, specificity, positive predictive value, and negative predictive value.

Hyperabduction Test

Gagey and Gagey[15] described this test for assessing the laxity of the inferior glenohumeral ligament (IGHL) as follows (Figure 4–33):

> To measure the range of passive abduction, the physician stood behind the patient with his forearm pushed down firmly on the shoulder girdle in its lowest position, while lifting the relaxed upper limb in abduction with the other hand. During the test, the elbow was flexed at 90 degrees and the forearm was horizontal. Under these conditions, the shoulder girdle should not move and any movement was measured by a goniometer.

Normal subjects were found to have between 85 and 90 degrees of abduction while patients with instability had more than 105 degrees of abduction. A positive test for laxity of the IGHL was a hyperabduction test greater than 105 degrees. Some patients were limited by apprehension which assists in the diagnosis of instability and may contribute to false interpretation of the test.

Tests for Labral Pathology

See Table 4–8.

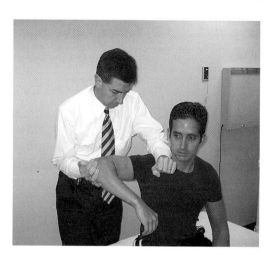

Figure 4–33. Hyperabduction test.

Table 4–8. LABRAL PATHOLOGY

Test	Description	Reliability/Validity Tests	Comments
Biceps load test	With the patient supine, an anterior apprehension test is performed. When the patient becomes apprehensive during the external rotation of the shoulder, external rotation is stopped. The patient is then asked to flex the elbow while the examiner resists the flexion with one hand and asks how the apprehension has changed, if at all. If the apprehension is lessened, or if the patient feels more comfortable than before the test, the test is negative for a superior labral, anterior–posterior (SLAP) lesion. If the apprehension has not changed, or if the shoulder becomes more painful, the test is positive. The test is repeated and the patient is instructed not to pull the whole upper extremity, but to bend the elbow against the examiner's resistance. The examiner should be sitting adjacent to the shoulder to be examined at the same height as the patient, and he should also face the patient at a right angle.	Kim et al.[39] Sensitivity: 90.9% Specificity: 96.9%	

Table 4–8. LABRAL PATHOLOGY—*cont'd*

Test	Description	Reliability/Validity Tests	Comments
Biceps load test II	This test is conducted with the patient in the supine position. The examiner sits adjacent to patient on the same side as the shoulder and grasps the patient's wrist and elbow gently. The arm to be examined is elevated to 120 degrees and externally rotated to its maximal point, with the elbow in the 90 degree flexion and the forearm in the supinated position. The patient is asked to flex the elbow while resisting the elbow flexion by the examiner. The test is considered positive if the patient complains of more pain from the resisted elbow flexion regardless of the degree of pain before the elbow flexion maneuver. The test is negative if pain is not elicited by the resisted flexion or if the pre-existing pain during the elevation and external rotation of the arm is unchanged or diminished by resisted elbow flexion.	Kim et al.[39] Sensitivity: 89.7% Specificity: 96.6%	
New pain provocation test	With the patient in a seated position, the abduction angle of the upper arm is maintained at 90–100 degrees, and the shoulder is rotated externally by the examiner. This maneuver is similar to the anterior apprehension test. The new pain provocation test is performed with the forearm in two different positions: maximum pronation and maximum supination. The test is described as positive for a superior labral tear when pain is provoked only with the forearm in the pronated position or when pain is more severe in this position [pronated] than with the forearm supinated.	Mimori et al.[55] Sensitivity: 100% Specificity: 90%	
Active compression test (O'Brien)	With the physician behind the patient, the patient is asked to forward flex the affected arm 90 degrees with the elbow in full extension. The patient then adducts the arm 10–15 degrees medial to the sagittal plane of the body. The arm is then internally rotated so the thumb is pointed	O'Brien and Pagnani[62] Sensitivity: 100% Specificity: 98.5% Burkhart et al.[8] Anterior Sensitivity: 88% Specificity: 42%	

Continued

Table 4–8. LABRAL PATHOLOGY—*cont'd*

Test	Description	Reliability/Validity Tests	Comments
	downward. The examiner then applies uniform downward force to the arm. With the arm in the same position, the palm is then fully supinated and the maneuver is repeated. The test is considered positive if pain is elicited with the first maneuver and is reduced or eliminated with the second maneuver. Pain localized to the acromioclavicular joint or on top of the shoulder was diagnostic of acromioclavicular joint abnormality. Pain or painful clicking described as inside the glenohumeral joint itself was indicative of labral abnormality.	Posterior Sensitivity: 32% Specificity: 13% Combined Sensitivity: 85% Specificity: 41% Holovacs and Osbahr[26] Sensitivity: 69% Specificity: 50% Stetson and Templin[78] Sensitivity: 67% Specificity: 41%	
Crank test	The crank test is performed with the patient in the upright position with the arm elevated to 160 degrees in the scapular plane. Joint load is applied along the axis of the humerus with one hand while the other performs humeral rotation. A positive test is determined by (a) pain during the maneuver usually during external rotation with or without click, or (b) reproduction of the symptoms usually pain or catching felt by the patient during athletic or work activities. The test should be repeated in the supine position where the patient is usually more relaxed.	Liu et al.[45] Sensitivity: 91% Specificity: 93% Liu and Henry[44] When combined with sulcus sign, apprehension and relocation tests in predicting labral tears: Sensitivity: 90% Specificity: 85% Mimori and Muneta[55] Sensitivity: 83% Specificity: 100% Stetson and Templin[79] Sensitivity: 64% Specificity: 67% Stetson and Templin[78] For superior labral tears: Sensitivity: 46% Specificity: 56%	
Anterior slide test	The patient is examined either standing or sitting, with their hands on the hips with thumbs pointing posteriorly. One of the examiner's hands is placed across the top of the shoulder from the posterior direction, with the last segment of the index finger extending over the anterior aspect of the acromion at the glenohumeral joint. The examiner's other hand is placed behind the	Kibler[35] Sensitivity: 78.4% Specificity: 91.5% McFarland et al.[53] Specificity: 84%	

Table 4–8. LABRAL PATHOLOGY—*cont'd*

Test	Description	Reliability/Validity Tests	Comments
	elbow and a forward and slightly superiorly directed force is applied to the elbow and upper arm. The patient is asked to push back against this force. Pain localized to the front of the shoulder under the examiner's hand, and/or a pop or click in the same area, is considered to be a positive test. This test is also positive if the athlete reports a subjective feeling that this testing maneuver reproduces the symptoms that occur during overhead activity.		
Compression–rotation test	The compression–joint rotation test is performed with the patient supine, the shoulder abducted 90 degrees, and the elbow flexed at 90 degrees. A compression force is applied to the humerus, which is then rotated, in an attempt to trap the torn labrum. Labral tears may be felt to catch and snap during the test, as meniscal tears do with McMurray's test.	Holovacs and Osbahr[26] Sensitivity: 80% Specificity: 19% McFarland et al.[53] Sensitivity: 49%	
Clunk test	The patient lies supine. The examiner places one hand on the posterior aspect of the shoulder over the humeral head while holding the humerus above the elbow and fully abducts the arm over the patient's head. The examiner then pushes anteriorly with the hand over the humeral head while the other hand rotates the humerus into lateral rotation. A clunk or grinding sound indicates a positive test and is indicative of a tear of the labrum. This test may also cause apprehension if anterior instability is present.	There are no studies assessing the sensitivity and specificity of the maneuver.	It is interesting to note that Hawkins et al.[22] described a palpable and often audible "clunk" to mean shoulder relocation in glenohumeral instability. There has been no validation of the test for this indication either.

See stability tests as some evaluated labral pathology.

The labrum provides an attachment site for the glenohumeral ligaments and the tendon of the long head of the biceps. Its principal function is to increase the depth of the glenoid socket and to act as a buttress preventing the humeral head from rolling over the anterior edge of the glenoid.[62] The labrum also prevents subluxation resulting from negative intra-articular pressure of approximately 20 to 30 pounds created by the coaptation of the labrum and humeral head acting as a "suction cup."[76] Lippit and Matsen[43] showed that the labrum is important in resisting subluxation in all directions. Many types of capsular lesions are associated with instability of the glenohumeral joint.[1,3,8,11,13]

Biceps Load Test

Kim et al.[39] described the biceps load test for evaluating the integrity of the superior glenoid labrum in shoulders with recurrent anterior dislocations. The test is performed as follows (Figure 4–34):

> The test is performed with the patient in the supine position. The examiner sits adjacent to the patient on the same side as the affected shoulder and gently grasps the patient's wrist and elbow. The arm to be examined is abducted at 90 degrees, with the forearm in the supinated position. The patient is allowed to relax, and an anterior apprehension test is performed. When the patient becomes apprehensive during the external rotation of the shoulder, external rotation is stopped. The patient is then asked to flex the elbow while the examiner resists the flexion with one hand and asks how the apprehension has changed, if at all. If the apprehension is lessened, or if the patient feels more comfortable than before the test, the test is negative for a superior labral, anterior–posterior (SLAP) lesion. If the apprehension has not changed, or if the shoulder becomes more painful, the test is positive. The test is repeated and the patient is instructed not to pull the whole upper extremity, but to bend the elbow against the examiner's resistance. The examiner should be sitting adjacent to the shoulder to be examined at the same height as the patient, and he or she should also face the patient at a right angle. The direction of the examiner's resistance should be in the

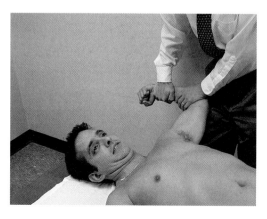

Figure 4–34. Biceps load test.

same plane as the patient's arm so as not to change the degree of abduction and rotation of the shoulder. The forearm should be kept in the supinated position during the test.

The authors noted that the test had a sensitivity of 90.9%, a specificity of 96.9%, positive predictive value of 83%, and negative predictive value of 98% when compared to findings at time of arthroscopy.

Biceps Load Test II

Kim et al.[38] also described a modified version of the biceps load test. The authors describe the new test as follows:

> This test is conducted with the patient in the supine position. The examiner sits adjacent to the patient on the same side as the shoulder and grasps the patient's wrist and elbow gently. The arm to be examined is elevated to 120 degrees and externally rotated to its maximal point, with the elbow in the 90 degree flexion and the forearm in the supinated position. The patient is asked to flex the elbow while resisting the elbow flexion by the examiner. The test is considered positive if the patient complains of more pain from the resisted elbow flexion regardless of the degree of pain before the elbow flexion maneuver. The test is negative if pain is not elicited by the resisted flexion or if the pre-existing pain during the elevation and external rotation of the arm is unchanged or diminished by resisted elbow flexion.

The authors found the test to have a sensitivity of 89.7%, a specificity of 96.6, and a negative predictive value of 95.5% when compared to arthroscopy. Compared to the first biceps load test described earlier, the positive predictive value improved to 92.1%.

New Pain Provocation Test

Mimori et al.[55] described the new pain provocation test for superior labral tears of the shoulder (Figure 4–35). The test was described as follows:

> The pain provocation test is performed with the patient in the sitting position. During the testing, the abduction angle of the upper arm is maintained at 90 degrees to 100 degrees, and the shoulder rotated externally by the examiner. This maneuver is similar to the anterior apprehension test. The new pain provocation test is performed with the forearm in two different positions: maximum pronation and maximum supination.
>
> The test is described as positive for a superior labral tear when pain is provoked only with the forearm in the pronated position or when pain is more severe in this position [pronated] than with the forearm supinated.

The authors found the test to have a sensitivity of 100%, a specificity of 90%, and an accuracy of 97% compared to MRI/arthrography (22 patients) and 15 patients who had arthroscopy.

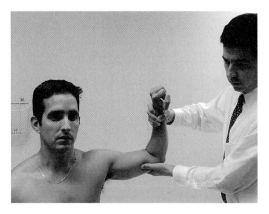 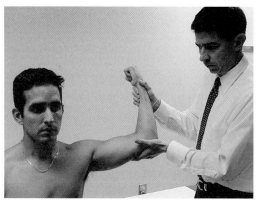

Figure 4–35. New pain provocation test.

Active Compression/O'Brien Test

O'Brien and Pagnani[62] introduced a test for diagnosing labral tears and acromioclavicular joint abnormalities. They termed this exam the active compression test and described it as follows (Figure 4–36):

> [With] the physician behind the patient, the patient is asked to forward flex the affected arm 90 degrees with the elbow in full extension. The patient then adducts the arm 10 to 15 degrees medial to the sagittal plane of the body. The arm is then internally rotated so the thumb is pointed downward. The examiner then applies uniform downward force to the arm. With the arm in the same position, the palm is then fully supinated and the maneuver is repeated. The test is considered positive if pain is elicited with the first maneuver and is reduced or eliminated with the second maneuver. Pain localized to the acromioclavicular joint or on top of the shoulder was diagnostic of acromioclavicular joint abnormality. Whereas pain or painful clicking described as inside the glenohumeral joint itself was indicative of labral abnormality.

In their study, O'Brien and Pagnani utilized a prospective protocol to determine the sensitivity, specificity, and positive and negative predictive values of the test. Verification of the results of the examination were determined by various combinations of radiography, MRI, and clinical data. The examination maneuver had 100% sensitivity, 98.5% specificity, 94.6% positive predictive value, and 100% negative predictive value in detecting labral tears; and 100% sensitivity, 95.2% specificity, 91.5% positive predictive value, and 100% negative predictive value for combined acromioclavicular joint and labral tears.

Burkhart et al.[8] found that, when compared to the findings at the time of arthroscopy, the O'Brien test had a sensitivity of 88% and a specificity of 42% for assessing anterior labral lesions, a sensitivity of 32% and a specificity of 13% for assessing

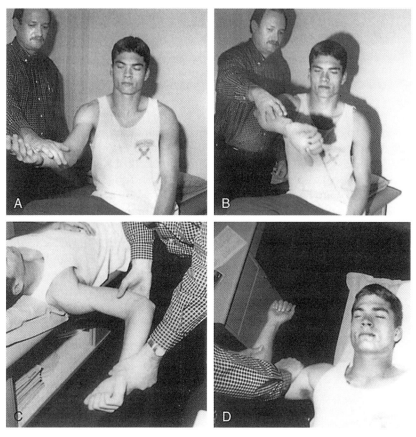

Figure 4–36. Active compression test/O'Brien's test. Reproduced with permission from Burkhart SS, Morgan CD, Kibler WB: Shoulder injuries in the overhead athlete. Clin Sports Med 2000;19:131.

posterior labral tears, and a sensitivity of 85% and specificity of 41% for assessing combined labral tears.

Holovacs and Osbahr[26] reported the test to have a sensitivity of 69% and specificity of 50% when compared with arthroscopy. Stetson and Templin[76] showed the test to have sensitivity of 67%, a specificity of 41%, and positive predictive value of 60% when compared to arthroscopy or open surgery.

Crank Test

Liu and Henry[44] utilized the crank test to assist in predicting the presence of labral tears. The crank test is performed as follows (Figure 4–37):

The crank test is performed with the patient in the upright position with the arm elevated to 160 degrees in the scapular plane. Joint load is applied along the axis of

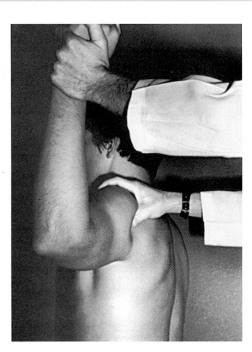

Figure 4–37. Crank test. Reproduced with permission from Matsen FA, et al: Glenohumeral instability. In Rockwood CA, Matsen FA (eds), The Shoulder, 2nd edn. Philadelphia: WB Saunders, 1998, p. 681.

the humerus with one hand while the other performs humeral rotation. A positive test is determined by (1) pain during the maneuver usually during external rotation with or without click or (2) reproduction of the symptoms usually pain or catching felt by the patient during athletic or work activities. The test should be repeated in the supine position where the patient is usually more relaxed. Frequently, a positive crank test in the upright position will also be positive in the supine position.

When comparing the results from the crank test to the findings on arthroscopy, the authors found the test to have a sensitivity of 91%, specificity of 93%, positive predictive value of 94%, and negative predictive value of 90%.

In a later study, the authors found that combining the crank test with the sulcus sign, apprehension, and relocation tests produced a sensitivity of 90% and specificity of 85% in predicting labral tears when comparing findings at the time of arthroscopy.[43]

Mimori et al.[55] found the crank test to have a sensitivity of 83% and specificity of 100% when compared to findings at arthroscopy. Stetson and Templin[79] reported a sensitivity of 64%, a specificity of 67%, and a positive predictive value of 53% when compared to arthroscopy. Stetson and Templin[78] also compared the crank test, O'Brien's test, and magnetic resonance imaging to arthroscopy for evaluation of superior labral tears. The crank test had a sensitivity of 46%, specificity of 56%, positive predictive value of 41%, and negative predictive value of 61%. The O'Brien's test had a sensitivity of 54%, specificity of 31%, positive predictive value of 34%, and negative predictive value of 50%. This demonstrated the physical exam to be poor compared to imaging.

Glasgow et al.[18] described patients with "functional instability" of the shoulder who failed conservative treatment and could not return to their overhead activities to monitor functional outcomes after labral resection. All of the patients had a palpable labral "click" when attempting to sublux the humerus either anteriorly or posteriorly on exam. They did not state a specific name for their exam maneuver, but all patients in the study were examined under anesthesia. The arm was examined in the plane of the scapula, abducted to 90 degrees with the humerus in the neutral position and anterior or posterior forces directed to the humeral head with and without axial loading to the elbow. It was noted that "various points of abduction, external rotation, and forward flexion" were used for instability testing. The definition of instability was not specified, but if a labral click was present when attempting subluxation (with the arm in the scapular plane at 90 degrees of abduction and neutral) a labral tear was felt to be present. This retrospective study documented that all the patients (29) with a click in their symptomatic shoulder had a longitudinal labral tear. Eight were superior, 19 anterior, and two posterior. It is unknown how many asymptomatic patients do have a click with this maneuver.

Anterior Slide Test

Kibler[35] described the anterior slide test for diagnosing labral tears, as follows (Figure 4–38):

> The patient is examined either standing or sitting, with their hands on the hips with thumbs pointing posteriorly. One of the examiner's hands is placed across the top of the shoulder from the posterior direction, with the last segment of the index finger

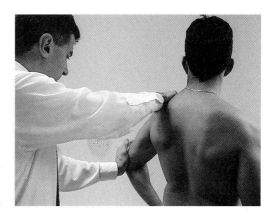

Figure 4–38. Anterior slide test.

extending over the anterior aspect of the acromion at the glenohumeral joint. The examiner's other hand is placed behind the elbow and a forward and slightly superiorly directed force is applied to the elbow and upper arm. The patient is asked to push back against this force. Pain localized to the front of the shoulder under the examiner's hand, and/or a pop or click in the same area, was considered to be a positive test. This test is also positive if the athlete reports a subjective feeling that this testing maneuver reproduces the symptoms that occur during overhead activity.

The author found the test to have a sensitivity of 78.4% and a specificity of 91.5% when compared to arthroscopy.

Compression–Rotation Test

Snyder et al.[75] described the compression-rotation test for diagnosing labral tears, as follows (Figure 4–39):

The compression–joint rotation test is performed with the patient supine, the shoulder abducted 90 degrees and the elbow flexed at 90 degrees. A compression force is applied to the humerus, which is then rotated, in an attempt to trap the torn labrum. Labral tears may be felt to catch and snap during the test, as meniscal tears do with McMurray's test.

Holovacs and Osbahr[26] reported the test to have a sensitivity of 80% and a specificity of 19% for labral pathology when compared to findings at time of arthroscopy.

McFarland et al.[53] compared the active compression test, anterior slide, and compression rotation for SLAP lesion to findings at time of arthroscopy. They identified the active compression test as the most sensitive at 47%, with the highest positive predictive value of 10%, and the anterior slide as the most specific test at 84%. They noted that clicking or pain location were not reliable portions of the tests.

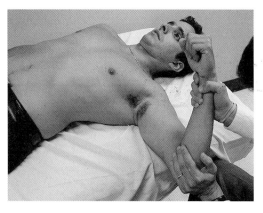

Figure 4–39. Compression–rotation test.

Clunk Test

Andrews and Gillogly[2] are given credit for developing the clunk test. They described it as follows (Figure 4–40):

> The patient lies supine. The examiner places one hand on the posterior aspect of the shoulder over the humeral head while holding the humerus above the elbow and fully abducts the arm over the patient's head. The examiner then pushes anteriorly with the hand over the humeral head while the other hand rotates the humerus into lateral rotation. A clunk or grinding sound indicates a positive test and is indicative of a tear of the labrum. This test may also cause apprehension if anterior instability is present.

There are no studies assessing the sensitivity, specificity, positive predictive value, or negative predictive value of the maneuver.

It is interesting to note that Hawkins and McCormack[24] described a palpable and often audible "clunk" to mean shoulder relocation in posterior glenohumeral instability. There has been no validation of the test for this indication either.

When studying Speed's maneuver, Burkhart et al.[8] noted a 100% sensitivity and 70% specificity for detecting anterior labral tears, 29% sensitivity and 11% specificity for posterior labral tears, and 78% sensitivity and 37% specificity for combined lesions.

Testing of the Acromioclavicular Joint

See Table 4–9.

The AC joint is a frequent source of shoulder pain. Osteoarthritis, osteolysis, ligament sprains, dislocations and fractures are possible causes. The joint is composed of the distal end of the clavicle medially and laterally by the acromion of the scapula. It is a diarthrodial joint, which usually contains an articular disc. The joint capsule is

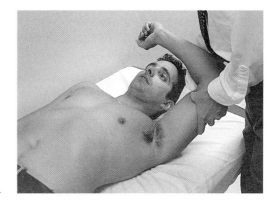

Figure 4–40. Clunk test.

Table 4–9. ACROMIOCLAVICULAR JOINT TESTS

Test	Description	Reliability/Validity Tests
Apley scarf test	The test is performed by passively adducting the arm across the body horizontally approximating the elbow to the contralateral shoulder. Pain at the acromioclavicular joint constitutes a positive test.	There are no studies assessing the sensitivity, specificity, positive predictive value, negative predictive value, or reliability of this exam maneuver.
Active compression test (O'Brien)	With the physician behind the patient, the patient is asked to forward flex the affected arm 90 degrees with the elbow in full extension. The patient then adducts the arm 10–15 degrees medial to the sagittal plane of the body. The arm is then internally rotated so the thumb is pointed downward. The examiner then applies uniform downward force to the arm. With the arm in the same position, the palm is then fully supinated and the maneuver is repeated. The test is considered positive if pain is elicited with the first maneuver and is reduced or eliminated with the second maneuver. Pain localized to the acromioclavicular joint or on top of the shoulder was diagnostic of acromioclavicular joint abnormality. Pain or painful clicking described as inside the glenohumeral joint itself was indicative of labral abnormality.	O'Brien and Pagnani[62] For detecting acromioclavicular joint pathology: Sensitivity: 100% Specificity: 96.6% For detecting both acromioclavicular joint pathology and labral tears: Sensitivity: 100% Specificity: 95.2% Chronopoulos et al.[10] Sensitivity: 41% Specificity: 95% Walton et al.[83] Sensitivity: 16% Specificity: 90%

quite thin, but surrounded by strong ligamentous support. Of the 45 degrees of rotation through the long axis of the clavicle, only 5–8 degrees occur through the acromioclavicular joint.[68]

Crossed-arm Adduction or (Apley) Scarf Test

The scarf test also known as the AC joint test, and the crossed-arm adduction test was first described by A. G. Apley in one of his books at some time in the late 1940s to determine the integrity of the acromioclavicular joint. The test is performed by passively adducting the arm across the body horizontally approximating the elbow to the contralateral shoulder (Figure 4–41). Pain at the acromioclavicular joint constitutes a positive test.[47,49,55]

Chronopoulos et al.[10] examined the clinical accuracy of several physical examination tests including the cross-body adduction test, resisted extension test, and active compression test. The diagnosis was based on localized AC joint pain, local tenderness at the AC joint, and pain resolution with a diagnostic injection and arthroscopic findings.

Figure 4–41. Scarf test.

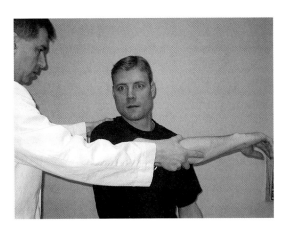

Active Compression Test

The active compression test developed by O'Brien and Pagnani[62] can be used to diagnose and differentiate acromioclavicular pathology and labral tears (Figure 4–36). A detailed description of this test can be found in the tests for the labrum section of this review. In their original study, O'Brien and Pagnani found that, when compared to various combinations of radiography, MRI, and clinical data, the test had a sensitivity of 100%, specificity of 96.6%, positive predictive value of 91.5%, and negative predictive value of 100% for detecting AC joint pathology. For determining both AC joint pathology and labral tears, the authors showed the test had a sensitivity of 100%, specificity of 95.2%, positive predictive value of 91.5%, and negative predictive value of 100%.

Chronopoulos et al.[10] found the active compression test had a sensitivity of 41%, specificity of 95%, positive predictive value of 29%, and negative predictive value of 97%. They noted an overall accuracy of 92% for AC joint pathology. Walton et al.[83] found the active compression test had a sensitivity of 16%, specificity of 90%, positive predictive value of 62%, and negative predictive value of 52%. They noted an overall accuracy of 53% for AC joint pathology.

Conclusion

Many physical examination tests of the shoulder have been described. It is important to know how to perform these tests properly and understand the sensitivity and specificity of each test when examining patients. The usefulness of these tests is enhanced when performed in conjunction with a careful history. The overall sensitivity and specificity of the individual tests may be enhanced by using them in combination rather than relying on the results of a single test in isolation. When adopted in this manner, physical examination of the shoulder can be extremely helpful in guiding appropriate treatment and eliminating unnecessary imaging studies.

REFERENCES

1. An YH, Friedman RJ. Multidirectional instability of the glenohumeral joint [review]. Orthop Clin N Am 2000;31:275–285.

2. Andrews JR, Gillogly S. Physical examination of the shoulder in throwing athletes. In Zarins B, Andrews JR, Carson WG (eds), Injuries to the Throwing Arm, based on the proceedings of the national conferences sponsored by the USOC sports medicine council. Philadelphia: WB Saunders, 1985.

3. Arroyo JS, Hershon SJ, Bigliani LU. Special considerations in the athletic throwing shoulder. Orthop Clin N Am 1997;28:69–78.

4. Bennett W. Specificity of Speed's test: arthroscopic technique for evaluating the biceps tendon at the level of the bicipital groove. Arthroscopy 1998;14:789–796.

5. Bergman AG, Fredericson M. Shoulder MRI after impingement test injection. Skeletal Radiol 1998;27:365–368.

6. Blackburn TA. Rehabilitation of the shoulder and elbow after arthroscopy. Clin Sports Med 1987;6:587–606.

7. Bryant L, Shnier R, Bryant C, Murrel GA. A comparison of clinical estimation, ultrasonography, magnetic resonance imaging, and arthroscopy in determining the size of rotator cuff tears. J Shoulder Elbow Surg 2002;11:219–224.

8. Burkhart SS, Morgan CD, Kibler WB. Shoulder injuries in overhead athletes: the "dead arm" revisited. Clin Sports Med 2000;19:125–158.

9. Calis M, Akgun K, Birtane M, et al. Diagnostic values of clinical diagnostic tests in subacromial impingement syndrome. Ann Rheum Dis 2000;59:44–47.

10. Chronopoulos E, Kim TK, Park HB, et al. Diagnostic value of physical tests for isolated chronic acromio-clavicular lesions. Am J Sports Med 2004;32:655–661.

11. Cleeman E, Flatow EL. Shoulder dislocations in the young patient. Orthop Clin N Am 2000;31:217–229.

12. Crenshaw AH, Kilgore WE. Surgical treatment of bicipital tenosynovitis. J Bone Joint Surg Am 1966;48:1496–1502.

13. Doukas WC, Speer KP. Anatomy, pathophysiology, and biomechanics of shoulder instability. Orthop Clin N Am 2001;32:381–391, vii.

14. Fuchs S, Chylarecki C, Langenbrink A. Incidence and symptoms of clinically manifest rotator cuff lesions. Int J Sports Med 1999;20:201–205.

15. Gagey OJ, Gagey N. The hyperaduction test. J Bone Joint Surg Br 2000;83:69–74.

16. Gerber C, Ganz R. Clinical assessment of instability of the shoulder. J Bone Joint Surg Br 1984;66:551–556.

17. Gerber C, Krushell R. Isolated rupture of the tendon of the subscapularis muscle. J Bone Joint Surg Br 1991;73:389–394.

18. Glasgow SG, Bruce RA, Yacobucci GN, Torg JS. Arthroscopic resection of glenoid labral tears in the athlete: a report of 29 cases. Arthroscopy 1992;8:48–54.

19. Greis P, Kuhn J. Validation of the lift-off test and analysis of subscapularis activity during maximal internal rotation. Am J Sports Med 1996;24:589–593.

20. Gross ML, Distefano MC. Anterior release test: a new test for occult shoulder instability. Clin Orthop Rel Res 1997;339:105–108.

21. Gross J, Fetto J, Rosen E. Musculoskeletal Examination. Cambridge: Blackwell Science, 1996.

22. Hawkins, Abrams JS, Schutte JP. Multidirectional instability of the shoulder: an approach to diagnosis. Orthop Trans 1987;11:246.

23. Hawkins RJ, Kennedy JC. Impingement syndrome in athletes. Am J Sports Med 1980;8:151–158.

24. Hawkins RJ, McCormack RG. Posterior shoulder instability: Orthopedics 1988;11(1).

25. Hawkins RJ, Schutte JP. The assessment of glenohumeral translation using manual and fluoroscopic techniques. Orthop Trans 1988;12:727–728.

26. Holovacs T, Osbahr D. The sensitivity and specificity of the physical examination to detecting glenoid labrum tears. Scientific Program AAOS 67th Annual Meeting, 2000.

27. Jenp YN, Malanga GA, Growney ES, An KN. Activation of the rotator cuff in generating isometric shoulder rotation torque. Am J Sports Med 1996;24:477–485.

28. Jobe FW, Bradley J. The diagnosis and nonoperative treatment of shoulder injuries in athletes. Clin Sports Med 1989;8:419–438.

29. Jobe FW, Jobe CM. Painful athletic injuries of the shoulder. Clin Orthop 1983;Mar;(173):117–124.

30. Jobe FW, Kvitne RS, Giangarra CE. Shoulder pain in the overhand or throwing athlete: the relationship of anterior instability and rotator cuff impingement. Orthop Rev 1989;18:963–975. [Published erratum Orthop Rev 1989;18:1268.]

31. Kelly BT, Kadrmas WR, Kirkendall DT, Speer KP. Optimal normalition tests for shoulder muscle activation: an electromyographic study. J Orthop Res 1996;14:647–653.

32. Kelly BT, Kadrmas WR, Kirkendall DT, Speer KP. The manual muscle examination for rotator cuff strength. Am J Sports Med 1996;24:581–588.

33. Kelly BT, Roskin LA, Kirkendall DT, Speer KP. Shoulder muscle activation during aquatic and dry land exercises in nonimpaired subjects. J Orthop Sports Phys Ther 2000;30:204–210.

34. Kibler WB. Role of the scapula in the overhead throwing motion. Contemp Orthop 1991;22:525–532.

35. Kibler WB. Specificity and sensitivity of the anterior slide test in throwing athletes with superior glenoid labrum tears. Arthroscopy 1995;11:296–300.

36. Kibler WB. The role of the scapula in athletic shoulder function. Am J Sports Med 1998;26:325–337.

37. Kibler WB, Burkhurt SS, Morgan CD. Shoulder injuries in overhead athletes. Clin Sports Med 2000;19:125–158.

38. Kim SH, Ha KI, Ahn JH, et al. Biceps load test. II: A clinical test for SLAP lesions of the shoulder. Arthroscopy 2001;17:160–164.

39. Kim SH, Ha KI, Han KY. Biceps load test: a clinical test for superior labrum anterior and posterior lesions in shoulders with recurrent anterior dislocations. Am J Sports Med 1999;27:300–303.

40. Kirkley A, Litchfield RB, Jackowski DM, Lo IK. The use of the impingement test as a predictor of outcome following subacromial decompression for rotator cuff tendinosis. Arthroscopy 2002;18:8–15.

41. Levy AS, Kelly BT, Linter SA, et al. Function of the long head of the biceps at the shoulder: electromyographic analysis. J Shoulder Elbow Surg 2001;May-Jun;10(3):250–255.

42. Levy AS, Lintner S, Kenter K, Speer KP. Intra- and interobserver reproducibility of the shoulder laxity examination. Am J Sports Med 1999;27:460–463.

43. Lippitt S, Matsen F. Mechanisms of glenohumeral joint stability. Clin Orthop 1993;291:20–28.

44. Liu S, Henry M. A prospective evaluation of a new physical examination in predicting glenoid labral tears. Am J Sports Med. 1996;24:721–725.

45. Liu SH, Henry MH, Nuccion S, Shapiro MS, Dorey F. Diagnosis of glenoid labral tears: a comparison between magnetic resonance imaging and clinical examinations. Am J Sports Med 1996;24:149–154.

46. Ludington NA. Rupture of the long head of the biceps flexor cubiti muscle. Ann Surg 1923;77:358–363.

47. MacDonald PB, Clark P, Sutherland K. An analysis of the diagnostic accuracy of the Hawkins and Neer subacromial impingement signs. J Shoulder Elbow Surg 2000;9:299–301.

48. Magee DJ. Orthopedic Physical Assessment, 2nd edn. Philadelphia: WB Saunders, 1997.

49. Malanga GA, Jenp YN, Growney ES, An KN. EMG analysis of shoulder positioning in testing and strengthening the supraspinatus. Med Sci Sport Exerc 1996;28:661–664.

50. Matsen F, Harryman D, Sidles J. Mechanics of glenohumeral instability. Clin J Sports Med 1991;10:783–788.

51. Matsen F, Kirby R. Office evaluation and management of shoulder pain. Orthop Clin N Am 1982;13(3):453–475.

52. Matsen FA, Thomas SC, Rockwood CA. Glenohumeral instability. In Rockwood CA, Matsen FA (eds), The Shoulder. Philadelphia: WB Saunders, 1990.

53. McFarland EG, Kim TK, Savino RM. Clinical assessment of three common tests for superior labral anterior-posterior lesions. Am J Sports Med 2002;30:810–815.

54. McLeod W, Blackburn TA, White B. EMG evaluations of rotator cuff exercises. Presented at the AOSSM meeting, Nashville, 1985.

55. Mimori K, Muneta T, Nakagawa T, Shinomiya K. A new pain provocation test for superior labral tears of the shoulder. Am J Sports Med 1999;27:137–142.

56. Moore KL. The upper limb. In Clinically Oriented Anatomy, 2nd edn. Baltimore: Williams & Wilkins, 1985.

57. Naredo E, Aguado P, De Miguel E, et al. Painful shoulder: comparison of physical examination and ultrasonographic findings. Ann Rheum Dis 2002;61:132–136.

58. Neer CS: Anterior acromioplasty of the chronic impingement syndrome in the shoulder. J Bone Joint Surg Am 1972;54:41–50.

59. Neer CS. The shoulder in sports. Orthop Clin N Am 1977;8:583–591.

60. Neer CS. Impingement lesions. Clin Orthop Rel Res 1983;173:70–77.

61. Neer CS, Foster CR. Inferior capsular shift for involuntary inferior and multidirectional instability of the shoulder. J Bone Joint Surg Am 1980;62:897–908.

62. O'Brien S, Pagnani M. The active compression test: a new and effective test for diagnosing labral tears and acromioclavicular joint abnormality. Am J Sports Med 1998;26:610–613.

63. O'Driscoll SW. A reliable and simple test for posterior instability of the shoulder. J Bone Joint Surg Br 1991;73(Suppl. 1):50.

64. Odom CJ, Taylor AB, Hurd CE, Denegar CR. Measurement of scapular asymmetry and assessment of shoulder dysfunction using the lateral scapular slide test: a reliability and validity study. Phys Ther 2001;Feb;81(2):799–809.

65. Patte D. The limits of repair (group IV) [in French]. Rev Chir Orthop Reparatrice de l'appareil Moteur 1988;74:321–323.

66. Poppen NK, Walker PS. Normal and abnormal motion of the shoulder. J Bone Joint Surg Am 1976;58:195–201.

67. Protzman R. Anterior instability of the shoulder. J Bone Joint Surg Am 1980;62:909–918.

68. Reid DC. Focusing on the diagnosis of shoulder pain: pearls for practice. Physician Sports Med 1994;22(6):28–37.

69. Renfree KJ, Wright TW. Anatomy and biomechanics of the acromioclavicular and sternoclavicular joints. Clin Sports Med 2003;22:219–237.

70. Rowe CR. Dislocations of the shoulder. In Rowe CR (ed.), The Shoulder. Edinburgh: Churchill Livingstone, 1988.

71. Rowe CR, Zarins B. Recurrent transient subluxation of the shoulder. J Bone Joint Surg Am 1981;63:863–872.

72. Saha AK. Mechanism of shoulder movements and a plea for the recognition of "zero position" of the gleno-humeral joint. Clin Orthop Rel Res 1983;173:3–10.

73. Silliman J, Hawkins R. Current concepts and recent advances in the athlete's shoulder. Clin Sports Med 1991;10:693–705.

74. Sillman JF, Hawkins RJ. Classification and physical diagnosis of instability of the shoulder. Clin Orthop 1993;291:7.

75. Snyder SJ, Karzel RP, Del Pizzo W, et al. SLAP lesions of the shoulder. Arthroscopy 1990;6:274–279.

76. Speer KP. Shoulder instability. Clin Sports Med 1995;14:751–758.

77. Speer KP, Hannafin JA, Altchek DW, Warren RF. An evaluation of the shoulder relocation test. Am J Sports Med 1994;22:177–183.

78. Stetson WB, Templin K. The crank test, the O'Brien test, and routine magnetic resonance imaging scans in the diagnosis of labral tears. Am J Sports Med 2002;30:806–809.

79. Stetson WB, Templin K. Sensitivity of the crank test vs. the O'Brien test in detecting SLAP lesions of the shoulder. Poster exhibit, AAOS 67th Annual Meeting, 2000.

80. Tennent TD, Beach WR, Meyers JF. A review of the special tests associated with shoulder examination. 1: The rotator cuff tests. Am J Sports Med 2003;31:154–160.

81. Tzannes A, Murrell GA. Clinical examination of the unstable shoulder. Sports Med 2002;32:447–457.

82. Walch G, Boulahia A, Calderone S, Robinson AHN. The "dropping" and "hornblower's" signs in evaluation of rotator-cuff tears. J Bone Joint Surg Br 1998;Jul;80(4):624–628.

83. Walton J, Mahajan S, Paxinos A, et al. Diagnostic values of tests for acromioclavicular joint pain. J Bone Joint Surg Am 2004;Apr;86-A(4):807–812.

84. Wright RW, Fritts HM, Tierney GS, Buss DD. MR imaging of the shoulder after an impingement test: how long to wait. Am J Roentgenol 1998;171:769–773.

85. Yergason RM. Supraspinatus sign. J Bone Joint Surg 1931;13:60.

86. Yocum LA. Assessing the shoulder. Clin Sports Med 1983;2:281–289.

Chapter 5

Physical Examination of the Elbow, Wrist, and Hand

THOMAS AGESEN, MD • SCOTT F. NADLER, DO •
JOHN WRIGHTSON, MD • JEFFREY MILLER, MD

Introduction

When a patient enters the examining room, the physical exam has begun. Any examination of the elbow, wrist, and hand requires examination of more proximal structures – specifically the shoulder and the neck (see corresponding chapters). The examiner must note any ecchymosis, rashes, or edema in the extremity. The elbow, wrist, hand, and fingers should be observed for evidence of local joint swelling or deformities. Local joint swelling and warmth may indicate synovitis or infection of the underlying joint. This chapter focuses on examination of the elbow, wrist, and hand.

Anatomy

The Elbow Joint

The elbow joint is a synovial hinged joint that flexes and extends in one plane (Figure 5–1). The major weight-bearing articulation is between the distal humerus and the proximal ulna.[14,31,37,38,45,63] The distal humeral articulating surface is called the *trochlea*, named for its shape. The articulating surface of the proximal ulna has undulations to match the humeral trochlea. The bony congruency of the ulna and humerus makes the forearm flex with respect to the humerus at a fixed angle called the *carrying angle of the arm*.[4] The proximal radius articulates with the capitellum of the humerus, located on

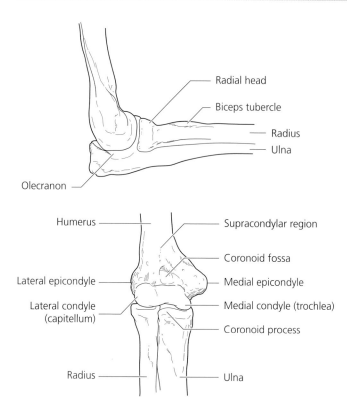

Figure 5–1. Osseous anatomy of the elbow joint. Adapted from Bennett JB: Acute injuries to the elbow. In Nicholas J, Hershman E (eds), The Upper Extremity in Sports Medicine, 2nd edn. St Louis: Mosby, 1995, p. 302.

the lateral side. The proximal radius also articulates with the proximal ulna, a synovial joint that allows rotation of the radial head within the annular ligament. There is also a synovial articulation between the proximal ulna and radius. In contrast to the knee, there are no intra-articular (cruciate) ligaments to offer stability to the elbow joint. The stability of the elbow arises from the bony congruency, medial (ulnar) collateral ligament, lateral (radial) collateral ligament, anterior ligament, posterior ligament, joint capsule, muscles, and tendons.

The medial collateral (ulnar) ligament runs from the medial condyle of the humerus to the ulna. The ulnar collateral ligament has three fibrous sections. Anterior fibers run from the medial humeral condyle to the medial side of the coronoid process of the ulna. Posterior fibers run from the medial condyle of the humerus to the medial portion of the olecranon process of the ulna. There are transverse fibers running from the olecranon to the coronoid process of the ulna. Between the anterior and posterior fibers are fibrous tissues that reinforce the underlying articular capsule.[14,31,37,38,45,63]

The lateral collateral (radial) ligament runs from the lateral condyle of the humerus to the annular ligament with some fibers extending to the radial neck (Figure 5–2). The annular ligament almost completely surrounds the radial head, allowing radial rotation

Figure 5–2. The lateral collateral ligament of the elbow. Adapted from Bennett JB: Acute injuries to the elbow. In Nicholas J, Hershman E (eds), The Upper Extremity in Sports Medicine, 2nd edn. St Louis: Mosby, 1995, p. 302.

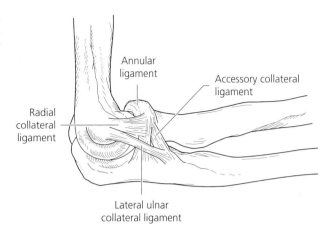

within, and attaches to the ulna anterior and posterior. Therefore, the annular ligament gives stability to the proximal radioulnar joint. The anterior capsule is thickened and is often considered the anterior ligament giving stability against hyperextension of the elbow. The posterior capsule also has thickened bands that are often considered the posterior ligament. The muscles and tendons that traverse the elbow also promote stability to the elbow.

The radius and ulna are held together by separate proximal and distal joints and by two fibrous interosseous structures. Inferiorly, the proximal radioulnar joint is stabilized by the quadrate ligament running from the radial head to the lateral side of the ulna. The proximal radioulnar joint is a pivot synovial joint, and the radial head articulates with the sigmoid cavity of the larger proximal ulna. The first of two interosseous fibrous structures is the oblique cord. The oblique cord fibers run proximal to distal from the ulna to radius (opposite the interosseous membrane fiber course). Next the strong fibrous interosseous membrane runs almost the entire length of the two bones. This interosseous membrane has fibers running obliquely, proximal attachment on the medial radius to distal attachment on the lateral ulna. Force transmission at the wrist drives proximal through the radius to the ulna via the interosseous membrane. In addition, the radius and ulna are held together by the distal radioulnar joint. The distal radioulnar joint has anterior and posterior radioulnar ligaments. These ligaments attach the distal radius and ulna offering stability. The distal radioulnar joint is a synovial pivot joint. The ulnar head articulates with the sigmoid cavity of the much larger distal radius.

The Wrist (Radiocarpal) Joint

As the name suggests, the wrist joint is the articulation between the distal radial bone and the proximal row of carpal bones.[14,31,37,38,45,63] However, the wrist encompasses

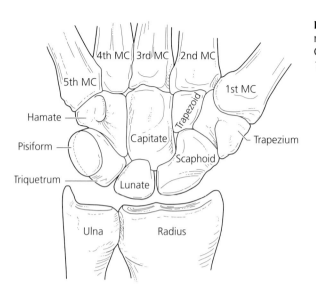

Figure 5–3. Skeletal anatomy of the wrist joint. MC, metacarpal. Adapted from Steinberg BD, Plancher KD: Clinical anatomy of the wrist and elbow. Clin Sports Med 1995;April;14:301.

the radiocarpal, midcarpal, intercarpal, carpometacarpal, and distal radioulnar joints. There are eight carpal bones in the wrist joint, arranged in a proximal and a distal row (Figure 5–3). The proximal-row carpal bones (lateral to medial) are the scaphoid, lunate, triquetrum, and pisiform. The pisiform bone lies on the palmer aspect of the triquetrum, so essentially there are functionally only three carpal bones in the proximal row. The distal-row carpal bones (lateral to medial) are the trapezium, trapezoid, capitate, and hamate. It follows that the distal radius articulates with the proximal row of carpal bones, the proximal row of carpal bones articulates with the distal row of carpal bones, the distal row of carpal bones articulates with the metacarpal heads. Each "row" of articulation has a separate compartment and is physically distinct from the next. In fact, there are five separate synovial cavities that do not communicate with each other in the wrist joint. Therefore, each synovial cavity has its own synovial fluid production and can have its own "effusion."

The wrist joint has a tremendous number of ligaments.[14,31,37,38,45,63] Palmar, dorsal, and interosseous ligaments connect the carpal bones together (Figure 5–4). The ulnar collateral ligament connects the ulnar head with the (proximal carpal row) triquetrum and pisiform. Then the ulnar collateral ligament sends fibers to the (distal carpal row) hamate, and finally fibers extend to the base of the fifth metacarpal. The ulnar head is separated from the trapezium by the triangular fibrocartilage (TFC), and forms one of the synovial compartments of the wrist. The TFC connects medially with the distal lateral radius and laterally with the ulnar collateral ligament (Figure 5–5). On the lateral side of the hand, the radial collateral ligament sends fibers from the distal radius to the (proximal carpal row) scaphoid and fibers continue to the (distal carpal row) trapezium.

Figure 5–4. Ligaments of the wrist. DIC, dorsal intercarpal; DRC, dorsal radiocapitate; DRU, dorso-radioulnar; DST, dorsal scaphotriquetral; LRL, long radiolunate; LT, lunotriquetral; RSC, radioscapho-capitate; SC, scaphocapitate; SRL, short radio-lunate; SL, scapholunate; TC, triquetrocapitate; TH, triquetrohamate; UC, ulnocapitate; UL, ulno-lunate; UT, ulnotriquetral. Adapted from Berger RA: The ligaments of the wrist: a current overview of anatomy with consideration of the potential functions. Hand Clin 1997;13:423.

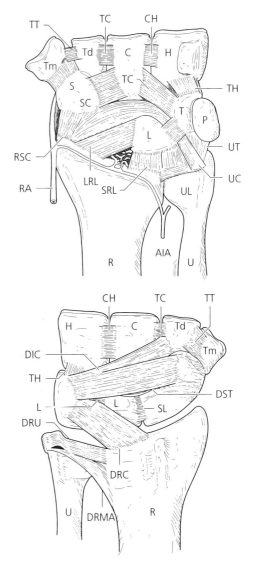

The radiocarpal joint or the proximal row of articulation is a condyloid joint. The joints between adjacent carpal bones are arthrodial joints. The distal radius articulates with the scaphoid, lunate and triquetrum. There are interosseous ligaments between the scaphoid and lunate, as well as between the lunate and triquetrum. Therefore, the second synovial cavity of the "wrist" is bounded: medially by the ulnar collateral ligament, laterally by the radial collateral, proximally the radius, distally by the first row of carpal bones and their interosseous ligaments. The third and largest synovial cavity of the wrist joint is distal to the proximal row of carpal bones and their interosseous ligaments. This synovial cavity includes the distal row of carpal bones and ends at the

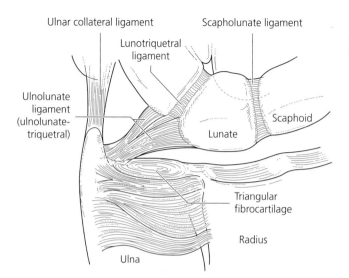

Ulnar collateral ligament

Scapholunate ligament

Lunotriquetral ligament

Ulnolunate ligament (ulnolunate-triquetral)

Scaphoid

Lunate

Triangular fibrocartilage

Radius

Ulna

Figure 5–5. The triangular fibrocartilage complex. Adapted from Steinberg BD, Plancher KD: Clinical anatomy of the wrist and elbow. Clin Sports Med 1995;April;14:300.

metacarpal heads and their interosseous ligaments. The fourth synovial cavity in the wrist region, bounded by carpometacarpal ligaments, is between the trapezium and the first metacarpal head (base of the thumb). The fifth and final synovial cavity in the wrist region is between pisiform and the triquetrum bones.

There are multiple ligaments, both palmar and dorsal, interconnecting the carpal bones. The palmar and dorsal radiocarpal ligaments require mentioning. These two ligaments extend from the distal radius to the proximal row of carpal bones on the respective sides of the wrist. The fibers run distally and medially (toward the ulnar side). When one supinates or pronates the wrist, these fibers pull the ulna with the radius.

Other important ligaments include the transverse carpal ligament or flexor retinaculum, which extends from the scaphoid and trapezoid bones on the radial or lateral side of the wrist to the hamate on the ulnar or medial side of the wrist (Figure 5–6). This ligament and the carpal bones beneath form the carpal tunnel. Nine tendons (flexor pollicis longus and four each from the flexor digitorum superficialis and profundus) and one nerve (median) pass beneath the transverse carpal ligament. Smaller ligaments that are clinically important include the pisohamate and pisometacarpal. As their names suggest, these ligaments run from the pisiform bone to the hamate and fifth metacarpal, respectively. The ligament from the pisiform to the hook of the hamate forms the roof of Guyon's canal. Both branches of the ulnar nerve enter this canal already divided into the deep and superficial palmer branches (see Ulnar Nerve below).

Understanding the underlying anatomy of the wrist region makes physical examination more rewarding. For example, knowing the number of synovial cavities allows one to appreciate the amount of destruction that rheumatoid arthritis can inflict to the

Figure 5–6. The median nerve under the flexor retinaculum. **A.** Palmar branch. **B.** Distal median nerve. Adapted from: Entrapment neuropathy. In Birch R, Bonney G, Wynn Parry CB (eds), Surgical Disorders of the Peripheral Nerves. Edinburgh: Churchill Livingstone, 1998, p. 269.

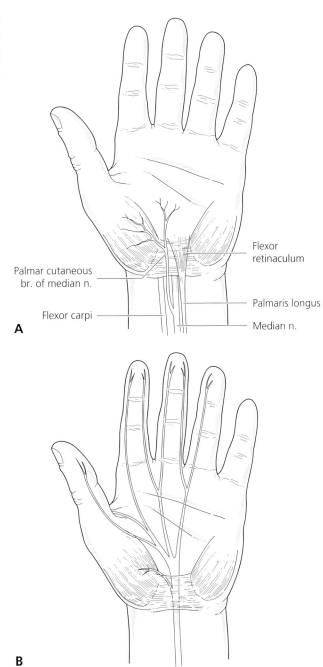

Flexor retinaculum

Palmar cutaneous br. of median n.

Palmaris longus

Flexor carpi

Median n.

A

B

wrist region and to the distal ulnar area where there are a tremendous number of synovial-lined joint cavities. The physical exam of the carpal bones themselves and their limited movement in relationship to each other becomes appreciated when the numbers of ligaments (palmar, dorsal and interosseous) in the wrist are known.

The metacarpal bones have interosseous, dorsal, and palmar ligaments connecting them to each other, to carpal bones, and to phalanges. The movements at the metacarpophalangeal (MCP) joints are slight gliding, flexion, and extension. The interphalangeal joints are pivot joints, allowing flexion and extension. Each proximal interphalangeal (PIP) and distal interphalangeal (DIP) joint is reinforced by palmar, medial, and lateral collateral ligaments. The first MCP joint is a saddle joint. This allows thumb apposition for gripping things more effectively. The first metacarpal articulates with the first phalanx and is stabilized by collateral ligaments.

Muscles About the Elbow

Biceps brachii has two origins called the short and long heads. The long-head origin is the supraglenoid tubercle of the scapula, intimately associated with the shoulder joint capsule and with the short-head origin from the coracoid process of the scapula. The two heads join on top of the brachialis muscle on the anterior portion of the arm. The insertion of the biceps is at the radial tuberosity and the biceps aponeurosis, which blends with the forearm flexor sheath on the medial forearm (Figure 5–7). The major action of the biceps is flexion of the elbow and supination of the forearm. The musculocutaneous nerve innervates the biceps brachii muscle from the root levels C5 and C6.

The supinator has multiple origins. It originates from the lateral, posterior aspect of the ulna distal to the olecranon, the lateral humeral epicondyle, the radial collateral ligament of the elbow, and the annular ligament of the radial head. It inserts on to the proximal, lateral radius (Figure 5–8). Supination of the forearm with respect to the arm is the major function of this muscle. It is most effectively tested with the elbow fully flexed to put the biceps at a mechanical disadvantage. The radial nerve innervates the supinator muscle from the root levels C6 and C7.

The brachialis muscle originates on the anterior aspect of the humerus distal to the deltoid and coracobrachialis muscle insertions. The insertion is on the lateral aspect of the proximal ulna called the ulnar tuberosity (see Figure 5–7). The major action of the brachialis is flexion of the elbow, regardless of forearm supination or pronation. The musculocutaneous nerve innervates the brachialis from the root levels C5 and C6.

The brachioradialis muscle originates from the lateral aspect of the humerus called the *supracondylar ridge* and the adjoining intermuscular septum (see Figure 5–7). It inserts at the distal, lateral aspect of the radius near the styloid process. The major action of the brachioradialis is elbow flexion with the forearm halfway between

Figure 5–7. Anterior approach to the anatomy of the elbow region. Adapted from Kaplan EB: Surgical Approaches to the Neck, Cervical Spine, and Upper Extremity. Philadelphia: WB Saunders, 1966, p. 77.

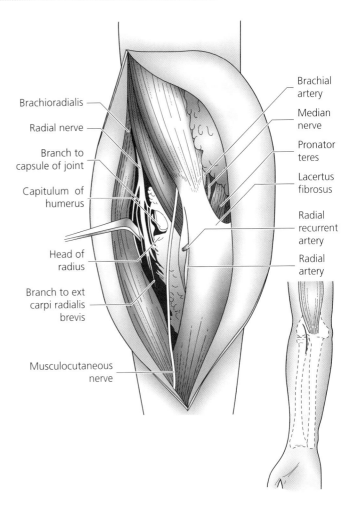

Brachioradialis

Radial nerve

Branch to capsule of joint

Capitulum of humerus

Head of radius

Branch to ext carpi radialis brevis

Musculocutaneous nerve

Brachial artery

Median nerve

Pronator teres

Lacertus fibrosus

Radial recurrent artery

Radial artery

pronation and supination (thumb up). The radial nerve innervates the brachioradialis from the root levels C5 and C6.

The triceps brachii muscle has three heads: the long head, medial head, and lateral head. The long head originates from the infraglenoid tubercle of the scapula. The medial head originates from the medial intermuscular septum and adjacent part of the distal humerus below the radial groove. The lateral head originates from the lateral intermuscular septum and the adjacent humerus proximal, but lateral to the radial groove. The three heads join in the posterior aspect of the arm and insert at the proximal olecranon of the ulna (Figure 5–9). The major action of the triceps brachii is extension of the elbow. The radial nerve innervates the triceps muscle from the root levels C6, C7, and C8.

The anconeus muscle is a small muscle originating on the lateral epicondyle of the humerus and inserts on to the lateral aspect of the olecranon of the ulna (see Figure 5–9).

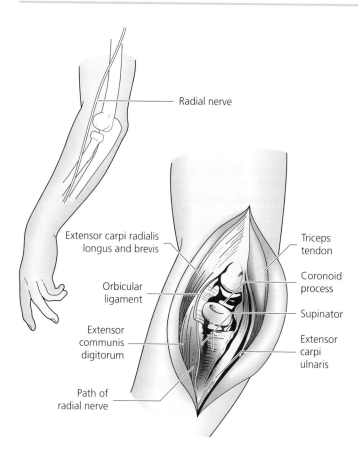

Figure 5–8. Lateral approach to the anatomy of the elbow region. Adapted from Kaplan EB: Surgical Approaches to the Neck, Cervical Spine, and Upper Extremity. Philadelphia: WB Saunders, 1966, p. 83.

Radial nerve

Extensor carpi radialis longus and brevis

Orbicular ligament

Extensor communis digitorum

Path of radial nerve

Triceps tendon

Coronoid process

Supinator

Extensor carpi ulnaris

The major action is extension of the elbow. The radial nerve innervates the anconeus muscle from the root levels C7 and C8.

Extrinsic Muscles of the Hand

Our discussion of the extrinsic and intrinsic muscles of the hands will focus on the major action and innervation.[14,31,37,38,45,63] A full discussion of each and every muscle, including origins and insertions of the muscles, should be sought in an anatomy text.

Flexor Group

Pronator teres (PT) arises from the medial epicondyle of the humerus and the medial coronoid process of the ulna (Figure 5–10). It inserts on to the lateral edge of the middle third of the radius. The median nerve innervates the PT, and the root levels are C6 and C7. The major action is forearm pronation with the elbow slightly flexed.

Figure 5–9. Posterior approach to the anatomy of the elbow region. Adapted from Kaplan EB: Surgical Approaches to the Neck, Cervical Spine, and Upper Extremity. Philadelphia: WB Saunders, 1966, p. 82.

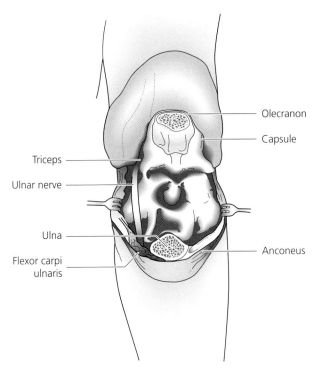

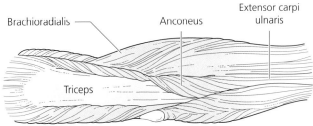

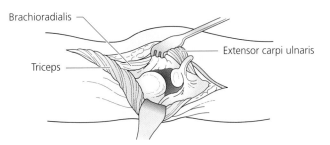

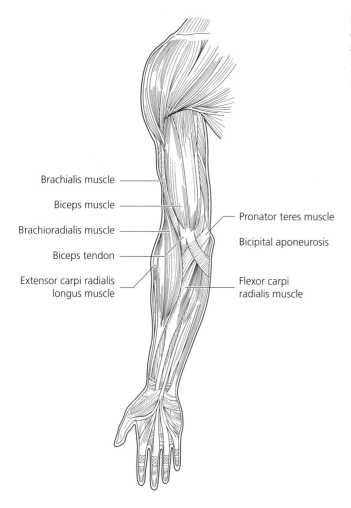

Figure 5–10. Superficial muscles of the anterior elbow region. Adapted from Anderson TE: Anatomy and physical examination of the elbow. In Nicholas J, Hershman E (eds), The Upper Extremity in Sports Medicine, 2nd edn. St Louis: Mosby, 1995, p. 262.

Brachialis muscle

Biceps muscle

Brachioradialis muscle

Biceps tendon

Extensor carpi radialis longus muscle

Pronator teres muscle

Bicipital aponeurosis

Flexor carpi radialis muscle

Pronator quadratus (PQ), as the name indicates, is a quadrangular shaped muscle with origin and insertion on the distal ulna and radius, respectively. The PQ assists pronation of the forearm and is the last muscle innervated by the anterior interosseous nerve (AIN), the root level most commonly sited at C7 and C8 (perhaps some T1).

Palmaris longus (PL) is absent in a certain percentage of the population, and does not travel beneath the flexor retinaculum at the wrist. The PL origin is at the medial epicondyle of the humerus from the common flexor tendon, and the insertion is at the palmar aponeurosis of the hand. The major action is assisting wrist flexion. The median nerve innervates the palmaris longus, and the root levels are C7, C8, and some T1.

Flexor carpi radialis (FCR) is medial to the pronator teres and lateral to the palmaris longus and flexor carpi ulnaris. The FCR muscle's origin is at the medial humeral epicondyle from the common flexor tendon, and the insertion is at the second and third metacarpal bones in the hand (see Figure 5–10). The flexor carpi radialis does not go deep to the flexor retinaculum at the wrist and, therefore, like the palmaris longus, is not within the carpal tunnel. The major action of the flexor carpi radialis is wrist flexion with a slight pronation component. The major innervation is from the median nerve from the root levels C6 and C7.

Flexor carpi ulnaris (FCU) has two heads of origin: from the medial humeral epicondyle and common flexor tendon and from the proximal posterior surface of the ulna just medial to the origin of the extensor carpi ulnaris. The major action of the flexor carpi ulnaris is wrist flexion with ulnar deviation. The major innervation is from the ulnar nerve from the root levels C8 and T1.

Flexor digitorum superficialis (FDS) has two heads of origin: from the medial to the humeral epicondyle at the common flexor tendon and coronoid process of the ulna and from the lateral radius just distal to the insertion of the supinator. The median nerve and the ulnar artery lie deep to this muscle and pass between the two heads of the FDS. The FDS muscle gives rise to four tendons in the distal forearm. These four tendons pass deep to the flexor retinaculum at the wrist, and therefore the FDS lies within the carpal tunnel at the wrist. The four tendons then continue on to each of digits two, three, four, and five. The final insertion of the tendons of the FDS is the middle phalanx of digits 2–5. Interestingly, each tendon splits just proximal to the final insertion to allow the tendon of the flexor digitorum profundus to pass through. Therefore, the tendons of the FDS insert on both the medial and lateral aspects of the middle phalanx of digits 2–5. The major action of the muscle is flexion of the middle phalanx of digits 2–5. In addition, this muscle can aid in flexion at the MCP and wrist joints. The median nerve innervates the flexor digitorum superficialis from the root levels C7, C8, and T1.

Flexor digitorum profundus (FDP) has extensive origin from the anterior and medial ulna and adjacent interosseous membrane. The FDP muscle then gives rise to four tendons that pass deep to the flexor retinaculum at the wrist. Therefore, like the flexor digitorum superficialis, the FDP tendons lie within the carpal tunnel. The four tendons of this muscle then divide, and one tendon goes to each of digits 2–5. The final insertion is the proximal distal phalanx, after passing through the split tendons of the flexor digitorum superficialis muscle. The major action of the FDP is flexion of the distal phalanx. The FDP can also secondarily aid more proximal phalangeal flexion and wrist flexion. The lateral portion of the FDP to digits two and three is innervated by the anterior interosseous nerve, whereas the medial portion to the fourth and fifth digits is innervated by the ulnar nerve. The root levels innervating the FDP are C7 and C8.

Flexor pollicis longus (FPL) originates just lateral to the flexor digitorum profundus on the interosseous membrane and the adjacent radial bone. In fact, the anterior interosseous nerve runs between the two muscles and innervates them both. The insertion of the FPL is at the base of the distal phalanx of the thumb. The FPL tendon passes within the carpal tunnel and is the most laterally situated tendon. The major action of the FPL is flexion of the distal phalanx of the thumb. The FPL can secondarily flex the more proximal phalanx and the wrist with radial deviation. It is innervated by the anterior interosseous nerve from root levels C7 and C8.

Extensor Group

Extensor carpi radialis longus (ECRL) originates at the lateral supracondylar ridge of the humerus, the adjacent intermuscular septum, and the lateral humeral epicondyle (Figure 5–11). It inserts at the base of the second metacarpal bone. The major action of the ECRL is extension of the wrist with a lateral or radial deviation. The innervation of the ECRL is from the radial nerve, root levels C7 and C8.

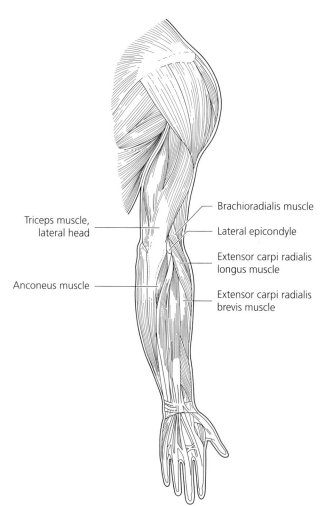

Triceps muscle, lateral head

Anconeus muscle

Brachioradialis muscle

Lateral epicondyle

Extensor carpi radialis longus muscle

Extensor carpi radialis brevis muscle

Figure 5–11. The superficial muscles of the posterior elbow region. Adapted from Anderson TE: Anatomy and physical examination of the elbow. In Nicholas J, Hershman E (eds), The Upper Extremity in Sports Medicine, 2nd edn. St Louis: Mosby, 1995, p. 262.

Extensor carpi radialis brevis (ECRB) originates at the lateral humeral epicondyle at the common extensor tendon (see Figure 5–11). The ECRB and the ECRL share a common tendon sheath and extensor compartment at the wrist. The ERCB inserts at the base of the third metacarpal. The major action of the ECRB is wrist extension. The radial nerve innervates the ECRB from the root levels C7 and C8.

Extensor digitorum communis (EDC) originates from the common extensor tendon at the lateral humeral epicondyle and inserts into the middle and distal phalanges of digits two, three, four, and five. The major action is extension of these digits. The radial nerve innervates the EDC from the root levels C7 and C8.

Extensor digiti minimi (EDM) is a small muscle originating at the common extensor tendon of the lateral humeral epicondyle and runs immediately adjacent to the EDC. The EDM has a separate extensor compartment at the wrist from the EDC and is considered a separate muscle from the EDC. It inserts at the middle and distal phalanx of the fifth digit (Figure 5–12). The major action is to extend the fifth digit. The radial nerve innervates the EDM from the root levels C7 and C8.

Extensor carpi ulnaris (ECU) originates from the lateral humeral epicondyle at the common extensor tendon and from the posterior surface of the proximal ulna. The ECU is the most medial muscle in the extensor group. It inserts at the base of the fifth metacarpal bone (see Figure 5–12). The major action is extension of the wrist with ulnar deviation. The radial nerve innervates the ECU from the root levels C7 and C8.

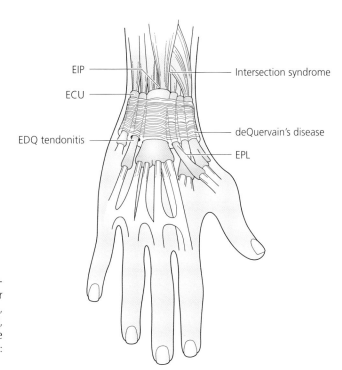

Figure 5–12. Extensor tendons and sites of overuse. ECU, extensor carpi ulnaris; EDM, extensor digiti minimi; EIP, extensor indicis proprius; EPL, extensor pollicis longus. Adapted from Kiefhaber TR, Stern PJ: Upper extremity tendinitis and overuse syndromes in athletes. Clin Sports Med 1992;11: 39–55.

Abductor pollicis longus (APL) originates on the proximal ulna, adjacent intermuscular septum and the radius, just distal and posterior to the insertion of the supinator. The insertion of the APL is at the base of the first metacarpal bone. The major action of the APL is abduction of the thumb. The radial nerve innervates the APL from the root levels C7 and C8.

Extensor pollicis longus (EPL) originates distal to the APL on the intermuscular septum and the ulna just lateral to the origin of the extensor carpi ulnaris. The insertion of the EPL is the proximal end of the first distal phalanx (see Figure 5–12). The major action is extension of the distal phalanx of the thumb. A secondary action of the EPL is wrist extension with radial deviation. The radial nerve innervates the EPL from root levels C7 and C8.

Extensor pollicis brevis (EPB) originates on the posterior surface of the radius and the adjacent intermuscular septum. The insertion is at the base of the proximal phalanx of the thumb. The major action is extension of the proximal phalanx of the thumb. The radial nerve innervates the EPB from root levels C7 and C8.

Extensor indicis (EI) originates on the distal posterior radius and inserts on the extensor surface of the index finger at the middle and distal phalanx (see Figure 5–12). The major action is extension of the index finger. The EI is the last muscle innervated by the radial nerve from root levels C7 and C8.

Intrinsic Muscles of the Hand

The following is a brief discussion of the muscles that have their origin and insertion entirely within the hand, distal to the wrist.[14,31,37,38,45,63]

Abductor pollicis brevis (APB) originates from the flexor retinaculum, trapezium, and scaphoid. The APB muscle inserts at the base of the proximal phalanx of the pollicis (thumb), with some fibers inserting on the adjacent extensor expansion (Figure 5–13). The major action of the APB muscle is abduction of the thumb. In addition, the fibers inserting on the extensor expansion can extend the thumb's interphalangeal joint. The median nerve innervates the APB muscle from root levels C8 and T1.

Flexor pollicis brevis (FPB) has superficial and deep heads. The superficial head originates from the flexor retinaculum and trapezium. The deep head originates from the trapezoid and the capitate. The two heads converge and insert on the base of the proximal phalanx just palmar to the insertion of the APB muscle (see Figure 5–13). The major action of the FPB is flexion of the first MCP and carpometacarpal joints. The FBP can also help in adduction and opposition of the thumb. The FPB has dual innervation with the median nerve innervating the superficial head from root levels C8 and T1. The ulnar nerve innervates the deep head from root levels C8 and T1.

Opponens pollicis (OP) originates from the flexor retinaculum and the adjacent trapezium. The OP inserts along the entire shaft of the first metacarpal on the radial side

Figure 5–13. Musculature about the thenar eminence. Adapted from Chase RA: Atlas of Hand Surgery, Vol. 2. Philadelphia: WB Saunders, 1984.

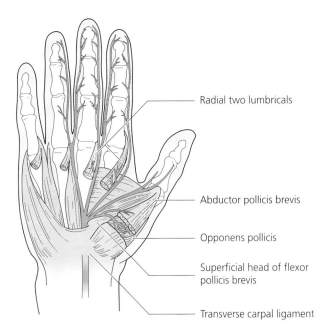

Radial two lumbricals

Abductor pollicis brevis

Opponens pollicis

Superficial head of flexor pollicis brevis

Transverse carpal ligament

(see Figure 5–13). The major action is opposition of the first metacarpal bone toward the other digits. The median nerve innervates the OP from root levels C8 and T1.

Adductor pollicis (AP) has an oblique head and a transverse head. The transverse head originates from the third metacarpal bone, and the oblique head originates from the adjacent carpal bones: capitate, trapezoid, trapezium, and probably a small slip from the base of the second metacarpal. The two heads converge and insert on the base of the first-digit's proximal phalanx. The major action of the adductor pollicis is adduction and flexion of the thumb. The ulnar nerve innervates the adductor pollicis from root levels C8 and T1.

Lumbrical muscles originate from the four tendons of the flexor digitorum profundus and insert on the extensor tendon hood of digits two, three, four, and five (see Figure 5–13). The major action of lumbricals is extension of the distal interphalangeal joints and flexion of the MCP joints. Lumbricals have dual innervation with the median nerve innervating the lateral two lumbricals (digits 2 and 3), whereas the ulnar nerve innervates the medial two lumbricals (digits 4 and 5).

Three palmar interosseous muscles are numbered 1, 2, and 3. They originate on the volar aspect of the shaft of the second, fourth, and fifth metacarpals. The palmar interosseous muscles insert on the lateral aspect of the base of the corresponding second, fourth, and fifth proximal phalanges and extensor expansion. The first palmar interosseous muscle inserts on the medial (ulnar) side of the second proximal phalanx and extensor expansion (index finger). The second and third insert on the lateral (radial) side of the proximal fourth and fifth phalanx and extensor expansions. It follows that the major action of the palmar interosseous muscles are adduction (bringing the fingers toward midline) of the phalanges. A secondary action is flexion of the metacarpal joints and extension of the interphalangeal joints. The ulnar nerve innervates all interossei muscles from root levels C8 and T1.

Four dorsal interosseous (DI) muscles are numbered 1, 2, 3, and 4. The dorsal interosseous muscles are larger than the palmar interosseous, have two head origins (bipennate), and lie between adjacent metacarpals. The first dorsal interosseous muscle (FDI) originates from both the first (thumb) and second metacarpals (index finger). At the base of the two heads of origin, the FDI has an opening through which the radial artery passes from dorsal to volar. The second dorsal interosseous muscle originates between the second (index) and third (middle) metacarpals. The third dorsal interosseous muscle originates from between the third (middle) and fourth (ring) metacarpals. The fourth dorsal interosseous muscle originates from between the fourth (ring) and fifth metacarpals. The second, third, and fourth dorsal interosseous muscles all have openings between their two heads through which pass bridging arteries from the dorsal to palmar blood supplies. All the dorsal interosseous muscles insert at the base of the corresponding proximal phalanx and extensor hood, opposite the palmar interosseous insertions. Phalangeal adduction, or movement of the fingers away from the middle finger, is the major action of these muscles. The ulnar nerve innervates the interosseous muscles from root levels C8 and T1.

Abductor digiti minimi (ADM) originates on the pisiform and the tendon of the flexor carpi ulnaris. The ADM inserts on the medial (ulnar) side of the base of the fifth proximal phalanx and the extensor expansion. The major action is abduction of the fifth digit. Secondarily, the ADM is responsible for flexion of the fifth MCP joint and extension of the fifth interphalangeal joints. The ulnar nerve innervates the ADM from root levels C8 and T1.

Flexor digiti minimi (FDM) originates from the hook of the hamate and the adjacent flexor retinaculum and inserts on the base of the proximal phalanx of the fifth digit. The major action is flexion of the MCP joint of the fifth digit. The ulnar nerve innervates the FDM muscle from root levels C8 and T1.

Opponens digiti minimi (OPM) muscle originates on the flexor retinaculum and the hook of the hamate and inserts along the medial (ulnar) shaft of the fifth metacarpal. The major action is flexion and rotation of the fifth metacarpal bone with respect to the plane of the other metacarpal bones. The ulnar nerve innervates the opponens digiti minimi muscle from root levels C8 and T1.

Palmaris brevis (PB) is a small muscle originating at the medial palmar aponeurosis that runs transversely across the palm and inserts into skin, as well as the pisiform. The palmaris brevis tightens the skin on the palm and may also protect the ulnar nerve and artery. The ulnar nerve innervates this muscle from root levels C8 and T1.

Nerves in the Upper Extremity

Four major nerves enter and innervate the upper extremity.[14,31,37,38,45,63] The following discussion gives a brief description of each nerve and the course the nerve takes to its final destination.

Musculocutaneous Nerve

The musculocutaneous nerve enters the arm as an extension of the lateral cord of the brachial plexus containing nerve fibers from cervical roots C5 and C6 (Figure 5–14).

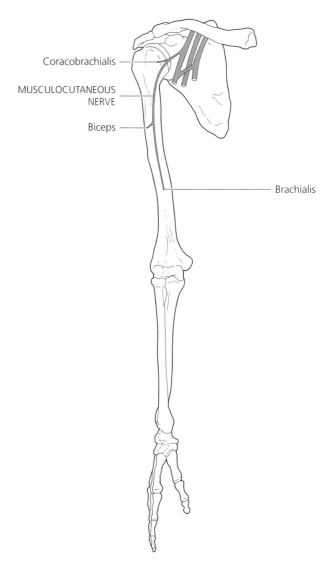

Coracobrachialis

MUSCULOCUTANEOUS NERVE

Biceps

Brachialis

Figure 5–14. The musculocutaneous nerve. Adapted from Birch R, Bonney G, Wynn Parry CB (eds): Surgical Disorders of the Peripheral Nerves. Edinburgh: Churchill Livingstone, 1998, p. 8.

The nerve enters the muscle belly of the coracobrachialis muscle and lies in the arm between the biceps and the brachialis muscles, innervating both. This nerve ends as a cutaneous nerve supplying the lateral forearm called the *lateral antebrachial cutaneus nerve*.

Median Nerve

The median nerve is formed by nerve fibers from the lateral and medial cords of the brachial plexus containing nerve fibers from the cervical root levels C6–T1 (Figure 5–15). This nerve enters the arm running with the ulnar nerve and the brachial artery and travels within the forearm just medial to the biceps tendon insertion and anterior to

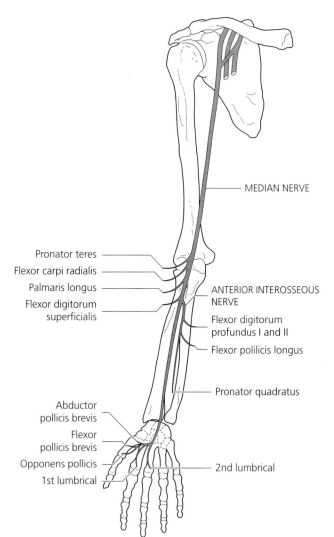

MEDIAN NERVE

Pronator teres
Flexor carpi radialis
Palmaris longus
Flexor digitorum superficialis

ANTERIOR INTEROSSEOUS NERVE

Flexor digitorum profundus I and II

Flexor polilicis longus

Pronator quadratus

Abductor pollicis brevis
Flexor pollicis brevis
Opponens pollicis
1st lumbrical

2nd lumbrical

Figure 5–15. The median nerve. Adapted from Birch R, Bonney G, Wynn Parry CB (eds): Surgical Disorders of the Peripheral Nerves. Edinburgh: Churchill Livingstone, 1998, p. 7.

the elbow joint. The median nerve dives deep to the PT, between its two heads, and runs between the FDS and FDP muscles. The median nerve innervates the PT, PL, FDS, and FCR in the forearm. The median nerve gives off the anterior interosseous nerve just after crossing the elbow joint. The AIN runs deep to the FDP and innervates the FDP to digits 1 and 2, FPL, and PQ. The median nerve continues between the tendons of the FDS and FDP at the wrist, just radial (lateral) to the superficialis tendon, ulnar (medial) to the FCR, and just deep (and lateral) to the PL tendon. The median nerve gives off the palmar cutaneous branch just proximal to the flexor retinaculum. It then passes deep to the flexor retinaculum and supplies the (superficial head) FPB, APB, OP, and lumbricals 1 and 2.

Ulnar Nerve

The ulnar nerve enters the arm as the extension of the medial cord of the brachial plexus with nerve fibers from the cervical root levels C8 and T1 (Figure 5–16). The nerve enters the arm slightly posterior to the brachial artery, innervating no muscles in the arm, and passes posterior to the medial humeral condyle in the ulnar groove. In the forearm, the ulnar nerve lies between the FCU and FDP and innervates the FDP to digits 3 and 4 and the FCU. Next, the ulnar nerve crosses the wrist joint medial to the FCU tendon and lateral to the ulnar artery. Once in the hand, the ulnar nerve passes medial to the pisiform bone, splitting into the superficial and deep palmar branches. These two branches enter the canal of Guyon together but exit to different endpoints. The space between the pisiform and the hook of the hamate forms the walls of Guyon's canal. The roof of Guyon's canal is the distal extension of the FCU tendon, and the floor is the pisohamate ligament. The superficial palmar branch supplies skin sensation to the medial half of the fourth and all of the fifth digits. The deep palmar branch travels (medial side) around the hook of the hamate and travels laterally to innervate the lumbricals 4 and 5, all interosseous muscles, all hypothenar muscles, the deep head of the FPB, and the adductor pollicis.

Radial Nerve

The radial nerve is the extension of the posterior cord of the brachial plexus with nerve fibers from the root levels C5–C8 (Figure 5–17). It enters the upper arm through the quadrangular space (borders teres major, minor, long head of the triceps and the humerus). In general, the radial nerve innervates all extensor muscles of the elbow, wrist, and fingers. The radial nerve has cutaneous innervation to the back of the arm, forearm, and hand. Once in the arm, the radial nerve lies against the humerus traveling distally and laterally in the spiral groove of the humerus, between the lateral and medial heads of the triceps. In the distal arm, the radial nerve lies between the anterior brachialis muscle and the posterior brachioradialis and ECRL muscles.

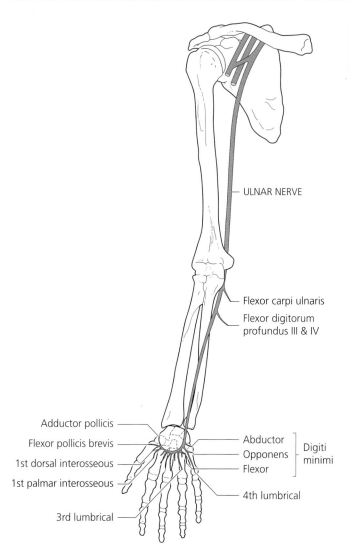

Figure 5–16. The ulnar nerve. Adapted from Birch R, Bonney G, Wynn Parry CB (eds): Surgical Disorders of the Peripheral Nerves. Edinburgh: Churchill Livingstone, 1998, p. 7.

ULNAR NERVE

Flexor carpi ulnaris

Flexor digitorum profundus III & IV

Adductor pollicis

Flexor pollicis brevis

1st dorsal interosseous

1st palmar interosseous

3rd lumbrical

Abductor
Opponens
Flexor

Digiti minimi

4th lumbrical

At the elbow, the radial nerve courses anterior to the lateral condyle of the humerus and splits into superficial and deep branches before entering the belly of the supinator. The superficial branch travels under the brachioradialis muscle becoming subcutaneous lateral to the tendon in the distal forearm. The superficial branch provides cutaneous innervation to the dorsum of the lateral hand and base of the thumb. The deep branch travels distally between the superficial and the deep extensor muscle groups. After innervating the supinator muscle, the radial nerve is called the *posterior interosseous nerve* (PIN). The deep branch (PIN) provides sensory input to the posterior of the wrist and carpal bones. The radial innervated muscles include triceps (all heads),

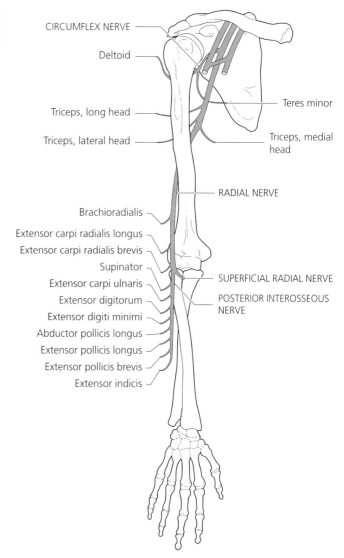

Figure 5–17. The radial nerve. Adapted from Birch R, Bonney G, Wynn Parry CB (eds): Surgical Disorders of the Peripheral Nerves. Edinburgh: Churchill Livingstone, 1998, p. 8.

CIRCUMFLEX NERVE

Deltoid

Teres minor

Triceps, long head

Triceps, lateral head

Triceps, medial head

RADIAL NERVE

Brachioradialis

Extensor carpi radialis longus

Extensor carpi radialis brevis

Supinator

Extensor carpi ulnaris

Extensor digitorum

Extensor digiti minimi

Abductor pollicis longus

Extensor pollicis longus

Extensor pollicis brevis

Extensor indicis

SUPERFICIAL RADIAL NERVE

POSTERIOR INTEROSSEOUS NERVE

brachioradialis, ECRL, ECRB, supinator, EDC, EDM, APL, EPL longus and brevis, and EI. The last radial innervated muscle is the EI.

Cutaneous Innervations in the Forearm and Hand

The lateral forearm from the elbow to the radial styloid has cutaneous innervation from the lateral antebrachial cutaneous (extension of the musculocutaneous nerve), nerve root level C5. Cutaneous branches of the median nerve innervate the lateral palm (thenar area). These branches from the C6 root leave the median nerve before the nerve enters the carpal tunnel. The rest of the palm, digits 1–3, and the lateral half of digit 4 are innervated by the digital branches of the median nerve after exiting from the carpal tunnel. The thumb is innervated from the C6 root level and the middle finger (digit 3) from C7. The ulnar nerve cutaneous branches, root level C8, innervate the hypothenar area and the medial dorsum of the hand (proximal to the DIP joint). These cutaneous branches leave the ulnar nerve prior to the wrist. The dorsal ulnar cutaneous nerve leaves the ulnar nerve 8 cm proximal to the wrist and loops around the medial aspect of the distal ulna head to reach the dorsum of the hand. The dorsal ulnar cutaneous nerve innervates the medial one-third of the dorsal hand. The medial antebrachial cutaneous nerve innervates the medial forearm from root level T1. This cutaneous nerve originates from the medial cord of the brachial plexus and travels with, but separate from, the ulnar nerve along the entire arm and forearm, providing cutaneous innervation to the medial forearm. The superficial radial nerve provides cutaneous innervation, from root levels C7 and C8, to the lateral dorsal three and a half digits proximal to the DIP joints. The posterior cutaneous nerve of the forearm supplying a small strip on the extensor forearm is a branch of the radial nerve.

Inspection

Visual inspection of the elbow, wrist, and hand requires proper exposure of the extremity from the shoulder to the hand. Such visualization allows the examiner to see any abnormality in the carry angle of the arm. As mentioned earlier, the bony congruency of the ulna and humerus makes the forearm flex with respect to the humerus at a fixed angle called the *carry angle of the arm*.[4] In the anatomic position, the anterior aspect of the elbow is covered by the biceps muscle and tendon, which are easily visualized. The anterior forearm just distal to the biceps muscle and tendon is called the *cubital fossa*. The cubital vein can be observed and palpated as it passes anterior to the elbow joint just lateral to the biceps tendon. The cephalic vein can be observed on the lateral side of the biceps muscle in the arm. The medial epicondyle of the elbow is the origin of the flexor/pronator muscle mass or the common flexor tendon. On the lateral aspect of the elbow can be seen the muscles that overlie the lateral epicondyle. The lateral epicondyle is the origin of the extensor muscle mass or the common extensor tendon. On the posterior elbow, a bony protuberance, the olecranon process of the ulna, is noted and is most obvious with the elbow flexed at 90 degrees. The olecranon bursa overlies the posterior elbow and is not observable in the normal state. However, a patient suffering from olecranon bursitis can have a golfball-sized swelling with tenderness and warmth over the olecranon.

Observing joint movements through their respective ranges of motion, both actively and passively, is part of inspection. The total joint motion is observed and documented from side to side with quality of movement also noted. Joint swelling or discoloration and any skin lesions or ecchymosis, hypertrophy, hypotrophy, or frank atrophy of muscles in the arm or forearm should also be documented. Other important observations include the presence of multiple healed scars of an occupational cause (e.g., cook or butcher), drug addiction, or physical abuse. Various injuries can be detected immediately through a comprehensive inspection of the extremity.

Distally, observation for asymmetry between the hand and wrist in both the supinated and pronated positions, comparing right to left sides, is essential. Any tumors, angular deformities, or soft tissue prominence should be noted. Swelling or enlargement of the joints should be noted. The digits should at rest be in a posture with slightly increased flexion noted from the index to the small finger. Any deviation from this normal cascade may be indicative of weakness of muscle groups or dysfunction of a tendon. Next, active flexion and extension of the digits should be observed for symmetric motion without triggering or limitation of motion. The forearm should be inspected for any gross asymmetry from side to side with pronation and supination assessed with the elbow flexed to 90 degrees, and this should be followed by measurement of elbow flexion and extension range.

Palpation

Palpation is a key aspect of the physical examination of any body part and is of critical importance when palpating for potential pathology around the elbow. Palpating the elbow requires pinpointing the exact area of tenderness or pathology.

The medial epicondyle is a bony protuberance that is easily palpable. Just anterior and distal to the medial epicondyle one can palpate from proximal to distal the muscle origins of the pronator teres, flexor carpi radialis, palmaris longus, FDS, and FCU.[39] Just posterior to the medial epicondyle, the ulnar groove can be palpated, as can the ulnar nerve traveling within. On the posterior aspect of the elbow, the olecranon process of the ulna is easily palpable, appreciating the triceps tendon insertion into the olecranon. Midway between the olecranon and the lateral epicondyle, one palpates the anconeus muscle. The lateral epicondyle is covered by a large mass of extensor muscle, called the *extensor bundle* or *wad*. From the lateral supracondylar ridge, to the lateral epicondyle one palpates a number of muscles. The muscles from proximal to distal are the brachioradialis, ECRL, ECRB, and EDC.

Deeper palpation about the lateral and medial elbow can reveal ligamentous and bony abnormalities. Deep palpation of the lateral, posterior elbow can reveal abnormalities in the capitellum of the humerus. About 2 cm distal to the capitellum, the radial head is palpated with the accompanying annular ligament that encircles the structure. Simple palpation of these structures while the patient pronates or supinates the forearm and flexes or extends the elbow may reveal crepitus. In the face of trauma, crepitus and pain while pronating or supinating the forearm in the region of the radial head area should raise suspicion for a radial head fracture. The lateral collateral ligament is difficult to directly palpate because of the overlying musculature; however, the anterior bundle of the medial collateral ligament is usually palpable with the elbow flexed from 30 to 60 degrees.[8]

Wrist and hand palpation is directed to the area of perceived pathology and can more precisely localize injury. Examination of the interphalangeal joints of the fingers is similar to that of other large hinge-type joints, although in many ways it is simpler. Testing for collateral ligament laxity followed by anterior posterior shifting and joint compression with rotation is utilized to detect arthropathy or instability. Detection of a synovial effusion in a small PIP joint may be more difficult than in a larger joint such as the knee, and, therefore, loss of mobility may be quite useful for screening. Palpation along the flexor tendon sheath is indicated in the diagnosis of trigger finger or tenosynovitis. A retinacular cyst is palpated generally between the level of A1 and A2 pulleys on the palmar aspect of the digits; because of their firmness these cysts are frequently mistaken for bony spurs.

Examination of the thumb MP joint deserves special consideration. A common injury involves rupture of the ulnar collateral ligament complex at this joint (skier's thumb). Stressing of the ulnar collateral complex with the MP joint in full extension will test the accessory component of the collateral ligament, whereas stressing of the joint at 30 degrees of flexion will test the true collateral ligament. Occasionally, the radial collateral ligament will be disrupted. Testing is performed in a similar fashion, stressing the radial side. Instability of the volar plate causing hyperextension at the MP joint is common. Unfortunately, this may be just a developmental variant in some patients whereas in others it is the result of an acute injury. Physical examination is limited with the history being more useful in differentiating the two.

Palpation in the wrist region must follow a logical sequence by the examiner so that some areas are not overlooked (Figure 5–18). The palmar aspect of the wrist is more difficult to palpate because of overlying soft tissues in the thenar and hypothenar areas. Medially, the first prominent tendon is the APL (insertion at the base of the first metacarpal). Palpation more medially reveals the pulsation of the radial artery with FCR tendon (insertion on the second metacarpal) situated medially. At the distal end of the FCR, the tuberosity of the trapezium forms a canal for the FCR tendon. Tenderness to palpation may indicate tendinitis of the FCR. Continuing more medially, one can feel the flexor retinaculum, the roof of the carpal tunnel. Provocative maneuvers are discussed later in this section. The next prominence palpated medially is the hook of the hamate on the hypothenar eminence. Just lateral and proximal to the hook

Figure 5–18. Surface anatomy of the wrist. Adapted from Nguyen DT, McCue FC, Urch SE: Evaluation of the injured wrist on the field and in the office. Clin Sports Med 1998;July;17:422.

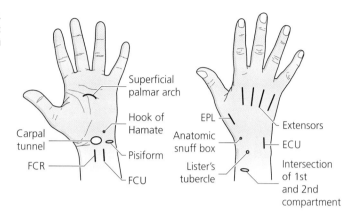

of the hamate, the pulsation of the ulnar artery is detected. Deep palpation to this area just at the distal palmer crease will reveal pain in the case of hamate fracture, though the pain is usually felt dorsally.[5] The FCU tendon surrounds the hamate as it inserts on the pisiform. As the examiner palpates more ulnarly, the pisiform bone is palpated, almost posterior and medial to the hamate. The pisiform may be fractured from a direct fall on the hypothenar aspect of the hand. Palpating the medial wrist one appreciates the distal end of the ulna, which actually ends proximal to the proximal wrist crease. Proximal to the pisiform and distal to the ulna lies the triangular fibrocartilage complex (TFCC), which can also be a source of pain on the medial aspect of the wrist. In 1981, Palmer and Werner described the TFCC as a "homogeneous structure composed of, but not dissectable into, the articular disc, the dorsal and volar radioulnar ligaments, the meniscus homologue, the ulnar collateral ligament and the sheath of the ECU."[72] There are no physical exam maneuvers to reliably test the TFCC, though direct palpation, forced ulnar deviation with rotation, and forearm supination, with the wrist ulnar deviated and extended may reproduce symptoms.

The dorsum of the wrist lacks significant subcutaneous tissue, and this potentially allows better palpation than the palmar aspect. In a wrist free of deformity, the ulnar styloid process is the most obvious structure on the dorsum of the wrist. In the ulnar notch on the extensor suface of the ulna is the ECU tendon (inserts on the base of the fifth metacarpal). On the dorsum of the distal radius is a bony prominence called *Lister's tubercle*. Medial to Lister's tubercle, lying sequentially more ulnar, are the EPL, EI, EDC, EDM, and ECU tendons, which also can palpated. Radial to Lister's tubercle and proceeding further radially, the ECRB, ECRL, EPB, and APL are palpated. On the radial aspect of the wrist, just distal to the radius and between the EPL and EPB tendons, lies the anatomic snuffbox. The EPB and APL are tender in deQuervain's stenosing tenosynovitis. At the base of the snuffbox, one can palpate the scaphoid bone, the radial artery extension, and, in the distal end of the snuffbox, the trapezoid. Tenderness at the base of the snuffbox is classic for scaphoid fractures, and tenderness more distal in the snuffbox suggests MCP arthrosis or possible radial collateral ligament injury.

Returning to the dorsum of the wrist, palpating distally from Lister's tubercle (see Figure 5–18) one can palpate the dorsal lunate, the capitate, and then the third metacarpal base. The adjacent metacarpal bases should also be palpated. Any tenderness over these structures suggests a sprain of the carpometacarpal joints with possible fracture, and the likely mechanism is forced wrist flexion. Tenderness over the lunate may indicate lunate fracture or Kienböck's disease (avascular necrosis of the lunate). The capitolunate ligament can be assessed along with the dorsal capitate-displacement apprehension test (see Special Tests below). Radial to the lunate, the scaphoid and the scapholunate ligament are appreciated. Laxity of the scapholunate ligament is evaluated using the scaphoid shift test (see Special Tests). Medial to the lunate one palpates the lunotriquetral ligament. Beckenbaugh coined the term *ulnar snuffbox* for the area distal to the ulna and between the flexor carpi ulnaris and the extensor carpi ulnaris.[5] In the floor of the ulnar snuffbox is the triquetrum. These lateral ligaments can be assessed with the ballottement and shear tests (see Special Tests). The findings on wrist examination help in planning for more focused radiologic assessment.

Arterial Palpation

- The *ulnar artery* lies distally between the tendons of the FCU and FDS. It is best palpated proximal to the pisiform bone in the medial forearm.
- The *radial artery* lies distally between the tendons of the brachioradialis muscle and FCR. It is best palpated medial to the radial styloid.

Common Finger Deformities

Mallet finger results when the extensor tendon of the distal phalanx is ruptured with or without bone avulsion from the distal phalanx (Figure 5–19). The deformity results in the inability to actively extend the distal phalanx. This deformity most commonly results from trauma with a mechanism of forced flexion of the DIP joint while the individual is actively trying to extend the finger.

Jersey finger results from rupture of the flexor tendon of the distal phalanx (Figure 5–20). As the name suggests, a common mechanism resulting in a jersey finger is the distal finger forcibly extended while trying to grab a shirt or jersey in

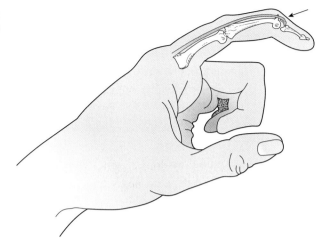

Figure 5–19. Mallet finger. Adapted from Mellion MB: *Office Sports Medicine*, 2nd edn. Philadelphia: Hanley & Belfus, 1996.

sports such as rugby or football. The patient is unable to flex the DIP of the affected finger against resistance.

Swan neck deformity is most often seen in rheumatoid arthritis or after trauma. The PIP joint is hyperextended while the MCP and DIP joints are in flexion. The swan neck deformity may also result from contractures of the hand intrinsics causing dorsal migration of the tendons.

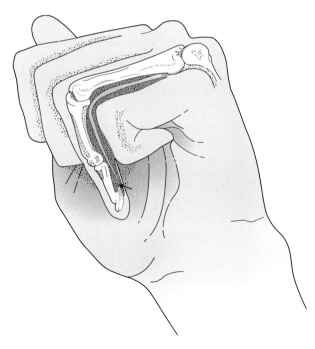

Figure 5–20. Jersey finger. Adapted from Mellion MB: *Office Sports Medicine*, 2nd edn. Philadelphia: Hanley & Belfus, 1996.

Boutonnière deformity is seen most frequently in rheumatoid arthritis and exists when there is rupture of the extensor hood over the proximal interphalangeal joint. Extensor hood rupture results in palmar migration of the lateral bands with extension noted at both the metacarpophalangeal and distal interphalangeal joints and flexion of the proximal interphalangeal joints.

Ulnar drift or ulnar deviation of the phalanges is commonly seen in subjects with late-stage rheumatoid arthritis. Ulnar drift occurs because the distal ulna suffers bony loss and resorption resulting in shortening of the ulna. The continuous pull of tendons crossing the wrist joint subsequently results in the ulnar drift.

Heberden's nodes and *Bouchard's nodes* are commonly seen in individuals with osteoarthritis. Heberden's nodes are characteristic nodules localized lateral and medial to the DIP joints on the dorsal surface. Nodules present on the proximal interphalangeal joint are called Bouchard's nodes. Osteoarthritis tends to spare the middle interphalangeal joints.[84]

Neurologic Examination

There are multiple possible sites for nerve entrapments in the upper extremity affecting any of the major nerves. It is key to remember that all the structures distal to an entrapment site are commonly affected. Understanding the anatomy and route of nerves becomes critically important so that lesions can be fully appreciated and identified.

Median Nerve Lesions

The median nerve innervates a number of key muscles in the upper extremity, and any lesion can be severely disabling. It can be compressed just proximal to the medial humeral condyle at an anomalous structure called the ligament of Struthers.[90] On physical exam, the wrist flexors, PT, and median innervated hand muscles are weak. The sensation on the thenar and first three and a half digits can be impaired. Wrist flexion occurs with ulnar deviation, as the FCU remains innervated. The patient should be asked to make a fist, because individuals with a high median nerve lesion will be unable to flex the index finger and, in many cases, middle finger actively or against resistance. When both the index and middle finger cannot be flexed, the hand forms the "active papal hand" or "benediction sign."[83] Over time, high median nerve injuries may result in "ape hand" deformity, because the radial nerve innervating APL, EPL, and EPB pull the first metacarpal into the plane of the palm.[38]

Entrapment may also occur under the lacertus fibrosus (Figure 5–21), between the two heads of the PT, or through its muscle belly; this is called the *pronator teres syndrome*. In this entity, pronator muscle function is spared, because its innervation is

Figure 5–21. Entrapment sites for the median nerve. Adapted from Santiago FH, Vallarino R: Median neuropathy. In Frontera WR, Silver JK (eds), Essentials of Physical Medicine and Rehabilitation. Philadelphia: Hanley & Belfus, 2002, p. 121.

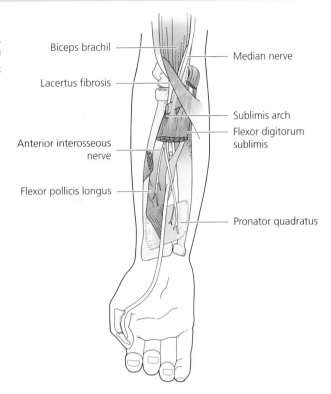

Biceps brachil

Median nerve

Lacertus fibrosis

Sublimis arch

Flexor digitorum sublimis

Anterior interosseous nerve

Flexor pollicis longus

Pronator quadratus

established prior to the median nerve being compressed. However, all muscles distal to the PT are affected and will result in wrist flexor weakness or lost or impaired sensation over the thenar and lateral three and a half digits. Symptoms of the pronator teres syndrome mimic carpal tunnel syndrome (CTS). In contrast to CTS, patients will often exhibit pain to palpation over the nerve entrapment site, which is proximal in the wrist.[47,60]

The anterior interosseous nerve may be compressed by a fibrous band from the muscle heads of either the FDS or FDP (see Figure 5–21). The anterior interosseous nerve (AIN) syndrome results in weakness of the AIN innervated FPL, FDP to digits 1 and 2, and the PQ.[16,46] The AIN is purely a motor nerve, and sensory findings are not part of the syndrome. However, patients often have dull ache in the forearm region, perhaps from sensory fibers going to the wrist joint. On physical exam, lack of flexion of the distal phalanx of the thumb and index finger result in the inability of the patient to make the "okay" sign (Figure 5–22). When pinching paper between the thumb and index finger, the patient uses the adductor pollicis (ulnar innervated muscle) to substitute for FPL weakness. Pronator quadratus weakness is tested with the elbow fully flexed placing the PT at a mechanical disadvantage.[43]

The most common nerve entrapment is that of the median nerve under the flexor retinaculum. Contained within the carpal tunnel are the four tendons of the FDP, FDS,

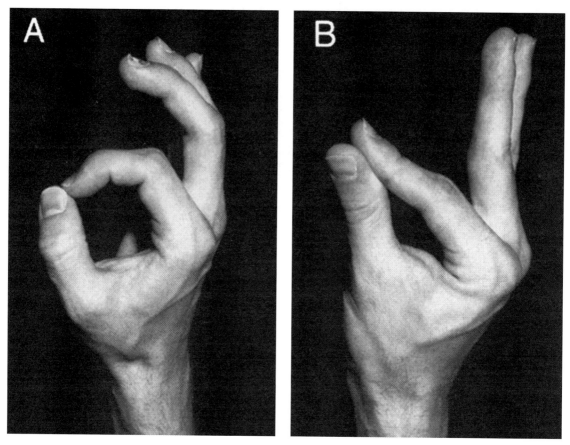

Figure 5–22. Injury to the anterior interosseous nerve with inability to form the "OK sign." Reproduced with permission from Concannon MJ: Common Hand Problems in Primary Care. Philadelphia: Hanley & Belfus, 1999, p. 137.

and FPL and the median nerve. Sensation over the thenar area is spared, but sensation to the first three and a half digits is impaired. Weakness of the APB and OP results in difficulty with abducting or opposing the thumb and may ultimately result in atrophy of the thenar.[44] Patients with CTS exhibit night-time exacerbations that are relieved by shaking the hands, a movement called the "flick sign." The flick sign is positive in 93% of individuals with CTS.[78] See below for common physical exam findings in carpal tunnel syndrome.

Ulnar Nerve Lesions

The ulnar nerve enters the arm as an extension of the medial cord of the brachial plexus with nerve fibers from the root levels C8 and T1. The most common site for

Figure 5–23. Entrapment of the ulnar nerve at the arcade of Struthers. Adapted from Spinner M: Injuries to the Major Branches of the Forearm, 2nd edn. Philadelphia: WB Saunders, 1978.

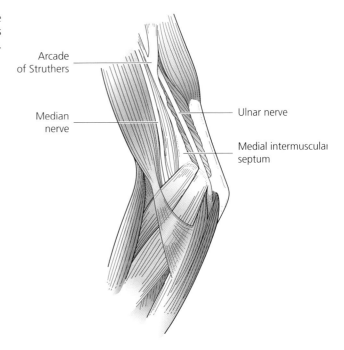

Arcade of Struthers

Median nerve

Ulnar nerve

Medial intermuscular septum

ulnar neuropathy in the arm is at the ulnar groove. However, just proximal to this site, another focus of entrapment termed the *arcade of Struthers* may occur and is present in up to 70% of people (Figure 5–23).[94] Ulnar nerve entrapments at the ulnar groove can spare the fibers innervating the FCU and FDP to digits 3 and 4. Proximal and distal ulnar nerve lesions have the same effect on the hand intrinsics. Proximal lesions denervating the forearm muscles allow the patient wrist flexion with radial deviation only, and wrist flexion strength is usually somewhat decreased. Ulnar deviation at the wrist will be lost. In chronic palsy, extension of the little finger at the interphalangeal joint is impossible with hyperextension at the metacarpophalangeal joints, flattening of the hypothenar eminence, and hollowing of the palm, termed *claw hand deformity*.[85] Interestingly, this hand deformity appears similar to the benediction sign.

Just distal to the elbow, the ulnar nerve lies between the two heads of the FCU, a potential entrapment point. Lesions at this site spare the FCU and usually the FDP with similar distal findings as noted with more proximal entrapment.

More distal ulnar nerve entrapment may occur at the wrist or hand (Guyon's canal). The deep motor and superficial sensory branches enter the canal together, and findings depend on what fibers have been affected. The sensation on the dorsum of the hand innervated by the dorsal ulnar cutaneous nerve is spared, and this sensory finding helps differentiate proximal from distal injury. The ulnar innervated hand intrinsics will be involved, and on examination the patient will be unable to success-fully grasp a piece of paper between the lateral side of the index finger and thumb.

The patient with an ulnar nerve lesion will substitute with the median innervated FPL and the Froment's sign is demonstrated, indicative of an ulnar nerve pathology. Patients with ulnar lesions may still be able to adduct and abduct the fingers weakly. The EDC, FDS, and FDP will adduct with activation.

Radial Nerve Lesions

The radial nerve can be injured proximally secondary to axillary crutch use or compression against the back of a chair – "bar stool neuropathy." Proximal injury will result in involvement of the triceps along with all other distally innervated muscles and cutaneous nerves. Injury along its course down the spiral groove, on the posterior aspect of the humerus, will result in sparing of the triceps. However, the remainder of muscles will be weakened, resulting in wrist drop and weakened grip strength secondary the mechanical disadvantage placed on the wrist and finger flexors. The radial nerve can also be entrapped as it enters the supinator muscle or at the arcade of Frohse, a fibrous arch at the origin of the supinator (Figure 5–24).[30] The supinator

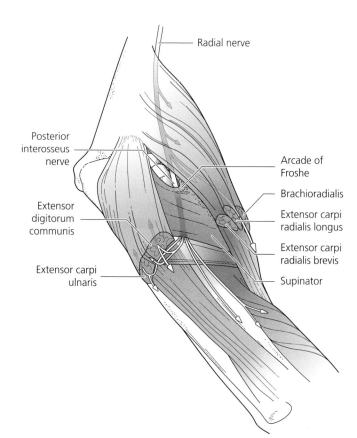

Radial nerve

Posterior interosseus nerve

Extensor digitorum communis

Extensor carpi ulnaris

Arcade of Froshe

Brachioradialis

Extensor carpi radialis longus

Extensor carpi radialis brevis

Supinator

Figure 5–24. Entrapment of the radial nerve at the arcade of Frohse. Adapted from Spinner M: Injuries to the Major Branches of the Forearm, 2nd edn. Philadelphia: WB Saunders, 1978.

Table 5–1. DERMATOMES, MYOTOMES, AND MUSCLE STRETCH REFLEXES IN THE UPPER EXTREMITY

Spinal Cord Level	Dermatomes	Myotomes	Deep Tendon Reflexes
C4	From midtrapezius to tip of acromion extending in a shawl like distribution to the other side	Non-specific	Non-specific
C5	Lateral arm from tip of acromion process to lateral humeral condyle	Elbow flexors	Bicipital aponeurosis
C6	Lateral forearm below the humeral condyle to the ventral and dorsal surfaces of the first and second digits	Wrist extensors	Non-specific
C7	Dorsum of third digit and corresponding metacarpal tapering to midline at wrist Ventrally from second, third, and fourth digits tapering to midline at wrist	Elbow extensors	Triceps tendon proximal to its insertion into the olecranon
C8	Ventrum and dorsum of fourth and fifth digits and corresponding metacarpals tapering to the ulnar styloid	Distal interphalangeal joint flexors	Non-specific
T1	Medial forearm from medial humeral condyle to ulna styloid	Fifth digit abductor	Non-specific
T2	Medial arm above the humeral condyles to above the axilla and across the chest to a contralateral corresponding distribution	Non-specific	Non-specific

Data from Magee[54] and ASIA SCI scales[81]

syndrome spares the fibers innervating the supinator muscle, but affects muscles innervated more distal by the posterior interosseous nerve (PIN). On physical exam, patients are able to extend the wrist. However, when asked to extend the wrist, there is radial deviation because of the unopposed ECR.[42] Placement of rope or handcuffs at the wrist may reveal more distal involvement at the wrist, in particular a condition termed *cheiralgia paresthetica*, which results in sensory loss on the dorsal thumb (Table 5–1).

Range of Motion

Range of motion (ROM) should be performed in any individual presenting for evaluation of hand, wrist, or elbow injury with any incongruency documented. The end-range feel for each of the joints of the upper extremity should also be noted (Figure 5–25).

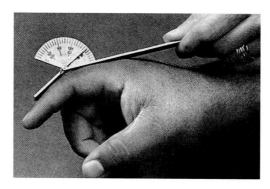

Figure 5–25. Range of motion of the proximal interphalangeal joints measured with a goniometer. Reproduced with permission from Hunter JM, Mackin EJ, Callahan AD (eds): Rehabilitation of the Hand: Surgery and Therapy, 4th edn. St Louis: Mosby, 1995, p. 56.

Elbow flexion should take into account the approximation of the forearm and arm muscles whose mass may prevent further motion. The end-range feel of finger extension should be more abrupt with bony and ligamentous endpoints. Table 5–2 lists the range of motions of the elbow, wrist, and digits.

Table 5–2. RANGE OF MOTION OF THE UPPER EXTREMITY

	Motion	Range (Degrees)
Elbow	Flexion	140–160
	Extension	0–10
	Pronation	80–90
	Supination	90
Wrist	Flexion	70–90
	Extension/hyperextension	60–70 hyperextension
	Abduction (radial deviation)	15–25
	Adduction (ulnar deviation)	20–35
Metacarpophalangeal (MCP) joints	Flexion digits II–V	70–90
	Extension digits II–V	20–30
	Abduction	15–20
	Digit 2 away from middle finger	
	Digits 4 and 5 away from middle finger	
	Adduction	Touches adjacent finger
	Digit 2 toward middle finger	
	Digits 4 and 5 toward middle finger	
Proximal interphalangeal (PIP) joints	Flexion digits 2–4	90–120
	Extension digits 2–4	Up to 10 degrees hyperextension
Distal interphalangeal (DIP) joints	Flexion digits 2–4	60–80
	Extension digits 2–4	Up to 10 degrees hyperextension

Data from Palmer[74] and Reese[80]

The thumb range of motion – and indeed the motions themselves – are unique. Thumb carpometacarpal (CMC) flexion occurs in the coronal plane, and requires the first metacarpal to glide over the palmar side of the second metacarpal (slightly out of plane with the palm). Thumb CMC joint extension returns the first metacarpal to the plane of the palm with radial abduction of the first metacarpal. Thumb opposition is a combination of movements of the CMC joint with flexion, medial rotation, and abduction of the first metacarpal in relation to the trapezium. Thumb opposition has no normal values to measure, but patients normally can touch the tip of the thumb to the little finger. Thumb carpometacarpal abduction (also called palmer abduction) and adduction occurs at 90 degrees to the plane of the palm. In abduction, the first metacarpal bone moves away from the plane of the palm at a right-angle. Adduction is a return to normal position from the abducted state.

Special Tests for the Elbow

Lateral and medial epicondylitis are extremely common and often painfully disabling conditions. The physical examination tests used to evaluate epicondylitis are therefore described and reviewed first (Table 5–3).

Lateral Epicondylitis ("Tennis Elbow")

The term *tennis elbow* developed out of the term used in 1883 by Winkworth – "lawn tennis arm."[105] Originally, Winkworth was describing medial epicondylitis. However, today, tennis elbow describes lateral epicondylitis, and "golfer's elbow" describes medial epicondylitis.[77]

There have been multiple descriptions of the physical exam findings in lateral epicondylitis, and the original descriptions are nearly impossible to locate. Individuals suffering this malady have tenderness over the lateral epicondyle that may radiate to the forearm.[9,49,77] Palpation 2–5 mm distal and anterior to the lateral epicondyle usually isolates the maximal tenderness.[49,77]

Resistant cases of lateral epicondylitis may be secondary to posterior interosseous nerve (PIN) entrapment at the radial tunnel.[52,82,99,101] Capener[13] observed a case of PIN entrapment by a lipoma causing symptoms similar to lateral epicondylitis. Roles and Maudsley[82] surgically treated resistant cases of tennis elbow to decompress the radial nerve and its branches within the forearm.

Resisted Wrist Extension Test

Although no original description can be located, multiple authors mention resisted wrist and finger extension.[9,49,77] According to Leach and Miller, "[with] pain on the

Table 5–3. TESTS FOR LATERAL AND MEDIAL EPICONDYLITIS

Test	Description	Reliability/Validity Tests	Comments
Resisted wrist extension	With pain on the lateral side (of the elbow), extending the wrist against resistance will increase the pain, and the more extended the elbow, the more likely wrist extension with resistance is to cause pain. Others state "resisting wrist and finger extension with the elbow in full extension will intensify the pain."	Not reported	
Extensor carpi radialis brevis test	The patient holds the elbow extended and the forearm pronated while he/she makes a fist and extends the wrist. The patient should hold this position while the examiner applies resistance (i.e., attempts to forcibly flex the wrist). Pain at the origin of the ECRB is highly suggestive of lateral tennis elbow. The test should be repeated with the elbow flexed 90 degrees. The pain will usually be worse with the elbow in extension and lessened with the elbow in flexion.	Not reported	
Resisted middle-finger extension	The clinical findings were fairly uniform. Pain radiated up and down the arm; the grip became weak; there were sometimes paresthesiae in the distribution of the superficial radial nerve; there was tenderness over the radial nerve and there was pain on resisted extension of the middle finger, which tightens the fascial origin of the extensor carpi radialis brevis. This last test could be elicited in all cases.	No formal studies to assess the sensitivity and specificity of this test	Lister et al.[52] reported 19 out of 19 cases of resistant tennis elbow relieved by radial tunnel release had positive resisted middle-finger tests. Werner[99] reported positive resisted middle-finger test in 67 out of 90 cases of resistant lateral elbow pain.
Resisted wrist flexion and pronation	Symptoms may be reproduced by resisted wrist flexion and pronation. With the elbow flexed to 90 degrees and the forearm supinated, the patient makes a fist and flexes maintaining that position as the the wrist, examiner attempts to forcibly extend the wrist. If resisted wrist flexion elicits pain at the origin of the flexor carpi radialis, this tendon is involved. This test should be repeated with the elbow fully extended and the amount of pain elicited with the elbow extended and flexed compared.	Not reported	

Table 5–3. TESTS FOR LATERAL AND MEDIAL EPICONDYLITIS—*cont'd*

Test	Description	Reliability/Validity Tests	Comments
	In contradistinction to lateral epicondylitis, medial tennis elbow usually hurts worst with the elbow flexed.		
Pronator syndrome	All showed local tenderness over the median nerve 4–5 cm distal to the elbow. Active forearm pronation against resistance, with the elbow in about 30 degrees of flexion, elicited pain in the proximal volar aspect of the forearm in all patients. In contrast, resisted active forearm supination with the elbow similarly flexed did not elicit pain.	Not reported	A positive Tinel's sign over the entrapment site (tapping the proximal edge of the pronator) was reported in 4 of 9 patients by Werner[100] and 20 of 39 patients by Hartz.[34]

lateral side (of the elbow), extending the wrist against resistance will increase the pain, and the more extended the elbow, the more likely wrist extension with resistance is to cause pain"[49] (Figure 5–26).

Others state "resisting wrist and finger extension with the elbow in full extension will intensify the pain."[49,77] There are no reliability or validity studies documenting the resisted wrist extension test. Further, there are no studies evaluating the specificity and sensitivity of this test.

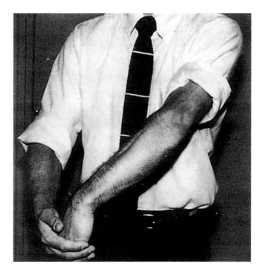

Figure 5–26. Resisted wrist extension. Reproduced with permission from Leach RE, Miller JK: Lateral and medial epicondylitis of the elbow. Clin Sports Med 1987;April;6:267.

Extensor Carpi Radialis Brevis Test, or Tennis Elbow Test

The ECRB test should be considered synonymous with the tennis elbow test. An original description could not be located, but the test maneuver is described in multiple sources. Budoff and Nirschl[9] describe the test as follows (Figure 5–27):

> Have the patient hold the elbow extended and the forearm pronated while he or she makes a fist and extends the wrist. The patient should hold this position while the examiner applies resistance (i.e., attempts to forcibly flex the wrist). Pain at the origin of the ECRB is highly suggestive of lateral tennis elbow. The test should be repeated with the elbow flexed 90 degrees. … The pain will usually be worse with the elbow in extension and lessened with elbow flexion.

Studies to corroborate the efficacy of the tennis elbow test could not be located. Most clinicians would argue that the symptoms associated with lateral epicondylitis and discomfort elicited with the tennis elbow test or resisted wrist extension are due primarily to inflammation of the ECRB tendon at or near its origin on the lateral humeral condyle.[29,64] Nirschl and Pettrone[64] noted 97% of 88 surgical cases revealed pathologic tissue at the origin of the ECRB tendon. Their findings support the initial work of Cyriax[18] and Goldie.[29] Interestingly, Greenbaum et al.[32] noted difficulty localizing pain to the ECRB or common extensor tendon. In fact, when attempting to dissect out the two tendons on a cadaver, it was extremely difficult, and the authors

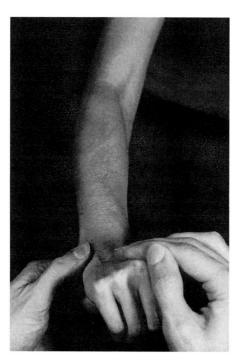

Figure 5–27. The extensor carpi radialis brevis test or "tennis elbow" test. Reproduced with permission from Anderson TE: Anatomy and physical examination of the elbow. In Nicholas J, Hershman E (eds), The Upper Extremity in Sports Medicine, 2nd edn. St Louis: Mosby, 1995, p. 273.

suggest that the symptoms may actually arise from the common extensor tendon and not the brevis tendon. Plancher et al.[77] described tenderness along the lateral supracondylar ridge, supporting involvement of the ECRL.

Resisted Middle-finger Extension Test

There is much controversy over the resisted middle-finger extension test. This test is often mentioned when discussing lateral epicondylitis, but the original description of the test was for the radial tunnel syndrome (Figure 5–28). Roles and Maudsley[82] described resistant cases of lateral epicondylitis, stating:

> The clinical findings were fairly uniform. ... Pain radiated up and down the arm; the grip became weak; there were sometimes paresthesias in the distribution of the superficial radial nerve; there was tenderness over the radial nerve and pain on resisted extension of the middle finger, which tightens the fascial origin of the extensor carpi radialis brevis. This last test could be elicited in all cases.

No formal studies assess the sensitivity and specificity of this test. Lister et al.[52] reported 19 out of 19 cases of resistant tennis elbow relieved by radial tunnel release had positive resisted middle-finger tests. Werner[99] reported a positive resisted middle-finger test in 67 out of 90 cases of resistant lateral elbow pain. In suspected radial tunnel syndrome, other physical exam findings include maximal tenderness at or just distal to the

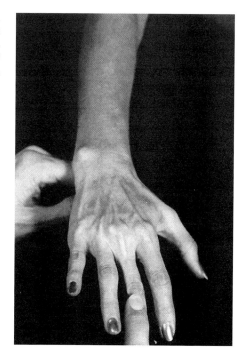

Figure 5–28. Resisted middle finger extension. Reproduced with permission from Anderson TE: Anatomy and physical examination of the elbow. In Nicholas J, Hershman E (eds), The Upper Extremity in Sports Medicine, 2nd edn. St Louis: Mosby, 1995, p. 273.

radial head (4–5 cm distal to the lateral epicondyle) and pain on resisted supination of the forearm.[99,101] A subsequent study by Werner[99] found elevated pressures over the PIN by the supinator muscle with both passive and active supination of the forearm.

Medial Epicondylitis

Although medial epicondylitis is far less common than lateral epicondylitis, it can cause significant morbidity (Figure 5–29). A comprehensive retrospective review by O'Dwyer[70] found lateral epicondylitis in 91%, medial epicondylitis in 8%, and both in 1% of individuals diagnosed with epicondylitis. Medial epicondylitis has been coined *golfer's elbow* because of the wrist flexion performed with the golf swing.[65] However, medial epicondylitis is most often seen in workers performing heavy or light manual labor.[48] Other activities implicated include rowing, baseball (pitching), javelin throwing, bricklaying, hammering, tennis (serving), and typing.[9,49,77,93]

Resisted Wrist Flexion and Pronation

There are no named tests for evaluating medial epicondylitis. However, the best description is by Budoff and Nirschl,[8] who state (Figure 5–30):

> Symptoms may be reproduced by resisted wrist flexion and pronation. With the elbow flexed to 90 degrees and the forearm supinated, the patient makes a fist and flexes the wrist, maintaining that position as the examiner attempts to forcibly extend the wrist. If resisted wrist flexion elicits pain at the origin of the flexor carpi radialis, this tendon is involved. This test should be repeated with the elbow fully extended and the amount of pain elicited with the elbow extended and flexed compared. In contradistinction to lateral epicondylitis, medial tennis elbow usually hurts worst with the elbow flexed.

There are no studies evaluating the specificity and sensitivity of the above test. Other findings include tenderness present 1–2 cm distal to the medial epicondyle.[70] The most likely muscles involved are the PT and FCR.[77,93] Individuals with suspected medial

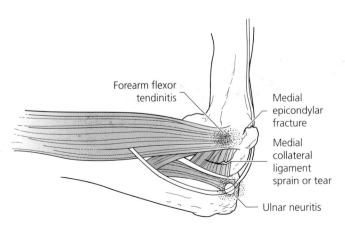

Forearm flexor tendinitis

Medial epicondylar fracture

Medial collateral ligament sprain or tear

Ulnar neuritis

Figure 5–29. Medial epicondylitis and related syndromes. Adapted from Bennett JB: Acute injuries to the elbow. In Nicholas J, Hershman E (eds), The Upper Extremity in Sports Medicine, 2nd edn. St Louis: Mosby, 1995, p. 307.

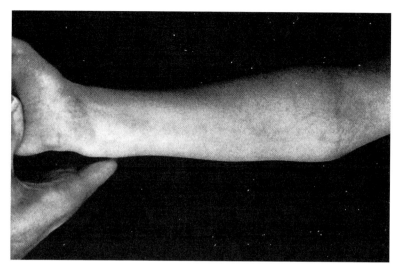

Figure 5–30. Resisted wrist flexion for medial epicondylitis. Reproduced with permission from Anderson TE: Anatomy and physical examination of the elbow. In Nicholas J, Hershman E (eds), The Upper Extremity in Sports Medicine, 2nd edn. St Louis: Mosby, 1995, p. 274.

epicondylitis need to be assessed for ulnar neuropathy at or near the elbow. Vangsness and Jobe[93] reported 23% and Nirschl[65] reported 50% ulnar nerve involvement with cases of medial epicondylitis. In contrast, a retrospective study by O'Dwyer reported zero percent nerve involvement with medial epicondylitis. Examiners must not forget to evaluate for instability of the medial collateral ligament in individuals with medial elbow pain.

Pronator Syndrome

A high median nerve compression has been coined the "pronator syndrome." First described by Seyffarth in 1951, as the name suggests, this lesion is higher (more proximal) than the much more common median nerve compression at the wrist (i.e., carpal tunnel syndrome). This nerve compression occurs as the median nerve passes between the two heads of the PT for which it gets its name.[34,88,100] Occasionally, a tight origin of the FDS is to blame.[100] In this syndrome, repetitive pronation and flexion of the wrist can trigger numbness and paresthesias in the forearm that are difficult to localize. Hartz et al.[34] described tenderness in the proximal part of the PT in 39 subjects with this condition. This finding is supported by Werner's 1985 results of 9 patients:

> All showed local tenderness over the median nerve 4–5 cm distal to the elbow. Active forearm pronation against resistance, with the elbow in about 30 degrees of flexion, elicited pain in the proximal volar aspect of the forearm in all patients. In contrast, resisted active forearm supination with the elbow similarly flexed did not elicit pain.

There are no named physical exam tests or maneuvers that have been reliably studied and validated. Similarly, there are no studies evaluating the sensitivity and specificity. A positive Tinel's sign (see section on Tinel's sign) over the entrapment site (tapping the proximal edge of the pronator) was reported in 4 of 9 patients by Werner and 20 of 39 patients by Hartz.[34,100]

Elbow Instability

The elbow has medial and lateral collateral ligaments as the main stabilizers. However, unlike in the knee, there are no cruciate ligaments to offer translational stability of the humerus in relation to the ulna. Elbow stability is offered mainly by the bony congruency between the humerus and ulna, muscles and their tendons, the joint capsule, and the collateral ligaments.

Posterolateral instability of the elbow can develop into a chronic condition following elbow dislocation or ligament sprain.[62,67] The symptoms of recurrent elbow instability are due to disruption of the ulnar fibers of the radial collateral ligament.[67] Clinically, individuals suffering from posterolateral instability have elbow locking, snapping, and subluxation that occur when the elbow is extended and the forearm supinated.[62,67,69] Subsequent studies have found that in addition to the lateral collateral ligament, the lateral muscles originating at the lateral humeral condyle must be disrupted for subluxation to occur (Table 5–4).[15]

Posterolateral Rotatory–Instability Test of the Elbow

O'Driscoll et al.[67] described the posterolateral rotatory–instability test of the elbow in the supine patient with the arm fully abducted and extended overhead (Figure 5–31). From this position they describe:

> The patient's forearm is fully supinated, and the examiner grasps the wrist/forearm and, starting from a position of full extension, slowly flexes the elbow while applying valgus and supination moments and axial compression force. This produces a rotary subluxation of the ulnohumeral joint. As the elbow is flexed to approximately 40 degrees, the posterolateral rotatory displacement increases to a maximum, creating a posterior prominence (the dislocated joint) associated with an obvious dimpling of the skin.

The authors admit that the test is best performed under general anesthesia. When performed in the conscious patient, a positive test is indicated by apprehension on the face of the patient, as subluxation is perceived. There are no studies evaluating the efficacy or assessing the specificity or sensitivity of this test.

VARUS STRESS TEST

The lateral ligamentous complex consists of three or four components, depending on which reference is cited. The first portion is the annular ligament as it attaches to the ulna laterally. Next is a poorly demarcated fan-shaped portion that takes origin from

Table 5–4. ELBOW STABILITY TESTS

Test	Description	Reliability/Validity Tests
Posterolateral rotatory– instability	The patient's forearm is fully supinated, and the examiner grasps the wrist of forearm and, starting from a position of full extension, slowly flexes the elbow while applying valgus and supination moments and axial compression force. This produces a rotary subluxation of the ulnohumeral joint. As the elbow is flexed to approximately 40 degrees, the posterolateral rotatory displacement increases to a maximum, creating a posterior prominence (the dislocated radiohumeral joint) associated with an obvious dimpling of the skin.	Not reported
Varus stress	The patient's arm is placed in 20 degrees of flexion and slight supination beyond neutral. The examiner then places one hand over the medial aspect of the distal humerus and the other hand lateral to the distal forearm. This is followed by a varus stress applied to the forearm with a concomitant counter force placed upon the humerus. This will create excessive gapping on the lateral aspect of the elbow joint when compared to the contralateral arm.	Not reported
Jobe's test (valgus stress)	Flex the elbow 25 degrees to unlock the olecranon from its fossa and gently stress the medial side of the elbow joint.	Not reported

the lateral epicondyle and inserts into and blends with the annular ligament. This structure has often been called the "radial collateral ligament" (Figure 5–2). Another component originates from the anterior, superior portion of the annular ligament to insert on the crista supinatoris. This segment is small and often inconspicuous from the other segments. The final component of the complex is often termed the "lateral ulnar collateral ligament" (LUCL) as it originates from the lateral humeral epicondyle

Figure 5–31. Examination for postero-lateral elbow instability.

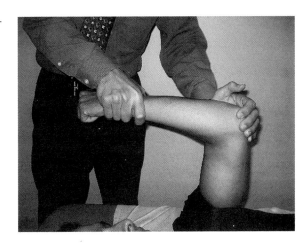

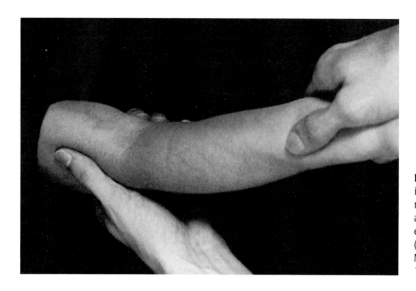

Figure 5–32. Varus/valgus stress testing of elbow. Reproduced with permission from Anderson TE: Anatomy and physical examination of the elbow. In Nicholas J, Hershman E (eds), The Upper Extremity in Sports Medicine, 2nd edn. St Louis: Mosby, 1995, p. 273.

to insert on the tubercle of the supinator crest.[51,59] The LUCL is a key component in preventing posterolateral or varus instability (Figure 5–32).[51]

As far as can be concluded from extensive search, a formal name has not been coined for testing the lateral collateral ligament. Nevertheless, the integrity of the radial collateral ligament is tested as follows:

> By placing the patient's arm in 20 degrees of flexion and slight supination beyond neutral, the examiner then places one hand over the medial aspect of the distal humerus and the other hand lateral to the distal forearm. This is followed by a varus stress applied to the forearm with a concomitant counterforce placed upon the humerus. This will create excessive gapping on the lateral aspect of the elbow joint when compared to the contralateral arm.[33]

These recommendations are based on the anatomic studies performed in large part by Morrey[59] and Lee.[51] Once again, a comprehensive literature review revealed no studies comparing the test results to cadaveric or surgical models. Therefore, the sensitivity and specificity of this physical exam maneuver cannot be confirmed.

Valgus Stress Test or Jobe's Test

Stressing of the medial collateral ligament has been called Jobe's test (see Figure 5–32). The original description by Jobe et al.[40] states that valgus instability can be demonstrated "[by] flexing the elbow 25 degrees to unlock the olecranon from its fossa and gently stressing the medial side of the elbow joint."

The medial collateral ligament (MCL) consists of three portions. The anterior bundle is anatomically most discrete, and functionally it provides the most stability to the medial aspect of the joint. It arises from the lateral 80% of the medial epicondyle to insert on the medial edge of the coronoid process.[51,59] The anterior ligament provides 70% of the valgus stability at the elbow, except in full extension where the radial head and anterior capsule provide the majority of valgus stability. The posterior portion of the MCL is a fan-shaped thickening of the posterior capsule, which originates from the posterior aspect of the medial epicondyle to insert on the medial semilunar notch.[51,59] This structure does not provide significant valgus stability until the arm is flexed beyond 90 degrees. The transverse oblique segment is composed of horizontally arranged medial capsule fibers that traverse from the tip of the olecranon to the coronoid process. No contribution to stability is derived from this portion of the MCL complex. Modest flexion of the arm will also minimize contributions of the capsular and osseous structures toward varus or valgus stability, and hence more effectively isolate the ligamentous structures' stabilizing capabilities.[51,59]

As previously mentioned, a search of medical journal databases did not elucidate any studies to validate the efficacy of Jobe's test in diagnosing excessive or abnormal MCL laxity.

Special Tests for the Wrist and Hand

See Table 5–5.

The history of the problem or injury is the most important factor in making the diagnosis of hand and wrist disorders. Nonetheless, a careful physical examination is necessary to confirm the diagnosis and rule out other problems.

Tests for Carpal Instability

Lunotriquetral Ballottement Test

This test has also been called Reagan's test. Reagan et al.[79] described the evaluation of lunotriquetral sprains as follows (Figure 5–33):

> [Fix] the lunate with the thumb and index finger of one hand while, with the other hand, displacing the triquetrum and pisiform first dorsally then palmarly.

A positive test result is confirmed if pain, crepitus and excessive laxity are elicited. The test is performed with the patient's hand palm down, and the examiner is observing the dorsal aspect of the wrist.

The usefulness of this test for determining lunotriquetral instability has been confirmed by others, but its efficacy has not been established.[1,96] Numerous authors have discussed this test, but few have performed controlled studies to determine the sensitivity or specificity of the test. Marx et al.[55] noted the sensitivity of this examination

Table 5–5. CARPAL LIGAMENT AND JOINT TESTS

Test	Description	Reliability/Validity Tests	Comments
Reagan's test (lunotriquetral ballottment test)	Fix the lunate with the thumb and index finger of one hand while, with the other hand, displacing the triquetrum and pisiform first dorsally then palmarly.	Marx et al.[55] Sensitivity: 64% Specificity: 44%	Results obtained from a comprehensive review of the literature.
Watson's test (scaphoid shift test)	The examiner sits face to face across a table with diagonally opposed hands raised (right to right or left to left) and elbows resting on the surface in between. With the patient's forearm slightly pronated, the examiner grasps the wrist from the radial side, placing his thumb on the palmar prominence of the scaphoid and wrapping his fingers around the distal radius. The examiner's other hand grasps at the metacarpal level, controlling wrist position. Starting in ulnar deviation and slight extension, the wrist is moved radially and slightly flexed, with constant pressure on the scaphoid.	Marx et al.[55] Sensitivity: 69% Specificity: 64–68%	Once again, based on the modest ability of the test to be both sensitive and specific, the results obtained must be interpreted cautiously. In light of this, it has limited clinical utility.
Shear test to assess the lunate triquetral ligament	The shear test is performed with the subject's forearm in neutral rotation and the elbow on the examination table. The examiner's contralateral fingers are placed over the dorsum of the lunate. With the lunate supported, the examiner's ipsilateral thumb loads the pisotriquetral joint from the palmar aspect, creating a shear force at the LT joint	Not reported	
Dorsal capitate-displacement apprehension test	The examiner's left hand grasps the distal end of the radius and ulna of the involved extremity, which are protected by lead gloves. With the examiner's right hand maintaining the patient's hand in neutral flexion and extension and in neutral radial and ulnar deviation, the examiner's right thumb is placed under the distal carpal row and is used to force the capitate dorsally. The test may be done under fluoroscopy. Apprehension and	Not reported	

Table 5–5. CARPAL LIGAMENT AND JOINT TESTS—*cont'd*

Test	Description	Reliability/Validity Tests	Comments
	discomfort with dorsal subluxation of the capitate from the lunate cup are considered a positive response to the test.		
Ulnocarpal stress	Generally chronic or subacute ulnar wrist pain, often exacerbated by activity and relieved by rest. Physical examination reveals swelling and tenderness that is usually localized to the region of the TFCC and lunotriquetral joint. Pronation and supination of the forearm with ulnar deviation of hand generally evokes the wrist symptoms.	Not reported	

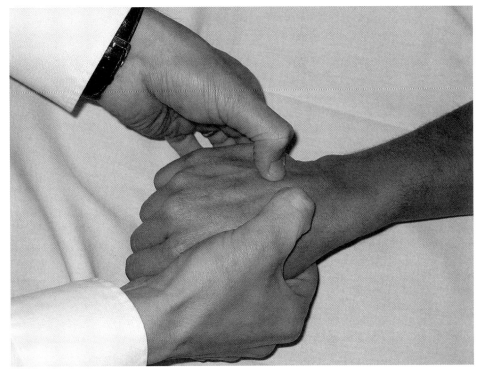

Figure 5–33. Lunotriquetral ballotment test.

maneuver to be 64% and the specificity to be 44%. As such, it would be difficult at best to base a diagnosis of instability primarily on a positive Reagen's test.

Scaphoid Shift Test, or Watson's Test

In 1978, H. K. Watson described one of the most widely utilized tests for carpal instability.[97] Watson's test, also known as the Scaphoid shift test, was originally used as an assessment tool to identify rotatory subluxation of the scaphoid. Proper performance of this test requires:

> The examiner as if to engage in arm wrestling, [sit] face to face across a table with diagonally opposed hands raised (right to right or left to left) and elbows resting on the surface in between. With the patient's forearm slightly pronated, the examiner grasps the wrist from the radial side, placing his thumb on the palmar prominence of the scaphoid and wrapping his fingers around the distal radius. ... The examiner's other hand grasps at the metacarpal level, controlling wrist position. Starting in ulnar deviation and slight extension, the wrist is moved radially and slightly flexed, with constant pressure on the scaphoid.[95]

If the scaphoid's supportive ligamentous structures are damaged, the scaphoid will palpably sublux. However, as with any diagnostic exam maneuver, the validity of the result is dependent on the interpretation of the examiner. In fact, Watson himself noted that the scaphoid shift "is not so much a test as a provocative maneuver. It does not offer a simple positive or negative result, but rather a variety of findings."[95]

In 1994, Wolfe and Crisco[106] evaluated the maneuver using an instrumented device to determine degrees of ligamentous laxity noted in asymptomatic individuals with a positive Watson test versus those with a negative scaphoid shift. Interestingly, high degrees of laxity may be associated with a positive scaphoid shift, but this is a result of generalized ligamentous hypermobility, hence giving a false positive result. This study cautions against making the diagnosis of carpal instability based on a hypermobile scaphoid and reiterates the necessity of concomitant pain for this to be recognized as a positive Watson's test.[106]

The sensitivity of the Watson test has been found to be 69%, and the specificity to range between 64% and 68%.[55] Once again, based on the modest ability of the test to be both sensitive and specific, the results obtained must be interpreted cautiously and therefore the test has limited clinical utility.

Shear Test for Lunotriquetral Ligament Instability

The shear test origin could not be determined, but it is used to stress the lunotriquetral ligament (similar to ballottement test above) (Figure 5–34). There are multiple sources that describe nearly the same way to perform this test.[3,89]

Figure 5–34. Shear test.

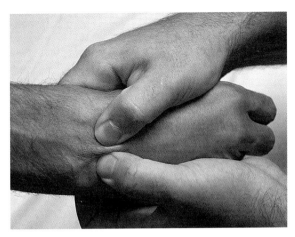

The shear test is performed with the subject's forearm in neutral rotation and the elbow on the examination table. The examiner's contralateral fingers are placed over the dorsum of the lunate. With the lunate supported, the examiner's ipsilateral thumb loads the pisotriquetral joint from the palmar aspect, creating a shear force at the lunotriquetral joint.[89]

Pain that is concordant or similar to the pain or discomfort of the patient is considered a positive test. Care should be made to compare the right and left wrist exams. There are no studies assessing the specificity or sensitivity of this test.

Dorsal Capitate-displacement Apprehension Test

Johnson and Carrera[41] gave a detailed description of this test for the first time (Figure 5–35). If performing on the patient's left hand:

> The examiner's left hand grasps the distal end of the radius and ulna of the involved extremity, which are protected by lead gloves. With the examiner's right hand maintaining the patient's hand in neutral flexion and extension and in neutral radial and ulnar deviation, the examiner's right thumb is placed under the distal carpal row and is used to force the capitate dorsally. The test may be done under fluoroscopy. Apprehension and discomfort with dorsal subluxation of the capitate from the lunate cup are considered a positive response to the test.

There are no studies evaluating this test's specificity and sensitivity.

Tests for Triangular Fibrocartilage Complex Tears

The triangular fibrocartilage complex (TFCC) can be a cause of ulnar-sided wrist pain.[72,73] The TFCC is difficult to test reliably with a physical exam, and radiologic

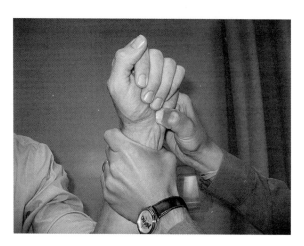

Figure 5–35. Dorsal capitate–displacement apprehension test.

studies are often negative. Westkaemper et al.[103] found an arthrogram was negative in 11 of 37 patients later found to have ulnar-sided wrist pathology at arthroscopy. In patients with chronic ulnar wrist pain, Shers and VanHeusden[86] found 31 out of 39 arthrograms correlated poorly with results of arthroscopy.

The use of magnetic resonance imaging for evaluating TFCC pathology depends on radiologist experience. Blazar et al.[6] compared MRI readings of two different radiologists finding sensitivities of 86% and 80% in detecting TFCC lesions with specificity rates of 96% and 80%.

The complexity of the TFCC increases as we realize the natural degenerative course the TFCC takes with aging. Mikic[57] studied the TFCC in a cadaveric model and found 38.4% had degenerative changes by the third decade of life, and no completely normal discs were found in individuals past their fifth decade. We, therefore, think that examiners should cautiously interpret the results of the physical exam of the TFCC.

Ulnocarpal Stress Test

This is a provocative test in which the examiner attempts to grind the TFCC between the ulnar-sided carpal bones and distal ulna. In 1991, Friedman and Palmer first described the ulnocarpal stress test (Figure 5–36). They found patients generally have

> ... chronic or subacute ulnar wrist pain, often exacerbated by activity and relieved by rest. Physical examination reveals swelling and tenderness that is usually localized to the region of the TFCC and lunotriquetral joint. Pronation and supination of the forearm with ulnar deviation of the wrist generally evokes increased symptoms.[25]

Nakamura et al.[61] noted "the test is positive when axial stress produces ulnar wrist pain during passive supination–pronation with the wrist in maximum ulnar deviation." When performed correctly, the test compresses the TFCC, eliciting clicking and pain in the face of a tear. It is essential to compare the symptomatic side to the uninvolved

Figure 5–36. Ulnocarpal stress test for TFCC tear.

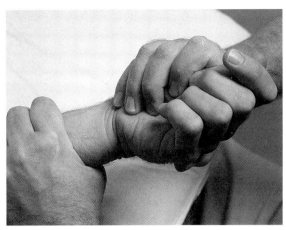

side, understanding that clicking and snapping may normally be present. There are no studies evaluating sensitivity, specificity and reliability.

TESTS FOR DEQUERVAIN'S TENOSYNOVITIS

Examining the first dorsal compartment for a suspected first compartment tendinitis (deQuervain's disease) is best performed with light tension on the first compartment tendons. It is important to rule out a ganglion cyst which may occur just volar to the first compartment, as well as tendinitis of the flexor carpi radialis which both may mimic deQuervain's disease.

Finkelstein Test

See Table 5–6.

In 1930, Finkelstein described a technique to ascertain the presence of "stenosing tenovaginitis" or tenosynovitis of the abductor pollicis longus (APL) and the extensor pollicis brevis (EPB) tendons. Anatomically, "the APL and EPB tendons lie in a groove on the dorsal lateral aspect of the radius ... It is frequently forgotten that these muscles are the chief radial deviators of the wrist."[53] In 1939, Finkelstein described his test as follows (Figure 5–37):

> On grasping the patient's thumb and quickly abducting the hand ulnarward, the pain over the styloid tip is excruciating.[24]

An error in performing the test has been perpetuated in the literature, and as a result, the test is commonly performed incorrectly. Dr Erich Eichhoff first described the test version used today in 1927:

> If one places the thumb within the hand and holds it tightly with the other fingers and then bends the hand severely in ulnar abduction, an intense pain is experienced on the styloid process of the radius, exactly at the place where the tendon sheath takes its course.[22]

Table 5–6. OTHER TESTS OF THE ELBOW AND WRIST

Test	Description	Reliability/Validity Tests	Comments
Finkelstein test	On grasping the patient's thumb and quickly abducting the hand ulnarward, the pain over the styloid tip is excruciating. If one places the thumb within the hand and holds it tightly with the other fingers and then bends the hand severely in ulnar abduction, an intense pain is experienced on the styloid process of the radius, exactly at the place where the tendon sheath takes its course.	Not reported	
Ulnar ligament of the thumb MCP joint	The integrity of the proper collateral ligament is assessed by carrying out valgus stress testing with the MCP joint in 30 degrees of flexion. To avoid a false interpretation, the examiner must prevent MCP rotation by grasping the thumb proximal to the joint. If there is more than 30 degrees of laxity (or 15 degrees more laxity than the noninjured side), rupture of the ligament proper is likely. The thumb is then positioned in extension for repeat valgus testing. If valgus laxity is less than 30 degrees (or 15 degrees less than the noninjured side), the accessory ligament is intact. If the valgus laxity is greater than 30 degrees (or 15 degrees of the noninjured side), the accessory ligament is also ruptured.	Not reported	
Thumb basilar joint grind test	The basal joint grind test is performed by stabilizing the triquetrum with the thumb and index finger and then dorsally subluxing the thumb metacarpal on the trapezium while providing compressive force with the other hand.	Not reported	

This maneuver with several variations has been further elucidated, but research supporting its sensitivity and specificity is lacking.[11,50,53] B. G. Elliott warns of performing the wrong maneuver as a source of a false-positive result.[23]

TESTS FOR THE THUMB METACARPOPHALANGEAL JOINT

See Table 5–6.

The thumb MCP joint suffers two common maladies: osteoarthritis and ulnar collateral ligament tears. The thumb MCP joint is a multiaxial diarthodial hinge joint

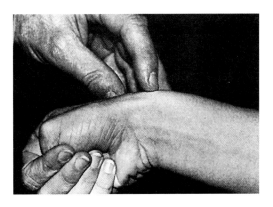

Figure 5–37. Finkelstein's test. Reproduced with permission from Hunter JM, Mackin EJ, Callahan AD (eds): Rehabilitation of the Hand: Surgery and Therapy, 4th edn. St Louis: Mosby, 1995, p. 60.

able to flex, extend, abduct, adduct, and circumduct.[17,91] There are static and dynamic stabilizers of the thumb MCP joint. The main static stabilizers are the radial and ulnar collateral ligaments, as well as the accessory collateral ligament.[91] The ulnar collateral ligament is taut at 30 degrees flexion at the MCP joint, and the ulnar accessory collateral ligament is taut in full extension at the MCP joint.[91] The joint capsule and the dorsal aponeurosis are the other static stabilizers. The dynamic stabilizers are muscles and tendons inserting to this area. Specifically, the adductor pollicis, abductor pollicis brevis and the flexor pollicis longus muscles add to the stability about the joint.[17,91]

Ulnar Collateral Ligament Instability

In 1955, Campbell described and coined the term *gamekeepers thumb*.[12] In his own words:

> The gamekeeper's method of killing a wounded rabbit is to hold the head in one hand and the rear legs in the other. A strong pull is then exerted while the neck is sharply extended. ... Invariably, a loose grip causes the neck to be stretched against the ulnar side of the thumb. It is the force of the pull, repeated manifold, which stretches the ulnar collateral ligament.

This mechanism of overuse injury is common to rabbit hunters, but traumatic injury is also seen, most commonly in skiers.[36] Therefore, gamekeeper's thumb is synonymous with skier's thumb (Figure 5–38).[36] The physical exam findings are really an extension of reproducing the valgus force that resulted in the original injury. An original description of testing the ulnar collateral ligament could not be found, but Heyman describes the maneuver (Figure 5–39) as follows:

> The integrity of the proper collateral ligament is assessed by carrying out valgus stress testing with the MCP joint in 30 degrees of flexion. To avoid a false interpretation, the examiner must prevent MCP rotation by grasping the thumb proximal to the joint.

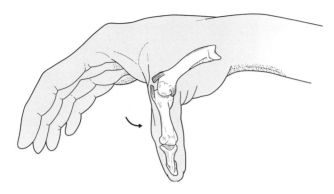

Figure 5–38. Skier's thumb. Adapted from Mellion MB: Office Sports Medicine, 2nd edn. Philadelphia: Hanley & Belfus, 1996.

If there is more than 30 degrees of laxity (or 15 degrees more laxity than the noninjured side), rupture of the ligament proper is likely. The thumb is then positioned in extension for repeat valgus testing. If valgus laxity is less than 30 degrees (or 15 degrees less than the noninjured side), the accessory ligament is intact. If the valgus laxity is greater than 30 degrees (or 15 degrees of the noninjured side), the accessory ligament is also ruptured.[36]

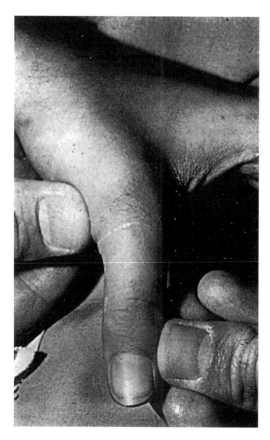

Figure 5–39. Valgus testing for ulnar collateral ligament stability. Reproduced with permission from Langford SA, Whitaker JH, Toby EB: Thumb injuries in the athlete. Clin Sports Med 1998;July;17:559.

As with many limb physical exam maneuvers, side to side comparison is important. There are no studies to evaluate the specificity and sensitivity of the above test. Heyman et al.[35] found that individuals with complete collateral ligament tears had greater than 35 degrees of valgus laxity, and 15 degrees greater than on the uninjured side. Stener[91] described anatomically the retraction of the collateral ligament in complete lesions which formed a small, palpable nodule; therefore a palpable mass at the proximal ulnar MCP joint is called a *Stener lesion*. Heyman et al.[35] found a similar palpable mass in 9 of 16 with ligament tears of which all had complete ligament tears (proper and accessory ligament tears) at operation. Therefore, the specificity of a palpable mass was 100%. On the other hand, there was no palpable mass in seven patients who had complete tears at operation, making the false negative rate 46%.

Basilar Joint Arthritis

The thumb MCP joint, like all synovial joints, is subject to arthritic changes. Arthritis of the thumb carpometacarpal joint will frequently present with pain in a similar region to deQuervain's disease. The basal joint grind test (Figure 5–40) is performed by stabilizing the triquetrum with the thumb and index finger and then dorsally subluxing the thumb metacarpal on the trapezium while providing compressive force with the other hand.

Arthritis of the scaphoid trapezoid trapezium joint (STT) joint may be confused with basal joint arthritis, but careful palpation over this joint just dorsal and radial to the scaphoid will help confirm the diagnosis. There are no tests that have been performed which have evaluated the sensitivity, specificity and reliability of the grind test.

Figure 5–40. Basal joint grind test.

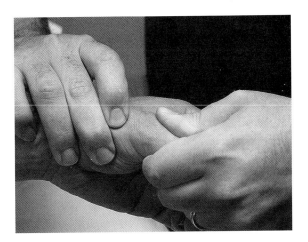

NERVE ENTRAPMENT

See Table 5–7.

Median Nerve Tests

Carpal Compression Test

Paley and McMurtry first described this test in 1985 (see Table 5–5).[71] The test is performed in the following manner (Figure 5–41):

> The examiner sits opposite the patient and holds the patient's hands such that his thumbs are over the course of the median nerve. ... The rest of the examiner's fingers are over the dorsum of the hand and wrist. The first phase consists of gentle, sustained, firm pressure applied by the examiner's thumbs to the median nerve of each hand simultaneously. Within a short time (15 seconds to two minutes), the patient will complain of reproduction of his pain, paresthesia and/or numbness in the symptomatic wrist(s).

Williams et al.[104] reported the sensitivity of the test to be 100%. Their data suggested that, in fact, the carpal compression test is more likely to be present in carpal tunnel syndrome (CTS) than Tinel's (sensitivity 67%) or Phalen's (sensitivity 88%) sign. A sensitivity of 87% and specificity of 90% has been reported for this test.[20,21] Once again, in comparison to Tinel and Phalen's signs, the carpal compression test was noted to be more sensitive and specific.

Wrist Flexion Test or Phalen's Test

In 1951, the wrist flexion test was introduced by G. S. Phalen and it now bears his name. To perform the test (Figure 5–42):

> The patient is asked to hold the forearms vertically and to allow both hands to drop into flexion at the wrist for approximately one minute. ... Compression by this maneuver causes almost immediate aggravation of the numbness and paresthesia in the fingers.[75]

Seror[87] studied the efficacy of Phalen's test in predicting the presence of carpal tunnel syndrome by comparing it with electromyographically obtained results. He found that as sensory nerve conduction velocity decreases, the percentage of patients with positive results using Phalen's test increases from 20% at 50 m/s to 78% at less than 30 m/s. Gerr and Letz[27] noted Phalen's test to be 75% sensitive when compared with electrophysiologic examination. Gellman et al.[26] noted the test to be 71% sensitive and 80% specific for carpal tunnel syndrome. In 1971, Phalen also reported similar results in a follow-up study, with sensitivity 80% and specificity 20%.[76] As with Tinel's sign, Phalen's test would be more effective during more advanced cases of median nerve compression.

Table 5–7. NERVE AND VASCULAR TESTS

Test	Description	Reliability/Validity Tests	Comments
Carpal compression	The examiner sits opposite the patient and holds the patient's hands such that his thumbs are over the course of the median nerve. The rest of the examiner's fingers are over the dorsum of the hand and wrist. The first phase consists of gentle, sustained, firm pressure applied by the examiner's thumbs to the median nerve of each hand simultaneously. Within a short time (15 seconds to two minutes) the patient will complain of reproduction of his pain, paresthesia and/or numbness in the symptomatic wrist(s).	Durkan[20] Sensitivity: 87% Specificity: 90%	
Phalen's test (wrist flexion)	The patient is asked to hold the forearms vertically and to allow both hands to drop into flexion at the wrist for approximately one minute. Compression by this maneuver causes almost immediate aggravation of the numbness and paresthesia in the fingers.	Gerr and Letz[27] Sensitivity: 75% Gellman et al.[26] Sensitivity: 71% Specificity: 80% Phalen[76] Sensitivity: 80% Specificity: 20%	When compared with electrophysiologic examination. As sensory nerve conduction velocity decreases, the percentage of patients with positive results using Phalen's test increases from 20% at 50 m/s to 78% at less than 30 m/s.
Wrist extension test (reverse Phalen's test)	The patient is asked to keep both hands with the wrist in complete dorsal extension for 1 minute. If numbness and tingling were produced or exaggerated in the median nerve distribution of the hand within 60 seconds, the test is judged to be positive.	DeKrom et al.[19] found only 45% of hands with electrodiagnostically confirmed CTS had a positive reverse Phalen's test. They found the reverse Phalen's positive in 49% of hands with negative electrodiagnostic testing for carpal tunnel syndrome. Ghavanini and Haghighat[28] Sensitivity: 43% Specificity: 74%	

Continued

Table 5–7. NERVE AND VASCULAR TESTS—*cont'd*

Test	Description	Reliability/Validity Tests	Comments
Tinel's sign at the wrist	Extend the wrist and tap in a proximal to distal direction over the median nerve as it passes through the carpal tunnel, from the area of the distal wrist crease, 2–3 cm toward the area between the thenar and hypothenar eminences.	Gellman et al.[26] Sensitivity: 44% Specificity: 94% Gerr and Letz[27] Sensitivity: 25% Specificity: 98%	Gerr and Letz compared positive Tinel's signs with patients complaining of CTS symptoms who also had confirmed carpal tunnel syndrome by electrophysiologic testing. Positive in only 32% of patients with carpal tunnel syndrome.[66]
Elbow flexion test for ulnar nerve entrapment at the cubital tunnel	Sitting with both arms and shoulders in the anatomic position, both elbows are fully but not forcefully flexed, with full extension of the wrist to maximize both compressive and tensile forces on the nerve. Elbows are kept off all surfaces to avoid external compression during the examination, and peripheral pulses checked to assure adequate tissue perfusion. Patients noted to the physician at 15-, 30-, 60-, 125- and 180 second intervals whether pain, numbness, or tingling occurred or increased.	Not reported	
Allen test	If obstruction of the ulnar artery is suspected, the radial arteries are located by their pulsations. See the text.	McGregor[56] used fluoroscein angiography to evaluate patients with a positive Allen test, and concluded "the Allen test is of no clinical value."	

Overall, analysis of the literature indicates that Tinel's sign is a less potent predictor than Phalen's test in detecting true positives, and the probability of obtaining a true negative with Phalen's test is much larger.[26,27] A comprehensive literature search places the sensitivity range from 67% to 88%, and the specificity ranges from 20% to 86%.

Figure 5–41. Carpal compression test.

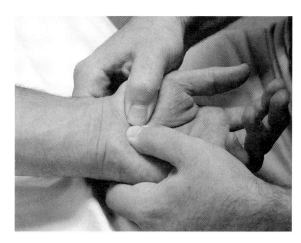

Wrist Extension Test or Reverse Phalen's Test

Pressures in the carpal tunnel increase with both wrist flexion and extension.[7,98] In fact, pressures in the carpal tunnel are greater with the wrist extended than with the wrist flexed.[98,102] Phalen himself was aware of this, stating: "although there is greater pressure within the carpal tunnel when the wrist is extended than when the wrist is flexed, sustained extension of the wrist seldom aggravates the symptoms of carpal tunnel syndrome."[76] The wrist extension maneuver is still one of the diagnostic tests for carpal tunnel syndrome.

An original description could not be located, but DeKrom et al.[19] described the following (Figure 5–43):

> The patient was asked to keep both hands with the wrist in complete dorsal extension for 1 minute. If numbness and tingling were produced or exaggerated in the median nerve distribution of the hand within 60 seconds, the test was judged to be positive.

Figure 5–42. Phalen's test.

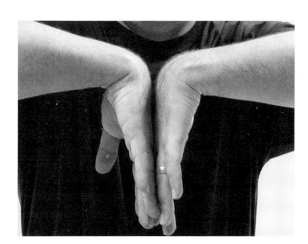

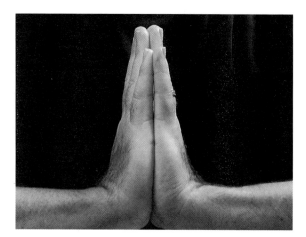

Figure 5–43. Reverse Phalen's test.

Phalen himself felt that wrist extension probably did not compress the median nerve at the site of inflammation.[76] Werner et al.[98,102] found carpal tunnel pressures from 30 to 40 mmHg with wrist extension. DeKrom et al.[19] found only 45% of hands with electrodiagnostically confirmed CTS had a positive reverse Phalen's test. In addition, they found the reverse Phalen's positive in 49% of hands with negative electrodiagnostic testing for carpal tunnel syndrome. Ghavanini and Haghighat[28] found the sensitivity to be 43% and the specificity to be 74%.

Tinel's Sign at the Wrist

In 1915 in *La Presse Medicale*, a French medical journal, Dr J. Tinel originally described the sign that now bears his name.[92] Tinel noted that tapping the proximal stump of an injured axon may create a tingling sensation, or *fourmillement* as Tinel called it, in the nerve's distal cutaneous distribution. In testing for CTS this test is performed as follows (Figure 5–44):

> [Extend] the wrist and [tap] in a proximal to distal direction over the median nerve as it passes through the carpal tunnel, from the area of the distal wrist crease, 2–3 cm toward the area between the Thenar and Hypothenar eminences.[92]

The maneuver was not initially used as a diagnostic sign of carpal tunnel syndrome, but rather, as a sign of axonal regeneration of peripheral nerves that had been transected.[58,92]

The sensitivity and specificity of Tinel's sign varies widely in the literature. Novak et al.[66] contend that, overall, Tinel's sign will be positive in only 32% of patients with carpal tunnel syndrome. The authors offer that a positive Tinel's sign is indicative of regenerating nerve fibers, which implies degeneration and then regeneration of

Figure 5–44. Tinel's sign.

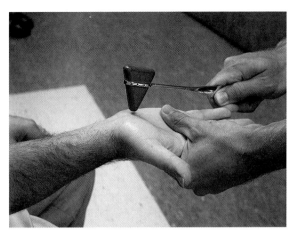

nerve fibers. Gellman et al.[26] found similar results with sensitivity and specificity of 44% and 94%, respectively. Gerr and Letz[27] compared the frequency of positive Tinel's signs with patients complaining of CTS symptoms who also had confirmed CTS by electrophysiologic testing. They found the sign to be 25% sensitive, but 98% specific for CTS. Therefore, a positive result will assure the examiner that CTS is present, but that one should not rely on the test as a diagnostic tool. This wide range, which seems to mirror the results noted for other studies noted in the literature, suggests that Tinel's sign, when used as a diagnostic tool, will only be minimally to moderately useful in detecting the presence of CTS accurately.

Ulnar Nerve Test

In 1986, Buehler and Thayer described a clinical test to help diagnose ulnar nerve entrapment about the elbow.[10] The *elbow flexion test* is performed as follows (Figure 5–45):

> Sitting with both arms and shoulders in the anatomic position, both elbows were fully but not forcefully flexed, with full extension of the wrist to maximize both compressive and tensile forces on the nerve. Elbows were kept off all surfaces to avoid external compression during the examination, and peripheral pulses were checked to assure adequate tissue perfusion. Patients noted to the physician at 15-, 30-, 60-, 125- and 180-second intervals whether pain, numbness, or tingling occurred or increased.

The ulnar nerve passes through the cubital tunnel which is a site for entrapment of the nerve.[10,68] In a cadaveric study, O'Driscoll et al.[68] classified the cubital tunnel into four classes: types 0, Ia, Ib, and II. In type 0, the cubital tunnel retinaculum (CTR)

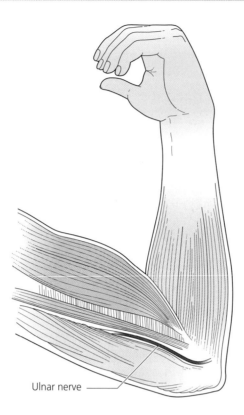

Figure 5–45. Elbow flexion test. Reproduced with permission from Stokes W: Ulnar neuropathy (elbow). In Frontera WR, Silver JK (eds), Essentials of Physical Medicine and Rehabilitation. Philadelphia: Hanley & Belfus, 2002, p. 139.

Ulnar nerve

was absent. Type Ia was considered normal, and the CTR was taut at full extension. In types Ib and II, the CTR is taut in 90–120 degrees of flexion; and in type II, the CTR contains muscle fibers and is bulky. There are no tests evaluating the specificity or sensitivity of the elbow flexion test. Care must be taken to maintain wrist neutrality during this test to prevent a false positive (i.e., positive Phalen's test for carpal tunnel syndrome).

Vascular Test for the Radial and Ulnar Arteries

See Table 5–7.

The blood supply to the hand comes from the radial artery on the lateral side of the wrist and the ulnar artery on the medial side of the wrist. In 1929, Allen described a physical exam maneuver testing the patency of the radial or ulnar artery in a paper on thromboangiitis obliterans. To perform the *Allen test* (Figure 5–46):

> If obstruction of the ulnar artery is suspected, the radial arteries are located by their pulsations; the examiner places one thumb lightly over radial, the four fingers of each hand behind the patient's wrist, thus holding the wrist lightly between the thumb

Figure 5–46. The Allen test. Reproduced with permission from Stokes W: Ulnar neuropathy (elbow). In Frontera WR, Silver JK (eds), Essentials of Physical Medicine and Rehabilitation. Philadelphia: Hanley & Belfus, 2002, p. 165.

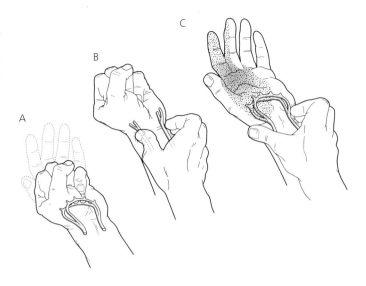

and fingers. The patient closes his hands as tightly as possible for a period of one minute in order to squeeze the blood out of the hand; the examiner compresses each wrist between his thumb and fingers, thus occluding the radial arteries; the patient quickly extends his fingers partially while compression of the radial artery is maintained by the examiner. The return of color to the hand and fingers is noted. In individuals with an intact arterial tree, the pallor is quickly replaced by rubor of a higher degree than normal, which gradually fades to normal color. If the ulnar artery is occluded, pallor is maintained for a variable period, due to the obstruction to arterial inflow in the two main channels; the radials are obstructed by the examiner's thumbs, the ulnars by the occlusive lesions.[2]

The above exam can be repeated to test the integrity of the radial arteries. To test the radial arteries, the examiner must compress the ulnar arteries. There are no studies to test the sensitivity, specificity, reliability or validity of this test. McGregor used fluoroscein angiography to evaluate patients with a positive Allen test, and concluded "the Allen test is of no clinical value."[56] However, use of the Allen test is still commonly taught and encouraged to be performed, prior to obtaining blood gases from the radial or ulnar arteries to avoid possible vascular compromise.

Conclusion

Physical examination of the hand, wrist, forearm, and elbow is vitally important in the diagnosis of common traumatic and overuse injuries of the upper extremity. Positive test results may support the use of further diagnostic testing, while negative results may further narrow the differential diagnosis. Understanding the true sensitivity, specificity, and reliability of these test maneuvers will help clinicians better evaluate the patients they treat.

REFERENCES

1. Alexander CE, Lichtman DL. Ulnar carpal instabilities. Orthop Clin N Am 1984;15:307–320.
2. Allen EV. Thromboangiitis obliterans: methods of diagnosis of chronic occlusive arterial lesions distal to the wrist with illustrative cases. Am J Med Sci 1929;178:237–244.
3. Ambroase L, Posner MA. Lunate-triquetral and midcarpal joint instability. Hand Clin 1992;8:653–668.
4. Beals RK. The normal carry angle of the elbow. Clin Orthop Relat Res 1976;119:194.
5. Beckenbaugh RD. Accurate evaluation and management of the painful wrist following injury: an approach to carpal instability. Orthop Clin N Am 1984;15:289–306.
6. Blazer PE, Chan PSH, Kneeland JB, et al. The effect of observer experience on magnetic resonance imaging interpretation and localization of triangular fibrocartilage complex lesions. J Hand Surg Am 2001;26:742–748.
7. Brain WR, Wright AD, Wilkinson M. Spontaneous compression of both median nerves in the carpal tunnel: six cases treated surgically. Lancet 1947;1:277–282.
8. Budoff JE, Nirschl RP. Tendinopathies about the elbow. In Garrett WE, Speer KP, Kirkendall DT (eds), Principles and Practice of Orthopedic Sports Medicine. Philadelphia: Lippincott Williams & Wilkins, 2000, p. 291.
9. Budoff JE, Nirschl RP. Tendinopathies about the elbow. In Garrett WE, Speer KP, Kirkendall DT (eds), Principles and Practice of Orthopedic Sports Medicine. Philadelphia: Lippincott Williams & Wilkins, 2000, p. 292.
10. Buehler MJ, Thayer DT. The elbow flexion test: A clinical test for the cubital tunnel syndrome. Clin Orthop Rel Res 1988;233:213–216.
11. Cameron J. Orthopaedic complications. In Schneider RC, Kennedy JC, Plant (eds), Sports Injuries: Mechanisms, Prevention, and Treatment. Baltimore: Williams and Wilkins, 1985.
12. Campbell CS. Gamekeeper's thumb. J Bone Joint Surg Br 1955;37:148–149.
13. Capener N. The vulnerability of the posterior interosseous nerve of the forearm: a case report and an anatomical study. J Bone Joint Surg Br 1966;48:770–773.
14. Clemente C. Anatomy: a Regional Atlas of the Human Body, 4th edn. Baltimore: Williams & Wilkins, 1997.
15. Cohen MS, Hastings H. Rotatory instability of the elbow: the anatomy and role of the lateral stabilizers. J Bone Joint Surg Am 1997;79:225–233.
16. Collins DN, Weber ER. Anterior interosseous nerve syndrome. South Med J 1983;76:1533.
17. Coonrad RW, Goldner JL. A study of the pathological findings and treatment in soft-tissue injury of the thumb metacarpophalangeal joint. J Bone J Surg Am 1968;50:439–451.
18. Cyriax JH. The pathology and treatment of tennis elbow. J Bone Joint Surg 1936;18:921–940.
19. DeKrom MCTFM, Knipschild PG, Kester ADM, Spaans F. Efficacy of provocative tests for diagnosis of carpal tunnel syndrome. Lancet 1990;335:393–396.
20. Durkan JA. A new diagnostic test for carpal tunnel syndrome. J Bone J Surg Am 1991;73:535–538.
21. Durkan JA. The carpal-compression test. Orthop Rev 1994;23:522–525.
22. Eichoff E. Zur pathogenese der Tenovaginitis stenosans. Bruns' Beitrage Zur Klinischen Chirurgie 1927:746–755.
23. Elliot BG. Finkelstien's test: a descriptive error that can produce a false positive. J Hand Surg Br 1992;17:481–482.
24. Finkelstien H. Stenosing tendovaginitis at the radial styloid process. J Bone Joint Surg 1939;12:509–540.
25. Friedman SL, Palmer AK. The ulnar impaction syndrome. Hand Clinics 1991;7:295–310.
26. Gellman H, et al. Carpal tunnel syndrome: an evaluation of the provocative diagnostic tests. J Bone Joint Surg Am 1986;68:735–737.
27. Gerr F, Letz R. The sensitivity and specificity of tests for carpal tunnel syndrome vary with the comparison subjects. J Hand Surg Br 1998;23(2):151–155.
28. Ghavanini MRA, Haghighat M. Carpal tunnel syndrome: reappraisal of five clinical tests. Electromyogr Clin Neurophysiol 1998;38:437–441.

29. Goldie I. Epicondylitis humeri (epicondylagia or tennis elbow): a pathologic study. Acta Chir Scand Supp. 1964;339.

30. Goldman S, et al. Posterior interosseous nerve palsy in the absence of trauma. Arch Neurol 1969; 21:435.

31. Gray H. Gray's Anatomy, eds Pick TP, Howden R. New York: Bounty Books, 1978; Figs 255–268.

32. Greenbaum B, et al. Extensor carpi radialis brevis: an anatomical analysis of its origin. J Bone Joint Surg Br 1999;81:926–929.

33. Gross J, Fetto J, Rosen E. Musculoskeletal Examination. Cambridge, MA: Blackwell Science, 1996, pp. 182–217.

34. Hartz CR, Linsheid RL, Gramse RR, Daube JR. The pronator teres syndrome: compressive neuropathy of the median nerve. J Bone J Surg Am 1981;63:885–890.

35. Heyman P, Gelberman RH, Duncan K, Hipp JA. Injuries of the ulnar collateral ligament of the thumb metacarpophalangeal joint: biomechanical and prospective clinical studies on the usefulness of valgus stress testing. Clin Orthop Rel Res 1993;292:165–171.

36. Heyman P. Injuries to the ulnar collateral ligament of the thumb metacarpophalangeal joint. J Am Acad Orthop Surg 1997;5:224–229.

37. Hollinshead WH, Rosse C. Textbook of Anatomy, 4th edn. Philadelphia: Harper & Row, 1985.

38. Jenkins DB. Hollinshead's functional anatomy of the limbs and back, 7th edn. Philadelphia: WB Saunders, 1998, 103–198.

39. Jobe FW, Ciccotti MG. Lateral and medial epicondylitis of the elbow. J Am Acad Orthop Surg 1994;2:1–8.

40. Jobe FW, et al. Reconstruction of the ulnar collateral ligament in athletes. J Bone Joint Surg Am 1986;68:1158–1163.

41. Johnson RP, Carrera GF. Chronic capitolunate instability. J Bone J Surg Am 1986;68:1164–1176.

42. Kaplan PE. Posterior interosseous neuropathies: a natural history. Arch Phys Med Rehabil 1984;65:399.

43. Kendall FP, McCreary EK, Provance PG. Muscle Testing and Function, 4th edn. Baltimore: Williams & Wilkins, 1993, p. 265.

44. Kendall FP, McCreary EK, Provance PG. Muscle Testing and Function, 4th edn. Baltimore: Williams & Wilkins, 1993, p. 238.

45. Kendall FP, McCreary EK, Provance PG. Muscle Testing and Function, 4th edn. Baltimore: Williams & Wilkins, 1993, pp. 235–298.

46. Kilof LG, Nevin S. Isolated neuritis of the anterior interosseous nerve. Br Med J 1952;1:850.

47. King D, Ashby P. The pronator syndrome. J R Coll Surg Edinb 1982;27:142.

48. Kurvers H, Verhaar J. The results of operative treatment of medial epicondylitis. J Bone J Surg Am 1995;77:1374–1379.

49. Leach RE, Miller JK. Lateral and medial epicondylitis of the elbow. Clin Sports Med 1987;6:259–272.

50. Leao L. De Quervain's disease: a clinical and anatomical study. J Bone Joint Surg Am 1958; 40:1063–1070.

51. Lee ML, Rosenwasser MP. Chronic elbow instability. Orthop Clin N Am 1999;30:81–89.

52. Lister GD, Belsole RB, Kleinert HE. The radial tunnel syndrome. J Hand Surg Am 1979;4:52–59.

53. Loomis LK. Variations of stenosing tenosynovitis at the radial styloid process. J Bone Joint Surg Am 1951;33:340–346.

54. Magee DJ. Orthopedic Physical Assessment, 4th edn. Philadelphia: WB Saunders, 2002, pp, 338–339, 402–403.

55. Marx RG, Bombardier C, Wright JG. What we know about the reliability and validity of physical examination tests used to examine the upper extremity. J Hand Surg Am 1999;24:185–192.

56. McGregor AD. The Allen test: an investigation of its accuracy by fluorescein angiography. J Hand Surg Br 1987;12:82–85.

57. Mikic ZDJ. Age changes in the triangular fibrocartilage of the wrist joint. J Anat 1978;126:367–384.

58. Moldaver J. Brief note: Tinel's sign. J Bone Joint Surg Am 1978;60:412–414.

59. Morrey BF, An KN. Functional anatomy of the ligaments of the elbow. Clin Orthop Rel Res 1985; 84:201.

60. Morris HH, Peters BH. Pronator syndrome: clinical and electrophysiological features in seven cases. J Neurol Neurosurg Psychiat 1976;39:461.

61. Nakamura R, Horii E, Imaeda T, et al. The ulnocarpal stress test in the diagnosis of ulnar-sided wrist pain. J Hand Surg Br 1997;22:719–723.

62. Nestor BJ, O'Driscoll SW, Morrey BF. Ligamentous reconstruction for posterolateral rotatory instability of the elbow. J Bone J Surg Am 1992;74:1235–1240.

63. Netter FH. Atlas of Human Anatomy. East Hanover: Novartis, 1989, plates 405–456.

64. Nirschl RP, Pettrone FA. Tennis elbow: the surgical treatment for lateral epicondylitis. J Bone Joint Surg Am 1979;61:832–839.

65. Nirschl RP. Sports and overuse injuries to the elbow. Muscle and tendon trauma: tennis elbow. In Morrey BF (ed.), The Elbow and Its Disorders, 2nd edn. Philadelphia: WB Saunders, 1985, pp. 537–552.

66. Novak CB, et al. Provocative sensory testing in a carpal tunnel syndrome. J Bone Joint Surg Br 1992;17:204–208.

67. O'Driscoll SW, Bell DF, Morrey BF. Posterolateral rotatory instability of the elbow. J Bone J Surg Am 1991;73:440–446.

68. O'Driscoll SW, Horii E, Carmichael SW, Morrey BF. The cubital tunnel and ulnar neuropathy. J Bone J Surg Br 1991;73:613–617.

69. O'Driscoll SW, Jupiter JB, King GJW, Hotchkiss RN, Morrey BF. The unstable elbow. In AAOS Instructional Course Lectures 2001;50:89–102.

70. O'Dwyer KJ, Howie CR. Medial epicondylitis of the elbow. Int Orthop 1995;19:69–71.

71. Paley D, McMurtry RY. Median nerve compression test in carpal tunnel syndrome diagnosis: reproduces signs and symptoms in affected wrist. Orthop Rev 1985;14(7):41–45.

72. Palmer AK, Werner FW. The triangular fibrocartilage complex of the wrist: anatomy and function. J Hand Surg Am 1981;6:153–162.

73. Palmer AK. Triangular fibrocartilage disorders: injury patterns and treatment. Arthroscopy 1990;6:125–132.

74. Palmer ML, Epler ME. Fundamentals of Musculoskeletal Assessment Techniques, 2nd edn. Philadelphia: Lippincott, Williams & Wilkins, 1998, pp. 127–196.

75. Phalen GS. Spontaneous compression of the median nerve at the wrist. J Am Med Assoc 1951;145:1128–1132.

76. Phalen GS. The carpal tunnel syndrome: clinical evaluation of 598 hands. Clin Orthop Rel Res 1972;83:29–40.

77. Plancher KD, Halbrecht J, Lourie GM. Medial and lateral epicondylitis in the athlete. Clin Sports Med 1996;15:283–304.

78. Pryse-Phillips W. Validation of a diagnostic sign in CTS J Neurol Neurosurg Psychiatr 1984;47:870–872.

79. Reagan DS, Linscheid RL, Dobyns JH. Lunotriquetral sprains. J Hand Surg Am 1984;9:502–514.

80. Reese NB, Bandy WD. Joint Range of Motion and Muscle Length Testing. Philadelphia: WB Saunders, 2002, pp. 79–126.

81. Reference Manual for the International Standards for Neurological and Function Classification of Spinal Cord Inury. Chicago: American Spinal Injury Association, 1994.

82. Roles NC, Maudsley RH. Radial tunnel syndrome: resistant tennis elbow as a nerve entrapment. J Bone Joint Surg Br 1972;54:499–508.

83. Sapira JD. The neurologic examination. In Sapira JD (ed.), The Art and Science of Bedside Diagnosis. Baltimore: Williams & Wilkins, 1990, pp. 506.

84. Sapira JD. The extremities. In Sapira JD (ed.), The Art and Science of Bedside Diagnosis. Baltimore: Williams & Wilkins, 1990, pp. 436.

85. Sapira JD. The extremities. In Sapira JD (ed.), The Art and Science of Bedside Diagnosis. Baltimore: Williams & Wilkins, 1990, pp. 505.

86. Schers TJ, VanHeusden HA. Evaluation of chronic wrist pain. Arthroscopy superior to arthrogram: comparison in 39 patients. Acta Orthop Scand 1995;66:540–542.

87. Seror P. Phalen's test in the diagnosis of carpal tunnel syndrome. J Hand Surg Br 1988;13:383–385.

88. Seyffarth H. Primary myosis in the pronator teres as a cause of lesion of the n. medianus (the pronator syndrome). Acta Psych Neurol Scand 1951;74:251–254.

89. Shin AY, Battaglia MJ, Bishop AT. Lunotriquetral instability: diagnosis and treatment. J Am Acad Orthop Surg 2000;8:170–179.

90. Smith RV, Fisher RG. Struthers ligament: a source of median nerve compression above the elbow. J Neurosurg 1973:38:778.

91. Stener B. Displacement of the ruptured ulnar collateral ligament of the metacarpo-phalangeal joint of the thumb. J Bone Joint Surg Br 1962;44:869–879.

92. Tinel J. Le signe "fourmillement" dans les lesions des nerfs peripheriques. La Presse Medicale 1915;23:388–389.

93. Vangsness CT, Jobe FW. Surgical treatment of medial epicondylitis. J Bone Joint Surg Br 1991;72:409–411.

94. Wadsworth TG, Williams JR. Cubital tunnel external compression syndrome. Br Med J 1973; 1:662–666.

95. Watson HK, et al. Examination of the scaphoid. J Hand Surg Am 1988;13:657–660.

96. Watson HK, Weinzweig J. Physical examination of the wrist. Hand Clinics 1997;13(1):17–34.

97. Watson HK. Triscaphe reconstruction. Presented at American Research in General Orthopedics, New Orleans, LA, March 1978.

98. Werner CO, Elmquist D, Ohlin P. Pressure and nerve lesion in the carpal tunnel. Acta Orthop Scand 1983;54:312–316.

99. Werner CO, Haeffner F, Rosen I. Direct recording of local pressure in the radial tunnel during passive stretch and active contraction of the supinator muscle. Arch Orthop Traumat Surg 1980;96:299–301.

100. Werner CO, Rosen I, Thorngren KG. Clinical and neurophysiologic characteristics of the pronator syndrome. Clin Orthop Rel Res 1984;197:231–236.

101. Werner CO. Lateral elbow pain and posterior interosseous nerve entrapment. Acta Orth Scand 1979;174:1–62.

102. Werner RA, Bir C, Armstrong TJ. Reverse Phalen's maneuver as an aid in diagnosing carpal tunnel syndrome. Arch Phys Med Rehabil 1994;75:783–786.

103. Westkaemper JG, Mitsionis G, Giannakopoulos PN, Sorteanos DG. Wrist arthroscopy for the treatment of ligament and triangular fibrocartilage complex injuries. Arthroscopy 1998;14:479–483.

104. Williams TM, Mackinnon SE, Novak CB, et al. Verification of the pressure provocative test in carpal tunnel syndrome. Ann Plastic Surg 1992;29:8–11.

105. Winkworth CE. Lawn-tennis elbow. Br Med J 1883:708.

106. Wolfe SW, Crisco JJ. Mechanical evaluation of the scaphoid shift test. J Hand Surg Am 1994; 19:762–768.

Chapter 6

Physical Examination of the Lumbar Spine

JENNIFER SOLOMON, MD • SCOTT F. NADLER, DO •
JOEL PRESS, MD

Patients with low back pain should undergo a detailed history and physical examination to establish an appropriate diagnosis and treatment plan. Non-specific diagnoses will lead to poorly directed treatment plans and may compromise patient outcomes. A comprehensive physical exam of a patient with low back pain (LBP) should include an in-depth evaluation of the neurologic, vascular, and musculoskeletal systems. To avoid missing key elements, it should be performed in a sequence: inspection, palpation, range of motion (ROM), flexibility, functional and neurologic assessments, and provocative maneuvers.

Inspection

The clinician should perform a general inspection of the patient's body habitus and posture during sitting, standing, and ambulating. The exam begins with observation of the patient during the history portion of the evaluation. Patients with low back pain often maintain a rigid posture to avoid bending, twisting, or other movements that may be painful. With acute symptoms, it is not uncommon to observe some degree of antalgic posturing. To ensure a complete examination the patient should disrobe completely.

Important bone landmarks include the anterior superior iliac spine at the level of the sacral promontory, and the posterior at the level of the spinous process of the second sacral vertebra.[52] A horizontal line through the highest points of the iliac crests passes also through the spinous process of the fourth lumbar vertebra. The trans-tubercular plane through the tubercles on the iliac crests cuts the body of the fifth lumbar vertebra. The upper margin of the greater sciatic notch is opposite the spinous process of the third sacral vertebra, and slightly below this level is the posterior inferior iliac spine. The surface markings of the posterior inferior iliac spine and the ischial spine are both situated in a line which joins the posterior superior iliac spine to the outer part of the ischial tuberosity; the posterior inferior spine is 5 cm and the ischial spine 10 cm below the posterior superior spine; the ischial spine is opposite the first portion of the coccyx. With the body erect, the line joining the pubic tubercle to the top of the greater trochanter is practically horizontal; the middle of this line overlies the acetabulum and the head of the femur.

Observation of the patient from the front involves several key components. The head should be straight on the shoulders. The shoulder height should be equal, although the dominant side may be slightly lower in an athletic individual who throws or uses a racquet (Figure 6–1A). The iliac crest height should be equal (Figure 6–1B). The patellae should be pointing anteriorly. The lower limbs should be straight and any deformity including valgus–varus misalignment should be noted.

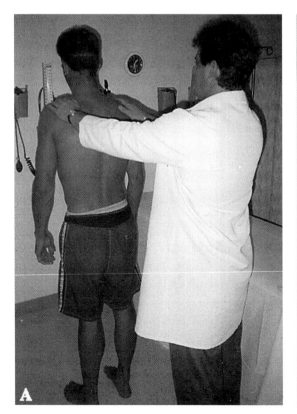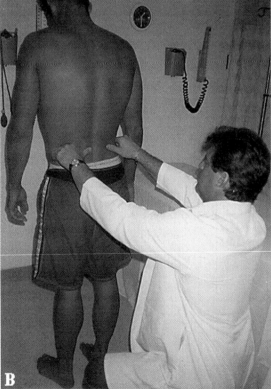

Figure 6–1. Inspection. **A:** Assessment of shoulder height. **B:** Assessment of iliac crest height. Reproduced with permission from Nadler S, Stitik T: Occupational low back pain: history and physical examination. Occup Med 1998;13(1):68.

Posterior observation involves inspection of bone and soft tissue alignment. Shifting of the pelvis or shoulders may be noted in the face of nerve root injury or gluteus medius weakness (Trendelenburg gait).[52] With a disc herniation lateral to the nerve roots, the patient will list away from the side of the irritated nerve root in an attempt to draw the nerve root away from the disc. Likewise, when the herniation is medial to the nerve root, the patient may list toward the side of the lesion. Underlying scoliotic curves may be evaluated by inspection of the height of the shoulders, scapula, and iliac crests. The spine of the scapula, which begins at the level of the third thoracic vertebra, should be at the same angle. The inferior angles of the scapula (T8) should be equidistant from the spine. Any curve in the spine should be noted, as well as muscular asymmetry. A rib hump deformity is often noted upon forward flexion of the trunk or may be identified through apparent scapular winging. The waist angles should be equal. Observation of the iliac crest heights for any differences may indicate a functional leg length discrepancy. The posterior superior iliac spines should be level and the relationship with the anterior superior iliac spines should be noted. In addition, the gluteal folds and popliteal creases should be level.

When examining a patient from the side, the ear lobe should be in line with the tip of the shoulder, and the peak of the iliac crest. A gentle lumbar lordotic curve is normal. Any exaggerated or increased curve should be noted. Exaggerated lordosis may be associated with a hip flexor contracture, weak hip extensors, or spondylolisthesis. The alignment of the lower extremities should also be observed.

The skin may reveal ecchymosis after blunt trauma, erythema with infection or inflammation, or rashes with shingles or infection. Atrophy of the tissues may be noted with the presence of nerve root or peripheral nerve injury.

Palpation

This part of the exam usually begins with the patient in the standing position. The examiner usually begins by placing fingers on the tops of the iliac crests, at the level of the L4/L5 interdisc space. Iliac crest height can be further evaluated as well as the scapulae and shoulder heights. While the patient is still standing, the examiner should palpate the spinous processes to evaluate a possible step-off from one level to the next. This may be an indication of spondylolisthesis of the posterior elements of the spine.

In the prone position, the L4/L5 interdisc space is again appreciated. The examiner then palpates the spinous processes and notes any tender areas. Palpation of the paraspinal musculature is essential to determine whether any tender or trigger points can be appreciated and whether muscle spasm is present. Tenderness may be present along muscles in which symptoms are referred, such as in the gluteal region and in the lower extremity. Palpation of the lumbar spine in the midline sometimes can elicit pain at the level of a symptomatic intervertebral disc. To complete the examination, palpation of the posterior superior iliac spines, iliac crests, the greater trochanters, and ischial tuberosities are all essential in determining the etiology of the patient's symptoms.

Deyo et al.[14] described palpation of soft tissue and bony tenderness as having both poor reproducibility (κ = 0.40) and specificity. However, bony tenderness may be suggestive of spinal infection.

Range of Motion

Lumbar ROM has been commonly used to measure impairment of patients with low back pain. Range of motion can be measured both passively and actively; however the literature supports greater accuracy of passive range assessment.[28] The motion of the lumbar spine must be assessed in all planes, including flexion, extension, side-bending, and rotation. When examining ROM, it is important to document any side-to-side differences as asymmetric movement may be one of the first findings in those with underlying disease entities. It is also important to note that the ROM may be affected by age and sex, whereas occupation and body mass index have little or no influence on motion.[56] It has also been determined that total sagittal ROM, flexion angle, and extension angle decline as age increases.[81] Normative values were determined by Ng et al. in 2001 (Table 6–1).[68]

Table 6–1. NORMATIVE VALUES OF LUMBAR RANGE OF MOTION

Direction of Motion	Mean Degrees of Motion
Flexion	59 ± 9
Extension	19 ± 9
Combined extension/flexion (sagittal)	71 ± 12
Right lateral flexion	31 ± 6
Left lateral flexion	30 ± 6
Coronal plane (lateral flexion)	60 ± 11
Right axial rotation	32 ± 9
Left axial rotation	33 ± 9
Transverse plan (axial rotation)	65 ± 17
Lumbar lordosis	24 ± 8

Reproduced with permission from Ng JK, Kippers V, Richardson CA, Parnianpour M. Range of motion and lordosis of the lumbar spine: reliability of measurement and normative values. Spine 2001;26:53–60.

Table 6–2. SEGMENTAL MOTION (IN DEGREES)

Level	Flexion	Extension	Lateral Bending	Axial Twist
L1/L2	8	5	6	2
L2/L3	10	3	6	2
L3/L4	12	1	8	2
L4/L5	13	2	6	2
L5/S1	9	5	3	5

Reproduced with permission from McGill SM. Low Back Disorders: Evidence-based Prevention and Rehabilitation. Champaign, IL, Human Kinetics, 2002.

Studies have measured lateral flexion from different reference points, which has led to differing normative data. Using T12/L1 to L5/S1 as the reference points for measuring lateral flexion, the range on both sides was 49–77 degrees. White and Panjabi[93] and Pearcy et al.[73,74] measured the segmental ROM of the spine (Table 6–2).

A key measurement is forward flexion because it is composed of both lumbar and pelvic movement.[66,67] The typical description of forward flexion suggests that the first 60 degrees takes place in the lumbar spine, while any further motion takes place in the hips; however, strict measurements validating this issue have not been performed.[57] When the lumbar spine and hip interplay is quantified, it is apparent that torso flexion is accomplished with a combination of hip and lumbar spine motion.[57] Caillet[7] has demonstrated that the initial 45 degrees of trunk flexion is essentially the reversal of lumbar lordosis and that the remainder of the motion is a result of pelvic rotation. It is also necessary to document the reversal of lumbar lordosis, as well as the amount of forward flexion when documenting this important assessment.

There is no gold standard to measure ROM of the lumbar spine in the peer-reviewed literature. Several studies have utilized external measurements with comparison to plain radiographs, though their findings have not been consistent.[6,76] Mayer et al.[55] and Saur et al.[78] have found good correlation between these measurements. Mayer et al. found no significant differences between radiographic range of motion measurements and non-invasive inclinometer techniques. Saur et al. found a very close correlation ($R = 0.93$) of range of motion taken with and without radiologic evaluation using an inclinometer.

Fingertips-to-Floor

A simple measurement of fingertip distance to the floor in flexion is commonly used in clinical practice. The subject is asked to stand erect with knees extended and to

bend forward as far as possible. The distance between the middle finger (at full extension) and the floor is measured with a measuring tape. The intra-tester reliability has
been shown to be 76%, and 83% for inter-tester reliability using this method.[62] The
specificity of this method has been shown to be 88.8% with a sensitivity of 45.3%.[85,86]
However, this test method is not specific for the lumbar spine as it assesses both hip
and lumbar spine range.

Right and left lateral flexion of the lumbar spine may also be assessed in a similar
manner utilizing no instrumentation and measuring fingertip distance. Thomas et al.[85]
compared spinal range of motion in 344 patients with new-onset LBP with 118 individuals without LBP. In right and left lateral flexion, the participant stood with head
and buttocks pressed against a wall, without any knee flexion, and was asked to bend
sideways. Lateral flexion was measured as the distance covered by the fingertips on the
lateral thigh. Right lateral flexion had a sensitivity of 23% and a specificity of 94%,
while left lateral flexion had a sensitivity of 26% and a specificity of 92%.

Schober Test

In 1937, Schober first described a test to measure segmental motion of the lumbar
spine.[79] It is described as follows:

> The first sacral spinous process is marked, and a mark is made about 10 cm above
> this mark. The patient then flexes forward, and the increased distance is measured.
> If there is normal motion of the lumbar spine with absence of disease, there should
> be an increase of 4–5 cm.

This test is used only to measure flexion, with intra-tester variation reported to be
just 4.8%.[5] The Schober test is not used to measure extension, lateral bending, or rotation, and it has been criticized because of the difficulty in isolating surface landmarks
through different depths of subcutaneous tissue.[65]

Modified Schober Test

In 1969, Wright and Moll[64] modified the Schober technique for the assessment of
patients with ankylosing spondylitis and others. It is described as follows:

> With the subject standing erect but relaxed, a point is drawn with a skin marker at
> the spinal intersection of a line joining the dimples of Venus (S1). Additional marks
> are made 10 cm above and 5 cm below S1. Subjects are asked to bend forward. The
> distance between the marks 10 cm above and 5 cm below S1 is measured.

The rationale for this modification was an observation that, on forward flexion,
both the lumbosacral junction and superiorly placed 10-cm skin marks tended to

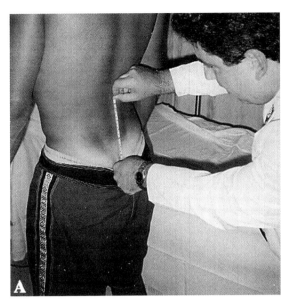 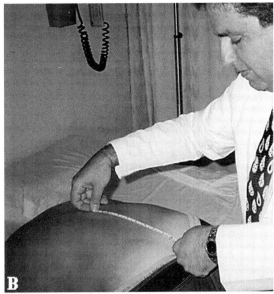

Figure 6–2. **A:** Modified Schober technique (neutral standing). **B:** Modified Schober technique (full flexion). Reproduced with permission from Nadler S, Stitik T: Occupational low back pain: history and physical examination. Occup Med 1998;13(1):69.

move less relative to the spinous processes and the skin than the previously used mark 5 cm inferior to the sacrum (Figure 6–2).[97]

Reynolds[77] found this measurement of motion to have good reliability, with Pearson correlation coefficients of 0.59 for lumbar flexion and 0.75 for extension. The coefficient of variation (COV) was reasonable at 11.65% for flexion, with greater variation for extension as demonstrated by a COV of 21.57%. Fitzgerald[23] reported a Pearson correlation coefficient of 1.0 for lumbar flexion and 0.88 for lumbar extension in a study of young healthy subjects; however, these results may not be applicable to older individuals.

Gill et al.[26] concluded that the modified Schober method was the most reproducible method of measurement between the fingertip-to-floor, modified Schober, dual inclinometer, and photometric techniques. The COV was excellent, ranging from 0.9% for flexion and 2.8% for extension.

Miller et al.[63] noted overall good inter-rater reliability ($R = 0.71$) of the modified Schober method. Potential errors that affect the reliability of this clinical test were (1) the presence or absence of dimples of Venus, (2) anatomic location of the dimples of Venus, (3) anatomic variability of the 10 cm line, (4) problems introduced by skin distraction, and (5) problems in developing a normative database. Stankovic[83] more recently noted an intra-rater correlation coefficient of 0.95 and an inter-rater correlation coefficient of 0.94 utilizing the modified Schober test. Thomas et al.[86] determined the specificity to be 95% and sensitivity to be 25% when comparing patients with and without low back pain.

Viitanen et al.[90] compared the modified Schober test to thoracolumbar flexion measure using a simple tape method and correlated the results with radiologic changes in patients with ankylosing spondylitis (AS). The Schober test and tape methods correlated fairly highly (modified Schober $R = 0.71, 0.62$; tape method $R = 0.49, 0.42$) with radiologic changes.

In conclusion, the modified Schober test has been found to be moderately reproducible and specific but not sensitive when examining patients with and without low back pain.[89]

Modified Modified Schober Test

The modified modified Schober technique was first described by Van Adrichmen and Van der Korst in 1973.[88] It is described as follows.

> The patient stands with feet 15 cm apart. The posterior superior iliac spines are identified and a mark is made on the midline of the lumbar spines horizontal to the PSIS. Another mark is placed on the spinous processes 15 cm superior to the PSIS line. A tape measure is aligned between the two marks, and the patient is asked to bend forward or backward depending on the motion being measured. The new distance between the markings is measured. The difference between the two measurements is recorded.

The Pearson correlation coefficient ranged from 0.78 and 0.89 for lumbar flexion and between 0.69 and 0.91 for lumbar extension. Inter-rater reliability was determined to be 0.72 for flexion and 0.76 for extension. Williams[96] reported similar values when evaluating inter-rater reliability, with 0.72 for flexion and 0.76 for extension, using the further modified Schober technique.

No studies have specifically evaluated the sensitivity or specificity of the modified modified Schober test in evaluating low back issues.

Inclinometer

The inclinometer method requires more specialized equipment, but it can be a useful tool for motion measurement. An inclinometer is a hand-held, circular, fluid-filled disc with a weighted gravity pendulum that remains vertically oriented.

The inclinometer technique has been described using single and dual techniques, with dual inclinometry demonstrating superior results. Dual inclinometry requires one inclinometer to be placed on the sacrum to measure hip motion and the other placed on the first lumbar vertebra to measure hip and lumbar range of motion. Loebl[51] described a method of measuring four spinal segments with one inclinometer placed on the T12 spinous process and the other at a point 15 cm above the S1 spinal level.

This test was based on the assumption that the curvature of the spine can be determined by the angle formed by the tangent of one point on the curve with the tangent of another point on the curve.[62] Range of motion is then measured by calculating the differences between angles measured while the back is in neutral, flexed, and extended positions.

The *AMA Guidelines for Impairment Evaluation, 5th edition,* recommends the use of dual inclinometry for measuring lumbar range of motion with techniques as described by Loebl.

Nattrass[68] evaluated the validity of spinal range of motion methods as outlined in the second and fourth editions of the *AMA Guidelines for Impairment and Disability.* Comparing goniometry and dual inclinometry, inter- and intra-rater reliability were found to be poor (Pearson correlation coefficient ranges from −0.38 to 0.54) with measurement error for thoracolumbar and lumbar movements as large as ±30 degrees, with the smallest error being 9 degrees. Reliability measures have varied greatly in the literature (Table 6–3).[68]

Table 6–3. TESTS OF LUMBAR SPINE MOTION

Test	Description	Reliability/Validity Tests	Comments
Finger tips to floor	The subject is asked to stand erect with knees extended and bend forward as far as possible. The distance between the middle finger and the floor is measured with a measuring tape. This method is not specific for the lumbar spine as it assesses both hip and lumbar spine.	Merrit 1986[62] Intra-tester reliability: 76% Inter-tester reliability: 83% The specificity of this method has been shown to be 88.8% with a sensitivity of 45.3%.[86,87]	
	Lateral flexion of the lumbar spine may be assessed in a similar manner.		

		Thomas 1998[86]
		Right lateral flexion:
		  Sensitivity: 23%
		  Specificity: 94%
		Left lateral flexion:
		  Sensitivity: 26%
		  Specificity: 92%
			Compared spinal range of motion in 344 patients with new-onset LBP with 118 individuals without LBP. In right and left lateral flexion, the participant stood with head and buttocks pressed against the wall, without any knee flexion, and was asked to bend sideways.[86]

Continued

Table 6–3. TESTS OF LUMBAR SPINE MOTION—*cont'd*

Test	Description	Reliability/Validity Tests	Comments
Schober test	The first sacral spinous process is marked, and a mark is made about 10 cm above this mark. The patient then flexes forward, and the increased distance is measured.[65]	Biering-Sorensen 1984[5] Intra-tester variation reported to be only 4.8%.	This test is used only to measure flexion. The Schober test is not used to measure extension, lateral bending, or rotation, and has been criticized because of the difficulty in isolating surface landmarks through different depths of subcutaneous tissue.

Modified Schober test	With the subject standing erect but relaxed, a point is drawn with a skin marker at the spinal intersection of a line joining the dimples of Venus (S1). Additional marks are made 10 cm above and 5 cm below S1. Subjects are asked to bend forward. The distance between the marks 10 cm above and 5 cm below S1 is measured.[52]	Reynolds 1975[77]
		Pearson correlation coefficients:
		  0.59 for lumbar flexion
		  0.75 for extension
		COV:
		  11.65% for flexion
		  21.57% for extension	

		Fitzgerald 1983[23]
		Pearson correlation coefficients:
		  Lumbar flexion: 1.00
		  Lumbar extension: 0.88
			Study was performed on young healthy subjects and may not be applicable to older individuals.

		Gill 1988[26]
		COV:
		  0.9% for flexion
		  2.8% for extension
			Concluded that the modified Schober method was the most reproducible method of measurement as compared to the fingertip-to-floor, modified Schober, dual inclinometer, and photometric techniques.

		Miller 1992[63] Inter-rater reliability: 0.71	Potential errors: (a) Presence or absence of dimples of Venus. (b) Anatomic location of dimples of Venus. (c) Anatomic variability of 10-cm line.

Table 6–3. TESTS OF LUMBAR SPINE MOTION—*cont'd*

Test	Description	Reliability/Validity Tests	Comments
			(d) Problems introduced by skin distraction. (e) Problems in developing a normative database.
		Stankovic 1999[83] Intra-rater CC: 0.95 Inter-rater CC: 0.94	
		Thomas 1998[86] Specificity: 95% Sensitivity: 25% Viitanen 1999[90] Correlation with radiographic data: Modified Schober, $R = 0.71, 0.62$ Tape method, $R = 0.49, 0.42$	When comparing patients with and without low back pain. Compared the modified Schober test to thoracolumbar flexion measure using a simple tape method and correlated the results with radiological changes in patients with ankylosing spondylitis (AS).
Modified modified Schober test	The posterior superior iliac spines are identified and a mark is made on the midline of the lumbar spines horizontal to the PSIS. Another mark is placed on the spinous processes 15 cm superior to the PSIS line. A tape measure is aligned between the two marks, and the patient is asked to bend forward or backward depending on the motion being measured. The new distance between the markings is measured. The difference between the two measurements is recorded.[88]	Van Adrichmen[88] Pearson correlation coefficient: Lumbar flexion: 0.78 and 0.89 Lumbar extension: 0.69 and 0.91 Inter-rater reliability: Flexion: 0.72 Extension: 0.76 Williams 1993[97] Inter-rater reliability: Lumbar flexion: 0.72 Lumbar extension: 0.76	
Inclinometer	Dual inclinometry requires one inclinometer to be placed on the sacrum to measure hip motion and the other placed on the first lumbar vertebra to measure hip and lumbar range of motion. Range of motion is then measured by calculating the differences between angles measured while the back is in neutral, flexed, and extended positions.[62]	Nattrass 1999[68] Pearson correlation coefficient ranged from −0.38 to 0.54 Measurement error for thoracolumbar and lumbar movements as large as ± 30 degrees, with the smallest error being 9 degrees.	Evaluated the validity of spinal range of motion methods as outlined in the second and fourth editions of the *AMA Guidelines for Impairment and Disability*. Compared goniometry and dual inclinometry.

Continued

Table 6–3. TESTS OF LUMBAR SPINE MOTION—*cont'd*

Test	Description	Reliability/Validity Tests	Comments

		Reynolds 1975[77]
		Inter-tester reliability:
		  Flexion, $R = 0.76$
		  Extension, $R = 0.87$
			Standard inclinometer

		Burdett 1986[6]
		Inter-tester reliability:
		  Flexion, $R = 0.73$
		  Extension $R = 0.15$
			Gravidity inclinometer

		Merrit 1986[62]
		Inter-tester reliability:
		  COV flexion: 9.6
		  COV extension: 65.4
		Intra-tester reliability:
		  COV flexion: 13.4
		  COV extension: 50.7
			Standard inclinometer

		Dillard 1991[15]
		Inter-tester reliability:
		  Flexion, $R = 0.78$
		  Extension, $R = 0.27$
		Intra-tester reliability:
		  Lateral flexion, $R = 0.66$
			Dual inclinometer

		Saur 1996[78]
		Inter-tester reliability:
		  Flexion, $R = 0.88$
		  Extension, $R = 0.94$
			Standard inclinometer

		Ng 2001[69]
		Intra-tester reliability:
		  Flexion, $R = 0.87$
		  Extension, $R = 0.92$
		  Right lateral flexion, $R = 0.96$
		  Left lateral flexion, $R = 0.94$
		  Right axial rotation, $R = 0.96$
		  Left axial rotation, $R = 0.94$
			Modified inclinometer with pelvic restraint

		Dopf 1994[16] Intra-tester reliability: $R = 0.93$	

		Nattrass 1999[68]
		Intra-tester reliability
		  Flexion, $R = 0.90$
		  Extension, $R = 0.70$
		  Lateral flexion,
		    $R = 0.89–0.90$
			Dual inclinometer

Table 6–3. TESTS OF LUMBAR SPINE MOTION—*cont'd*

Test	Description	Reliability/Validity Tests	Comments
		Williams 1993[97] Intra-tester reliability: Flexion, $R = 0.13–0.87$ Extension, $R = 0.28–0.66$	
		Keely 1985[40] Intra-tester reliability: Extension, $R = 0.90–0.96$	Dual inclinometer
		Portek 1983[76] Intra-tester reliability: Flexion, $R = 0.86$	Standard inclinometer
		Mellin 1986,87,88,91[59-61] Intra-tester reliability: Flexion, $R = 0.86$ Extension, $R = 0.93$ Lateral flexion, $R = 0.6–0.85$	Dual inclinometer
		Gill 1994[26] Intra-tester reliability: COV flexion: 9.3–33.9 COV extension: 3.6–4.7	Dual inclinometer

The inclinometer can be used to measure lateral flexion with the individual asked to bend laterally.[65] The degree of lateral flexion for the lumbar spine is determined by subtracting measurements from the sacral inclinometer to that placed at T12. Intra-rater reliability has ranged from good to excellent (0.60–0.96).[60,68,69] Ohlen et al.[71] noted an average of 88 degrees of lateral flexion in healthy subjects, using a Debrunner kyphometer (a protractor with an attached degree scale with two movable arms), with a COV of 4.3% while using an inclinometer; 82 degrees of lateral flexion was measured with a coefficient of variation of 19%.

In conclusion, the inclinometer is moderately reliable but is not consistent in patients with LBP.

Neurologic Examination

Manual Motor Testing

The assessment of strength must be performed in a sequential manner, evaluating muscle groups innervated by different peripheral nerves and nerve roots. Lumbar radiculopathy is usually characterized by weaknesses affecting two or more muscles from the same spinal segment but different peripheral nerves. For example, an L5 radiculopathy may affect both the dorsiflexors of the foot and toes (peroneal nerve) and abduction of the hip (superior gluteal nerve). The strength examination should include the assessment of hip flexors (L1–L3), quadriceps (L2–L4), tibialis anterior (L4–L5), extensor hallucis longus (L5), and the gastrocnemius-soleus (S1). The latter muscle may be assessed via the performance of 10 toe raises or the ability to ambulate on toes.[66,67] Functional testing of the hip abductors should be performed with the patient standing on one leg to evaluate for the presence of a Trendelenburg sign.

Several studies have looked at the sensitivity and specificity of muscle strength testing in patients with lumbar radiculopathy (Table 6–4). Kerr et al.[41] demonstrated reduced ankle dorsiflexion in 54% and plantar flexion in 13% of those with lumbar

Table 6–4. NEUROLOGIC EXAM AS A TEST FOR LUMBAR DISC HERNIATION

Test	Description	Reliability/Validity Tests	Comments

Muscle strength testing	Assessment of strength must be performed in a sequential manner, evaluating muscle groups innervated by different peripheral nerves and nerve roots. Radiculopathy is characterized by weaknesses affecting two or more muscles from the same spinal segment but different peripheral nerves.
	
	The examination should include hip flexors (L1–L3), quadriceps (L2–L4), tibialis anterior (L4–L5), extensor hallucis longus (L5), and the gastrocnemius/soleus complex (S1).
		Spangfort 1971[81]
		Ankledorsiflexor weakness:
		  Sensitivity: 49%
		  Specificity: 54%
		
		Hakelius 1970,72[30,31]
		Ankle dorsiflexor weakness:
		  Sensitivity: 20%
		  Specificity: 82%
		Ankle plantar flexor weakness:
		  Sensitivity: 6%
		  Specificity: 95%
		Great-toe extensor weakness:
		  Sensitivity: 37%
		  Specificity: 71%
		Quadriceps weakness:
		  Sensitivity: <1%
		  Specificity: 99%
		
		Kerr 1988[41]
		Ankle dorsiflexor weakness:
		  Sensitivity: 54%
		  Specificity: 89%
		Ankle plantar flexor weakness:
		  Sensitivity: 13%
		  Specificity: 100%
		
		Kortelainen 1985[44]
		Ankle dorsiflexor weakness:
		  Sensitivity: 57%
			Tested ankle dorsiflexor in 2504 patients; 70–90% of pts with weakness had HNP at L4/L5 level.
			
			32% HNP at L4/L5
			57% HNP at L5/S1

Table 6–4. NEUROLOGIC EXAM AS A TEST FOR LUMBAR DISC HERNIATION—*cont'd*

Test	Description	Reliability/Validity Tests	Comments
		Knutsson 1961[43] Ankle dorsiflexor weakness: Sensitivity: 63% Specificity: 52%	For L5 root specifically, the sensitivity was 76% and the specificity was 52%.
		Lauder 2002[49] Great-toe extensor weakness: Sensitivity: 61% Specificity: 55% Quadriceps weakness: Sensitivity: 40% Specificity: 89% Ankle plantar flexor weakness: Sensitivity: 47% Specificity: 76%	
Muscle stretch reflex	Tapping the test tendon stretches the spindle and activates its fibers. Afferent projections from these fibers synapse with the alpha motor neurons, which in turn send impulses to the skeletal muscles, resulting in a brief muscle contraction. This contraction is graded on a standard scale.	Spangfort 1971[81] Ankle: Sensitivity: 50% Specificity: 62% Patella: Sensitivity: 4% Specificity: 97% Hakelius 1970,72[30,31] Ankle: Sensitivity: 52% Specificity: 63% Patella: Sensitivity: 7% Specificity: 93%	Ankle: HNP at L5/S1 level in 80–90% for ages 20–45, and 60% older than 50. Patella: Sensitivity of 50% in L3/L4 HNP. In 67% of cases of impairment, HNP is at L4/L5 and L5/S1 levels.
		Knutsson 1961[43] Ankle: Sensitivity: 56% Specificity: 57% Patella: Sensitivity: 15% Specificity: 67%	For S1 the sensitivity was 79% and the specificity was 62%.

For L3/L4 the sensitivity was 10% and the specificity was 85%. |
| | | Kerr 1988[41] Sensitivity: 48% Specificity: 89% | For L5/S1 the sensitivity was 78% and the specificity was 88%. |
| | | Lauder 2002[49] Ankle: Sensitivity: 47% Specificity: 90% | |

Continued

Table 6–4. NEUROLOGIC EXAM AS A TEST FOR LUMBAR DISC HERNIATION—*cont'd*

Test	Description	Reliability/Validity Tests	Comments
		Patella: Sensitivity: 50% Specificity: 93%	
		Kortelainen 1985[44] Sensitivity: 7%	In 85% of cases of impairment, HNP is at L4/L5 and L5/S1.
Sensory exam	The sensory examination should cover the bilateral lower extremities to evaluate for dermatomal or diffuse sensory loss. Sensation is evaluated using different modalities, including vibration, proprioception, temperature, light touch, and pinprick.	Kerr 1988[41] Sensitivity: 16% Specificity: 86% Knutsson 1961[43] Sensitivity: 29% Specificity: 67% Kosteljanetz 1984[46] Sensitivity: 66% Specificity: 51% Kortelainen 1985[44] Sensitivity: 38% Lauder 2002[49] Sensitivity: 50% Specificity: 62%	

disc protrusions from L4 to S1 with an overall specificity of 89%. Weakness of the extensor hallucis longus had a sensitivity of 12–51% with a specificity of 72–91% for detecting L5 radiculopathy, whereas weak ankle plantar flexors had an overall specificity between 26% and 99% in detecting S1 radiculopathy.

Sensory Examination

The sensory exam should cover the bilateral lower extremities to evaluate for true dermatomal or more diffuse sensory loss as seen in peripheral neuropathies with a "stocking" distribution of loss. Dermatomes may define the area of skin innervated by a single nerve root or peripheral nerve (Figure 6–3). Sensation is evaluated using many different modalities, including vibration, proprioception, temperature, light touch, and pinprick. The latter two are more commonly used in the neurologic evaluation, although vibration may be more sensitive for injury to large-diameter sensory nerves and proprioception loss may be indicative of posterior column dysfunction such as is

Figure 6–3. Dermatomes and peripheral nerve distribution of the lower extremities. Adapted with permission from Borenstein and Weisel, p. 67, Figure 4-6.

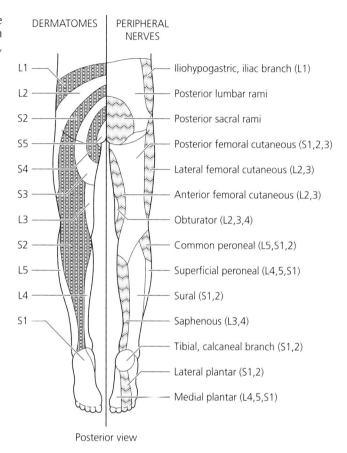

DERMATOMES | PERIPHERAL NERVES

L1 — Iliohypogastric, iliac branch (L1)
L2 — Posterior lumbar rami
S2 — Posterior sacral rami
S5 — Posterior femoral cutaneous (S1,2,3)
S4 — Lateral femoral cutaneous (L2,3)
S3 — Anterior femoral cutaneous (L2,3)
L3 — Obturator (L2,3,4)
S2 — Common peroneal (L5,S1,2)
L5 — Superficial peroneal (L4,5,S1)
L4 — Sural (S1,2)
S1 — Saphenous (L3,4)
Tibial, calcaneal branch (S1,2)
Lateral plantar (S1,2)
Medial plantar (L4,5,S1)

Posterior view

seen in B_{12} deficiency and syphilis.[88] The sensitivity and specificity of the sensory examination in the diagnosis of lumbar disc herniation has been described in the literature (Table 6–4).

Reflex Examination

The definition of a reflex is the involuntary contraction of muscles, induced by a specific stimulus. Tendon reflex activity depends on the status of the alpha motor neurons, the muscle spindles and their afferent fibers, and the gamma neurons whose axons terminate on intrafusal muscle fibers within the spindles. A tap on the tendon stretches the spindle and activates its fibers. Afferent projections form these fiber synapses with the alpha motor neurons, which in turn send impulses to the skeletal muscles resulting in the familiar brief muscle contraction or monophasic stretch reflex.

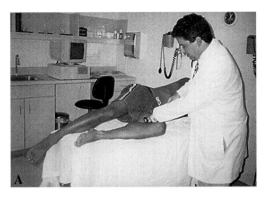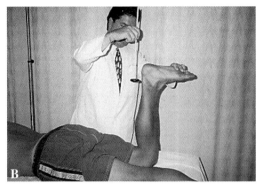

Figure 6–4. *A:* Medial hamstring reflex. ***B:*** Prone technique for eliciting Achilles reflex. Reproduced with permission from Nadler S, Stitik T: Occupational low back pain: history and physical examination. Occup Med 1998;13(1):74.

The reflex is usually named after the muscle being tested. Common stretch reflexes include the quadriceps or patellar reflex involving the L2–L4 spinal levels, medial hamstring reflex at the L5 level, and Achilles reflex involving the S1 level (Figure 6–4). A 5-point grading system recommended by the National Institute of Neurological Disorders and Stroke is the most commonly used scale (Table 6–5).[88] Eliciting reflexes may be difficult in the patient who is unable to relax. In 1885, Jendrassik described a technique to elicit reflexes by having the patient "hook together the flexed fingers of his right and left hands and pull them apart as strongly as possible" while the clinician taps on the tendon; this enhances the reflexes of normal patients.

Absent or exaggerated reflexes by themselves do not signify neurologic disease. In the elderly, up to 50% without neurologic disease lack an Achilles reflex bilaterally.[88] Small percentages (3–5%) of normal individuals have generalized hyperreflexia.[70]

Table 6–5. MUSCLE STRETCH REFLEX SCALE

Grade	Finding
0	Reflex absent
1	Reflex small, less than normal, includes trace response or a response only brought out with reinforcement
2	Reflex in the lower half of normal
3	Reflex in the upper half of normal
4	Reflex more than normal; includes clonus if present

Reproduced with permission from Victor M, Ropper AH, Adams RD. Adams & Victor's Principles of Neurology, 7th edn. New York: McGraw-Hill Professional, 2001.

Table 6–6. PHYSICAL SIGNS IN PATIENTS WITH LUMBAR DISC HERNIATIONS

Study	Positive SRL	Positive CSRL	Paresis	Achilles Areflexia	Patellar Areflexia	Decreased Lumbar ROM	No Neurologic Signs
Spengler et al.[82]	96%	60%	37%	41%	–	–	22%
Jonsson and Stromqvist[37,38]	88%	23%	50%	49%	11%	96%	–
Kortelainen et al.[44]	94%	–	38%	52%	7%	–	20%
Vucetic and Svensson[91]	85%	30%	28%	29%	11%	–	30%

Reproduced with permission from Vucetic N, Svensson O. Physical signs in lumbar disc hernia. Clin Orthop 1996;(333):192–201.

Absent or exaggerated reflex is significant only when it is associated with one of the following clinical settings:

1. The absent reflex is associated with other findings of lower motor neuron disease.
2. The exaggerated reflex is associated with other findings of upper motor neuron disease.
3. The reflex amplitude is asymmetric.
4. The reflex is unusually brisk compared with reflexes from a higher spinal level.[88]

Deyo et al.[14] reviewed the relevance of the physical examination in patients with low back pain (see Table 6–4). Andersson and Deyo[3] noted a specificity of 0.60 and a sensitivity of 0.50 for the Achilles reflex in diagnosing lumbar disc injury. In patients with a high probability (greater than 60%) of a herniated disc (which is based upon the clinicians' patient population and the prevalence of low back pain), the positive predictive value for an impaired Achilles reflex was 0.65 with a negative predictive value of 0.44. However, in patients with a low probability of a herniated disc, the positive predictive value was 0.04 with a negative predictive value of 0.98.

Vucetic et al.[91] found only lumbar range of motion and the crossed Lasègue sign to have any predictive ability in regard to determining the severity of disc injury. These signs could correctly classify 74% of uncontained hernias and 68% of contained hernias (Table 6–6).

Provocative Maneuvers

Numerous provocative maneuvers have been described in the literature in order to diagnose pathology of the lumbosacral spine. These maneuvers are not stand-alone tests and should always be used in conjunction with the history and remainder of the musculoskeletal evaluation.

Straight-leg Raising Test

The Lasègue sign or straight-leg raising (SLR) test was initially described by J. J. Frost, a student of Charles Lasègue in 1881, who memorialized his mentor through the naming of this test. In the described test, pain was induced in the distribution of the sciatic nerve upon lifting the leg while maintaining it extended via pressure on the knee. Frost suspected that the activation of pain during this maneuver was the result of pressure from the hamstring on the nerve.[41] Lazarevic described this test in 1880, one year earlier than Frost, after he observed 6 patients to have increased pain during stretching of the sciatic nerve.[24]

Lazarevic described a 3-step approach to the test[50]:

In the first step, the patient was asked to flex forward, maintaining his knees straight. In step 2, the patient was asked to lie supine and his trunk was slowly brought into flexion, maintaining his knees extended. In step 3, the supine patient had his leg raised with the knee extended. Elevation of the leg was stopped when the patient began to feel pain, and the angle of elevation and amount of pelvic movement was recorded. The patient was then asked to indicate the distribution of pain. All three maneuvers were noted to reproduce discomfort in the sciatic nerve distribution.

In 1884, Lucien de Beurmann concluded that during the lifting of a stretched leg, pain is evoked by stretching of the nerve rather than from the compression of the muscle.[39] Inman and Saunders[36] noted a 2- to 7-mm distal migration of the spinal nerve roots during performance of straight leg raising. Falconer et al.[22] described a 2- to 6-mm downward migration of the nerve roots through their respective foramen during the test. Goddard and Reid[27] noted the L5 nerve root to move 3 mm and the S1 nerve root to move 4–5 mm during performance of SLR.

The classic straight-leg raising test is considered positive when the supine leg is elevated to between 30 and 70 degrees and pain is reproduced down to the posterior thigh below the knee.[52] Pain below 30 degrees is not considered to be related to nerve root irritation.[20] Kosteljanetz et al.[45] noted prolapsed discs in 45 of 52 individuals diagnosed during surgery with a positive straight-leg raise on physical examination. In addition, no "typical" Lasègue's sign with pain into the leg was noted beyond 70 degrees of leg elevation.

Straight-leg raises with pain induced beyond 70 degrees of leg elevation is not believed to be due to nerve root tension. Rather it is thought likely to be related to tightness within the hamstrings or gluteal muscles (Figure 6–5).[80]

Several studies have looked at the sensitivity and specificity of the SLR on physical examination and have compared preoperative results with confirmation at surgery.

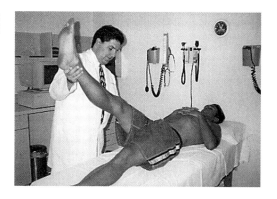

Figure 6–5. Straight leg raising test. Reproduced with permission from Nadler S, Stitik T: Occupational low back pain: history and physical examination. Occup Med 1998;13(1):74.

Spangfort[81] studied 2504 lumbar disc herniation operations and related the incidence of Lasègue's sign to the findings at surgery. He noted that 96.8% of patients with surgically confirmed disc herniations had a positive straight-leg test on physical examination. In patients with herniations from L4 to S1, positive straight-leg raise was noted in 96–98% of cases, while in those with herniations from L1/L2 to L3/L4 it was positive in only 73%. Of note, 88% of those patients with negative exploration had a positive SLR on examination.

Thomas et al.[86,87] found that SLR did not predict the likelihood of disc herniation at operation, though positive straight-leg raise was present in 87% of those with prolapsed discs. The specificity of SLR was 87% with a sensitivity of only 33%. Shiqing et al.[80] noted that 98.2% of patients with a positive SLR test had a disc protrusion at a lower lumbar level. In this study, the combination of SLR with ankle dorsiflexion, compression of the peroneal nerve, and flexion of the neck were positive in 70.8%, 73.5%, and 54.8% of subjects, respectively (Figure 6–6). Kosteljanetz et al.[45,46] found the positive SLR to be present in 49 of 55 patients with unilateral sciatica, 43 of whom

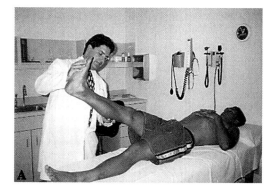
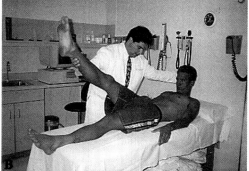

Figure 6–6. Straight-leg-raising provocation with ankle dorsiflexion (**A**) and head flexion (**B**). Reproduced with permission from Nadler S, Stitik T: Occupational low back pain: history and physical examination. Occup Med 1998;13(1):75.

had disc pathology at surgery, although the absence of positive SLR did not preclude the presence of a herniated lumbar disc.

Table 6–7 reviews clinical studies that have examined the prevalence, sensitivity, and specificity of the SLR in lumbar disc herniations. The literature has shown that a positive ipsilateral straight leg-raising test is a sensitive (72–97%) though non-specific (11–66%) test.[3]

Table 6–7. PROVOCATIVE MANEUVER FOR DIAGNOSIS OF LUMBAR DISC HERNIATION

Test	Description	Reliability/Validity Tests	Comments
Straight-leg raise	The supine patient has his/her leg raised with the knee extended. Elevation of the leg is stopped when the patient begins to feel pain, and the type and distribution of the pain as well as the angle of elevation is recorded.	Charnely 1951[8] Sensitivity: 72% Specificity: 66% Prevalence: 84%	N = 88
		Spangfort 1972[81] Sensitivity: 97% Specificity: 11% Prevalence: 88%	N = 2504 Criteria: leg pain
	The test is positive when the angle is between 30 and 70 degrees and pain is reproduced down to the posterior thigh below the knee.[53]	Hakelius 1970,72[30,31] Sensitivity: 96% Specificity: 14% Prevalence: 75%	N = 1986 Criteria: leg pain
		Kosteljanetz 1988[45] Leg pain, Leg or back pain Sensitivity: 76%, 91% Specificity: 45%, 21% Prevalence: 58%, 58%	N = 100
		Kosteljanetz 1984[46] Leg pain, Leg or back pain Sensitivity: 89%, 95% Specificity: 17%, 14% Prevalence: 86%, 86%	N = 52
		Deville 2000[13] Pooled data Sensitivity: 91% Specificity: 26%	Data compiled from the following: Edgar[18], Kosteljanetz[45,46], Gurdjian[29], Jönsson[37], Shiqing[80], Spangfort[81], Kerr[41], Knuttson[42], Aronson[4], Kortelainen[44], Albeck[2], Charnley[8], Hakelius[31], Hirsch[32]

Table 6–7. PROVOCATIVE MANEUVER FOR DIAGNOSIS OF LUMBAR DISC HERNIATION—*cont'd*

Test	Description	Reliability/Validity Tests	Comments
Crossed straight-leg raise	Same as above, with a pain elicited on raising the contralateral leg to the lesion.	Spangfort 1972[81] Sensitivity: 23% Specificity: 88% Prevalence: 86%	$N = 2504$ Criteria: contralateral leg pain
		Hakelius 1972[31] Sensitivity: 27% Specificity: 88% Prevalence: 85%	$N = 1986$ Criteria: contralateral leg pain
		Hudgins 1979[35] Sensitivity: 24% Specificity: 96% Prevalence: 83%	$N = 274$ Criteria: contralateral leg pain
		Kosteljanetz 1984[46] Contralateral leg pain, Contralateral leg or back pain Sensitivity: 24%, 42% Specificity: 100%, 85% Prevalence: 86%, 86%	$N = 52$
		Deville 2000[13] Pooled data Sensitivity: 29% Specificity: 88%	Data compiled from the following: Edgar[18], Kosteljanetz[46], Jönsson[37], Shiqing[80], Spangfort[81], Kerr[41], Knuttson[43], Hakelius[31]
Bowstring sign	After a positive straight-leg raise, slightly flex the knee and apply pressure to the tibial nerve in the popliteal fossa. Compression of the sciatic nerve reproduces leg pain.[12]	Supik 1994[85] Positive in 71% of patients with known lumbar disc herniation.	
Slump test	The patient is seated with legs together and knees against the examining table. The patient slumps forward as far as possible, and the examiner applies firm pressure to bow the subject's back while keeping sacrum vertical. The patient is then asked to flex the head, and pressure added to the neck flexion. Lastly the examiner asks the subject to	No data	

Continued

Table 6–7. PROVOCATIVE MANEUVER FOR DIAGNOSIS OF LUMBAR DISC HERNIATION—*cont'd*

Test	Description	Reliability/Validity Tests	Comments
	extend the knee and dorsiflexion at the ankle is added.[12]		
Ankle dorsiflexion test (Braggard's sign)	Elevate the leg as in SLR to the point of pain provocation. Drop the leg to a non-painful range, and dorsiflex the ipsilateral ankle.[53]	Stankovic 1999[83] 94.2% positive slump test in patients with frank disc herniation 78% in those with bulging discs 75% with no disc findings	
Femoral nerve stretch test	With the patient prone, the examiner places a palm at the popliteal fossa as the knee is dorsiflexed. Pain is produced in the anterior aspect of the thigh and/or back. For the results to be positive, the test should produce pain in the distribution of the patient's complaints.[95]	Positive in 84–95% of patients with a high lumbar disc[1,9,75]	Possibly best test for clinical diagnosis of high lumbar disc herniation.
Crossed femoral nerve stretch test	With the patient prone, the examiner places a palm at the popliteal fossa as the asymptomatic knee is dorsiflexed. Pain is produced in the anterior aspect of the symptomatic thigh and/or back. For the results to be positive, the test should produce pain in the distribution of the patient's complaints.[47]	No data	
Waddell signs	Distraction tests: Once a positive physical finding is demonstrated; this finding is then checked with the patient distracted. Findings that are present only on formal examination and not at other times may have non-organic component.	McCombe 1989[56] Reliability data, k coefficients: Distraction: –0.16 to 0.40 Over-reaction: 0.29 to 0.46 Abnormal sensory/motor: -0.03 to 0.26	Kappa agreement coefficients in which a score of 1 signified complete agreement, 0 signified no agreement, and –1 signified complete disagreement of several physical examination signs. A coefficient of 0.4 was selected for the "cutoff" point for reliability.
	Over-reaction: May take the form of extremes of verbalization,	Simulation: 0.25 to 0.48	Kummel[48] assessed limitation of shoulder

Table 6–7. PROVOCATIVE MANEUVER FOR DIAGNOSIS OF LUMBAR DISC HERNIATION—*cont'd*

Test	Description	Reliability/Validity Tests	Comments
	facial expression, muscle tension and tremor, collapsing, or sweating.	Superficial tenderness: 0.17 to 0.29	motion with production of low back pain and low back pain resulting from active cervical motion in addition to Waddell's signs. Prognosis for return to work was poor in subjects with positive Waddell signs; 52.9% did not return to work.
	Regional disturbances: Involving a widespread region of neighboring parts such as the leg below the knee, entire leg, or quarter or half of the body. The essential feature is divergence from the accepted neuroanatomy.		
	Simulation tests: On formal exam, a particular movement causes the patient to report pain. The movement is then simulated without being performed. If pain is reported, a non-organic influence is suggested.		
	Tenderness: Non-organic tenderness may be either superficial or non-anatomic. Superficial: The skin is tender to light pinch over a wide area of lumbar skin. Non-anatomic: Deep tenderness is felt over a wide area, is not localized to one structure, and often extends to the thoracic spine, sacrum, or pelvis[92].		
Hoover test	Performed to assess the patient's voluntary effort. The patient's heels are cupped by the clinician and the patient is instructed to individually raise his/her legs. Increased pressure should be felt on the untested cupped heel if true volitional effort is provided.	No study has been performed to formally evaluate the sensitivity, specificity, and reliability.	

Andersson and Deyo[3] reported the positive predictive value of the straight-leg test in individuals with a great probability of having a disc herniation to be 67%, whereas the negative predictive value was determined to be 57%. The positive predictive value in patients with a low probability – including patients with no sciatica or neurologic signs or symptoms – was determined to be 4% with a negative predictive value of 99%.

Deville et al.[13] determined that the pooled sensitivity for straight-leg raising test was 91% (95% confidence interval [CI]: 0.82–0.94), and the pooled specificity was 26% (95% CI: 0.16–0.38). The mean predictive value of a positive was 89%, and the negative predictive value was 33%. Deville and colleagues concluded that the studies evaluated were not representative of the general population, with high prevalence resulting in consequentially higher positive predictive values for SLR. It was also suggested that these studies were prone to verification bias, as nearly all studies were retrospective and based on data obtained on surgical patients. Flaws in the design of these studies – including independency of interpretation, verification bias, and retrospective design – were also noted.

Supik and Broom[85] compared the results of straight-leg raising, Lasègue's, and ankle dorsiflexion and crossed SLR (see below) with their patients' postoperative findings. The straight-leg lift was considered positive if hip, buttock, and leg pain were elicited, while Lasègue's sign was performed by raising the leg until pain was elicited then lowering the leg 10–15 degrees to reduce discomfort with subsequent ankle dorsiflexion intensifying the pain. The straight-leg lift was positive in 96% of patients and Lasègue's sign was positive 71% of the time. In this study of patients, the straight-leg sign was more sensitive than the other maneuvers, independent of level or location of the disc.

Jönsson and Strömqvist[37,38] graded the SLR depending on whether it was positive at 0–30 degrees, positive at 30–60 degrees, positive at greater than 60 degrees, or negative. In this study, 86% of patients had a positive SLR preoperatively, 42% occurred below 30 degrees, 26% between 30 and 60 degrees, and 18% above 60 degrees. The authors found an almost linear correlation between a positive SLR and pain at rest, pain at night, pain upon coughing, and reduction of walking capacity.

Crossed Straight-leg Raising Test

In 1901, Fajersztajn first described the crossed straight-leg raising test after noting on cadaveric study that SLR not only stretched the ipsilateral root, but also pulled laterally on the dural sac, stretching the opposite root.[21] Woodhall and Hayes[98] demonstrated the crossed straight-leg raise (CSLR) to be strongly predictive for a disc herniation, noting its presence in 92 of 95 subjects with large disc herniations. Hudgins[35] evaluated 351 patients thought to have a herniated disc on physical exam and found the CSLR test to be positive in 97% of those with a herniated disc; only 64% of subjects with SLR alone had a herniated disc.

Kosteljanetz et al.[45] also noted a significant propensity for the CSLR test to be positive, because 19 of 20 patients with this finding were noted to have disc herniations at surgery. The CSLR has also been correlated with outcome of treatment. Woodall and Hayes[97] and Edgar and Park[18] noted 32% and 44% of patients with positive findings, respectively, required surgical intervention.

Khuffash and Porter[42] examined the prognostic significance of the CSLR in 113 patients who had root tension signs from a lumbar disc lesion. A positive CSLR sign was found to be associated with poor prognosis for conservative management. Thirty percent of patients who presented with asymptomatic disc protrusion and 59% of those requiring surgery had positive crossed-leg pain, with 58% of patients with crossed-leg pain ultimately requiring discectomy. Certainly, there may have been some selection bias involved in choosing those who would require operative treatment.

Several studies have looked at the specificity and sensitivity of the CSLR. Thomas et al.[86,87] determined that the crossed Lasègue sign had a specificity of 100% with a low sensitivity.

Andersson and Deyo[3] examined the prevalence, sensitivity, and specificity of the CSLR. They showed that the CSLR is less sensitive (23–42%), but much more specific (85–100%) compared with the SLR, with a positive predictive value of 79% and a negative predictive value of 44%. The positive predictive value in patients with a low probability including patients with no sciatica or neurological signs or symptoms was determined to be 7%, with a negative predictive value of 98%.

Deville et al.[13] determined that the pooled sensitivity of CSLR was 29% (95% CI: 0.24–0.34), and the pooled specificity was 88% (95% CI: 0.86–0.90) with a positive predictive value of 92% at a prevalence of 0.82, and a negative predictive value of 22%.

Bowstring Sign

In 1888, Gower described the bowstring sign or posterior tibial nerve sign (Figure 6–7)[11]:

> In this test, when a positive straight leg raising test was noted, the leg was slightly flexed and pressure was applied to the tibial nerve in the popliteal fossa. Popliteal space compression was noted to be anatomically correlated with stretch of the sciatic nerve.

Supik and Broom[85] examined the sensitivity of several diagnostic signs of lower lumbar nerve root compression associated with disc herniation and found the bowstring test to be positive 71% of the time.

The Slump Test

The slump test appears to have been initially described by Cyriax in 1942, who noted that sciatic pain was reproduced in the seated individual with the knee of the painful

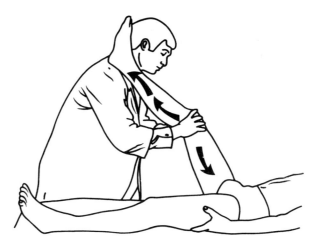

Figure 6–7. The bowstring sign. From MacNab I, Backache. Baltimore, Williams & Wilkins, 1977, with permission.

leg extended with the addition of cervical spine and trunk flexion.[12] It is described as follows (Figure 6–8):

> The subject sits straight with arms behind back, legs together, and posterior aspect of knees against the edge of the couch. The subject slumps as far as possible, producing full trunk flexion; the examiner applies firm pressure to bow the subject's back, and being careful to keep sacrum vertical. The subject is asked to flex his or her head, and over-pressure is then added to the neck flexion. While maintaining full spinal and neck flexion with over-pressure, the examiner asks the subject to extend the knee. Dorsiflexion is then added to knees extension. Neck flexion is then released, and the subject is asked to further extend the knee.

The Ankle Dorsiflexion Test (Braggard's Sign)

Straight-leg raising can be further enhanced by different variations, including the ankle dorsiflexion test (see Figure 6–6A). In 1884, Fajersztajn added the foot dorsiflexion test and neck flexion test, two provocative maneuvers that exacerbate leg pain by further increasing the pressure on the dura around the nerve root.[21] The ankle dorsiflexion test, or Braggard's sign, involves elevating the leg to the point of pain provocation, dropping the leg down to a non-painful range, and subsequent dorsiflexion of the ipsilateral ankle, increasing tension in the sciatic nerve distribution.[52]

Stankovic et al.[83] noted that 94.2% of patients with frank disc herniation had pain reproduction with slump testing compared with 78% of those with bulging discs and 75% with no positive findings.

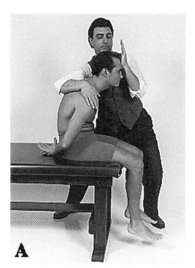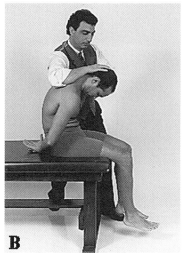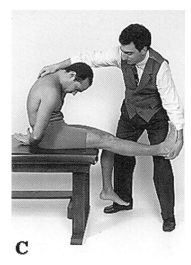

Figure 6–8. Slump test. **A:** Stage I. **B:** Stage II. **C:** Stage III. Reproduced with permission from Geraci MC, Alleva JT, McAdam FB. The physical examination of the spine and its functional kinetic chain. In Cole AJ, Herring SA (eds), The Low Back Pain Handbook: a Guide for the Practicing Clinician, 2nd edn. Philadelphia: Hanley & Belfus, 2003, p. 87.

Femoral Nerve Stretch Test

In 1918, Wassermann described the femoral stretching test after a systematic search for an objective physical sign in soldiers who complained of pain in the anterior thigh and shin when Lasègue's sign was absent:[95]

> With the patient prone, the examiner places a palm at the popliteal fossa as the knee is strongly dorsiflexed. Excruciating pain is produced in the anterior aspect of the thigh and/or back. Pain was apparent by facial grimacing, loud outcries, and reflex reaching for the groin area. For the results to be positive, the test should produce pain, usually very severe, in the distribution of the patient's complaints.

The pathophysiologic response is incompletely understood, but the pain is assumed to be caused by stretching of an irritable femoral nerve when there is compression of the L2, L3, or L4 nerve roots.[17] It has been observed that these traction forces result in a 2-mm movement of the L4 root.[19]

Overall, high lumbar disc herniations affecting these upper nerve roots are more challenging to diagnose owing to their unusual clinical presentation and overall rarity in comparison to those affecting the L4/L5 and L5/S1 levels.[1,9,75] The femoral nerve stretch test is probably the single best screening test to evaluate lumbar radiculopathy secondary to an upper lumbar disc herniation. It has been shown to be positive in 84–95% of patients with a high lumbar disc.[1,9,75] Estridge[19] demonstrated a strong correlation with L3/L4 disc herniation and a positive femoral stretch test, and Christodoulides[9] noted lateral L4/L5 disc protrusions causing L4 nerve root involvement in 95% of patients with a positive femoral nerve stretch test. Geraci and Alleva[25] reported increased sensitivity with the addition of hip extension to the femoral nerve stretch test, though no specific research protocol was utilized to support this assertion (Figure 6–9). Penning and Wilmink[72] showed that, with extension of the spine, the anterior dural surface at the L3/L4 and L4/L5 levels were indented by posterior bulging of the discs, which may lend support to the added benefit of extension during the femoral nerve stretch test.

The femoral stretching test is not pathognomonic for an upper lumbar disc herniation. It is likely to be positive in several conditions, including all forms of femoral neuropathy, tight iliopsoas or rectus femoris muscles, or pathology in or about the hip joint.[66]

The Crossed Femoral Nerve Test

The crossed femoral stretch test (CFST) was first described by Cyriax in 1947 (the original description is unavailable).[47] Crossed femoral stretch testing has received very little attention in the literature. Dyck[17] suggested that stretching of the psoas and quadriceps femoris muscles puts traction on the third and fourth lumbar nerve roots. Kreitz et al.[47] reported a case in which the CFST was positive in a patient with an L3/L4 lateral disc herniation. Nadler et al.[67] reported the presence of the crossed femoral nerve stretch test in two cases of high lumbar radiculopathies who presented with a positive femoral nerve stretch test along with a CSFT; however, unlike the

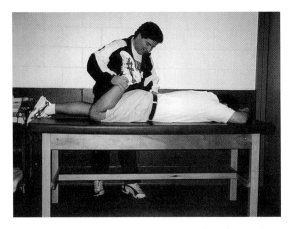
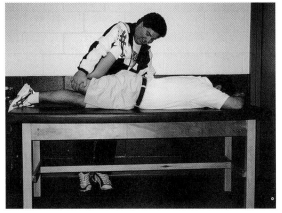

Figure 6–9. A: Femoral nerve stretch test (FNST). **B:** Enhancement of FNST with hip extension. Reproduced with permission from Nadler SF, Malanga GA, Stitik TP, et al. The crossed femoral nerve stretch test to improve the diagnostic sensitivity for the high lumbar radiculopathy: two case reports. Arch Phys Med Rehabil 2001;82:522–523.

previous cases described in the literature, both patients responded well to conservative treatment.

A CSFT may further support the diagnosis of a high lumbar radiculopathy, and possibly enhance the specificity of the femoral nerve stretch test.[67] Further study is needed to identify the prevalence of the CSFT in patients with upper lumbar radiculopathies and in patients with confirmed herniated lumbar intervertebral discs.

Waddell Signs

In 1980, Waddell et al.[92] described a standardized group of five types of physical signs: tenderness, simulation, distraction, regional, and over-reaction (Figure 6–10). The acronym DORST is used to identify the five nonorganic signs:

- **D**istraction: A positive physical finding is demonstrated in the routine manner; this finding is then checked while the patient's attention is distracted. Findings that are present only on formal examination and disappear at other times may have a non-organic component.
- **O**ver-reaction: During the examination, these reactions may take the form of disproportionate verbalization, facial expressions, muscle tension and tremor, collapsing, or sweating.

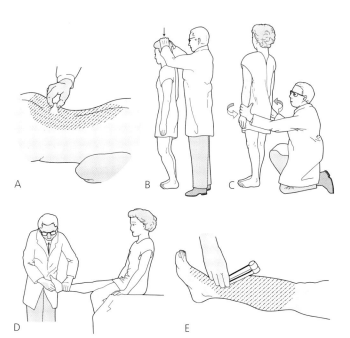

Figure 6–10. Waddell signs. **A:** Superficial sensitivity to light pinch. **B:** Axial loading causing low back pain. **C:** Passive rotation of the shoulders and pelvis in the same plane causing back pain. **D:** Straight-leg raising test in the seated position. **E:** Stocking distribution of sensory deficit. Adapted with permission.

- Regional disturbances: These involve a widespread region of neighboring parts such as the leg below the knee, entire leg, or quarter or half of the body. The essential feature is divergence from the accepted neuroanatomy.
- Simulation tests: These give the patient the impression that a particular examination is being carried out when in fact it is not. On formal examination, a particular movement causes the patient to report pain. The movement is then simulated without actually being performed. If pain is reported, a non-organic influence is suggested.
- Tenderness: Related to physical disease, this is usually localized to a particular neuromuscular structure. Non-organic tenderness may be either superficial or non-anatomic:
  Superficial – The skin is tender to light pinch over a wide area of lumbar skin.
  Nonanatomic – Deep tenderness is felt over a wide area, is not localized to one structure, and often extends to the thoracic spine, sacrum, or pelvis.

These provocative maneuvers aid in the identification of individuals who have physical findings without anatomic cause.[66] Three or more of the five types is considered clinically significant and is correlated with a significant psychological overlay consisting of hypochondriasis, hysteria, and depression utilizing the MMPI psychological screening tool.[91–93] These signs were found to be more than 80% reproducible with a κ coefficient between 0.55 and 0.71. Multiple positive signs should be considered a "yellow flag" and suggest that the patient does not have a straightforward physical problem, and psychological factors need to be considered.[53] Multiple positive signs should not be used to indicate that a subject is malingering. Repeated testing and numerous questions in combination with the results of the entire physical examination will improve reliability.[3]

The Hoover Test

The Hoover test may be performed to assess the patient's voluntary effort. The patient's heels are cupped by the clinician, and the patient is instructed to individually raise his or her legs. Increased pressure should be felt on the untested cupped heal if true volitional effort is provided. No study has been performed to formally evaluate the sensitivity, specificity, and reliability of the Hoover test.

Other Tests

Kummel[48] assessed the prognostic value of the limitation of shoulder motion with production of low back pain, as well as low back pain resulting from active cervical motion in addition to Waddell's signs. Prognosis for return to work was poor in subjects with positive Waddell signs – 52.9% did not return to work. However, with the additional finding of limitation of shoulder motion resulting in low back pain, the prognosis was worse – 69.6% did not return to work. If cervical motion additionally produced low back pain, the outlook was even poorer, with no return to work in 73.1%.

Inter-tester and Intra-tester Reliability Studies for LBP Maneuvers

Waddell et al.[93] noted moderate reliability (0.56) between examiners performing SLR on patients with low back injury. McCombe et al.[56] used κ agreement coefficients in which a score of 1 signified complete agreement, 0 signified no agreement, and −1 signified complete disagreement of several physical examination signs. A κ coefficient of 0.4 was selected for the "cutoff" point for reliability (Table 6–8).

Deyo et al.[14] reviewed the inter-observer agreement of several common tests performed in patients with low back pain (Table 6–9).

Table 6–8. INTER-RATER RELIABILITY FOR LOW BACK EXAMINATION

Sign	Kappa Coefficient
Bowstring sign	0.11–0.49
Femoral stretch sign	0.27–0.77
CSLR test	0.02–0.74
SLR test reproducing patient symptoms	0.36–0.81
SLR test reproducing back and leg pain	0.44–0.81
MMT	0.04–1.0
Waddell signs: superficial tenderness	0.17–0.29
Waddell signs: simulation	0.25–0.48
Waddell signs: distraction	−0.16–0.40
Waddell signs: over-reaction	0.29–0.46
Waddell signs: abnormal sensory/motor	−0.03–0.26
ROM – flexion	0.78–0.91
Movement – rotation pain	0.10–0.58
Movement – extension pain	0.31–0.57
Movement – flexion pain	0.52–0.56
Tenderness on palpation	0.28–0.50

Reproduced with permission from McCombe PF, Fairbank JCt, Cockersole BC, Pynsent PB. Volvo Award in Clinical Sciences. Reproducibility of physical signs in low-back. Spine 1989;14:908–918.

Table 6–9. INTER-OBSERVER AGREEMENT OF THE SEVERAL CLINICAL EXAMINATIONS IN PATIENTS WITH LOW BACK PAIN

SLR	Inter-Observer Agreement	Author
SLR with inclinometer	0.78–0.97 (R)	Hoeler and Tobis[33] Hsieh et al[34]
SLR with goniometer	0.69 (R)	McCombe et al.[56]
SLR causes leg pain	0.66 (κ)	McCombe et al.[56]
SLR visual <75	0.56 (κ)	Waddell et al.[92]
CSLR	0.74 (κ)	McCombe et al.[56]
Ankle dorsiflexion weakness	1.00 (κ)	McCombe et al.[56]
Great toe extensor weakness	0.65 (κ)	McCombe et al.[56]
Ankle reflexes normal *Inappropiate signs*	0.39–0.50 (κ)	McCombe et al.[56]
Superficial tenderness	0.29 (κ)	McCombe et al.[56]
Axial loading	0.25 (κ)	McCombe et al.[56]
SLR with distraction causing pain	0.40 (κ)	McCombe et al.[56]
Unexplainable neurologic exam	0.03 (κ)	McCombe et al.[56]
Over-reaction	0.29 (κ)	McCombe et al.[56]

Reproduced with permission from Deyo RA, Rainville J, Kent DL. What can the history and physical examination tell us about low back pain? JAMA 1992; 268:760–765.

Conclusion

In contrast to physical examination of the extremities, the specialized provocative tests have been well studied for the lumbar spine. Some tests, such as straight-leg raising, are highly sensitive but have only fair specificity. Other tests, such as the crossed SLR, are highly specific but have low sensitivity. This information is valuable to the clinician assessing individuals with LBP with and without radicular complaints in order to better understand the results of their physical exam. Knowledge of the varying reliability of the individual maneuvers raises some questions and answers others. Overall, it is important to understand how a test is performed, but it is equally important to understand what it truly means in the context of the entire clinical exam.

REFERENCES

1. Abdullah AF, Wolber PG, Warfield JR, Gunadi IK. Surgical management of extreme lateral lumbar disc herniations. Neurosurgery 1988;22:648–653.
2. Albeck MJ. A critical assessment of clinical diagnosis of disc herniation in patients with monoradicular sciatica. Acta Neurochir (Wien) 1996;138:40–44.
3. Andersson GB, Deyo RA. History and physical examination in patients with herniated lumbar discs. Spine 1996;21(suppl. 24):10–18S.
4. Aronson HA, et al. Herniated upper lumbar discs. J Bone Joint Surg Am 1963;45:311–317.
5. Biering-Sorensen F. Physical measurements as risk indicators for low-back trouble over a one-year period. Spine 1984;9:106–119.
6. Burdett RGh, Brown KE, Fall MP. Reliability and validity of our instruments for measuring lumbar spine and pelvic positions. Phys Ther 1986;66:677–684.
7. Caillet R. Low Back Pain Syndrome, 4th edn. Philadelphia: FA Davis, 1988.
8. Charnley J. Orthopaedic signs in the diagnosis of disc protrusion, with special reference to the straight leg raising test. Lancet 1951;260:186–192.
9. Christodoulides AN. Ipsilateral sciatica on the femoral nerve stretch test is pathognomonic of an L4/5 disc protrusion. J Bone Joint Surg Br 1989;71:88–89.
10. Cozen LN. Tests for chronic back pain. Contemp Orthopaed 1992;24:405–408.
11. Cram RH. A sign of the sciatic nerve root pressure. J Bone Joint Surg [Br] 1953;35:192–195.
12. Cyriax J. Perineuritis. Br Med J 1942;1:578–580.
13. Deville WL, van der Windt DA, Dzaferagic A, Bezemer PD, Bouter LM. The test of Lasègue: systematic review of the accuracy in diagnosing herniated discs. Spine 2000;25:1140–1147.
14. Deyo RA, Rainville J, Kent DL. What can the history and physical examination tell us about low back pain? JAMA 1992;268:760–765.
15. Dillard J, et al. Motion of the lumbar spine: reliability of two measurement techniques. Spine 1991; 16:321–324.
16. Dopf CA, et al. Analysis of spine motion variability using a computerized goniometer compared to physical examination: a prospective clinical study. Spine 1994;19:586–595.
17. Dyck P. The femoral nerve traction test with lumbar disc protrusions. Surg Neurol 1976;6:163–166.
18. Edgar MA, Park WM. Induced pain patterns on passive straight leg raising in lower lumbar disc protrusion. J Bone Joint Surg 1974;56B:658–666.
19. Estridge MN, Rothe SA, Johnson NG. The femoral stretching test: a valuable sign in diagnosing upper lumbar disc herniation. J Neurosurg 1982;57:813–817.
20. Fahrni WH. Observation on straight leg raising with special reference to nerve root adhesions. Can J Surg 1966;9:44–48.
21. Fajersztajn J. Ueber das gekreutzte ischiaphanomen. Wiener Klinische Wochenschrift 1901;14:41–47.
22. Falconer MA, McGeorge M, Begg AC. Observations on the cause and mechanism of symptom production in sciatica and low back pain. J Neurol Neurosurg Psychiat 1948;11:13–26.
23. Fitzgerald GK, Wynveen KJ, Rheault W, Rothschild B. Objective assessment with establishment of normal values for lumbar spinal range of motion. Phys Ther 1983;63:1776–1781.
24. Frost JJ. Contribution a l'étude clinique de la sciatique. Thèse no. 33, Faculté de Médecine, Paris, 1881.
25. Geraci MC, Alleva JT. Physical examination of the spine and its functional kinetic chain. In Cole AJ, Herrring SA (eds), The Low Back Pain Handbook. Philadelphia: Hanley & Belfus, 1996, p. 60.
26. Gill K, Krag MH, Johnson GB, Haugh LD, Pope MH. Repeatability of four clinical methods for assessment of lumbar spinal motion. Spine 1988;13:50–53.
27. Goddard MD, Reid JD. Movements induced by straight leg raising in the lumbosacral roots, nerves and plexus and in the intrapelvic section of the sciatic nerve. J Neurol Neurosurg Psychiat 1965;28:12–18.
28. Gonnella C, et al. Reliability in evaluating passive intervertebral motion. Phys Ther 1982;62:436–444.
29. Gurdjian ES, Webster JE, Ostrowski AZ, et al. Herniated lumbar intervertebral discs: an analysis of 1176 operated cases. J Trauma 1961;1:158–176.
30. Hakelius A. Prognosis in sciatica. Acta Orthop Scand 1970;129(suppl.):1–70.
31. Hakelius A, et al. The comparative reliability of preoperative diagnostic methods in lumbar disc surgery. Acta Orthop Scand 1972;43:234–238.

32. Hirsch C, Nachemson A. The reliability of lumbar disk surgery. Clin Orthop 1963;29:189–195.

33. Hoehler FK, Tobis JS. Low back pain and its treatment by spinal manipulation: measures of flexibility and asymmetry. Rhematol Rehabil 1982;21:21–26.

34. Hseih CY, et al. Straight leg raising test: compression of three instruments. Phys Ther 1983;63:1429–1432.

35. Hudgins WR. The crossed straight leg raising test: a diagnostic sign of herniated disc. J Occup Med 1979;21:407–408.

36. Inman VT, Saunders JB. The clinico-anatomical aspects of the lumbosacral region. Radiology 1942; 38:669–678.

37. Jönsson B, Strömqvist B. The straight leg raising test and the severity of symptoms in lumbar disc herniation. Spine 1995;20:27–30.

38. Jönsson B, Strömquvist B. Symptoms and signs in degeneration of the lumbar spine: a prospective, consecutive study of 300 operated patients. J Bone Joint Surg 1993;75B:381–385.

39. Karbowski K, Radanov BP. Historical perspective: the history of the discovery of the sciatica stretching phenomenon. Spine 1995;20:1315–1317.

40. Keely J, et al. Quantification of lumbar function. 5: Reliability of range-of-motion measures in the sagittal plane and in-vivo torso rotation measurement technique. Spine 1986;11:31–35.

41. Kerr RSC, et al. The value of accurate clinical assessment in the surgical management of the lumbar disc protrusion. J Neurol Neurosurg Psych 1988;51:169–173.

42. Khuffash B, Porter RW. Cross leg pain and trunk list. Spine 1989;14:602–603.

43. Knutsson B. Comparative value of electromyographic, myelographic and clinical–neurological examinations in diagnosis of lumbar root compression syndrome. Acta Orthop Scand 1961;49(suppl.):1–134.

44. Kortelainen P, Puranen J, Koivisto E, Lahde S. Symptoms and signs of sciatica and their relation to the localization of the lumbar disc herniation. Spine 1985;10:8–92.

45. Kosteljanetz M, Bang F, Schmidt-Olsen S. The clinical significance of straight leg raising (Lasègue's sign) in the diagnosis of prolapsed lumbar disc: interobserver variation and correlation with surgical findings. Spine 1988;13:393–395.

46. Kosteljanetz M, Esperen JO, Halburt H, Miletic T. Predictive value of clinical and surgical findings in patients with lumbago-sciatica: a prospective study (part 1). Acta Neurochirurgica 1984;73:67–76.

47. Kreitz BG, Cote P, Yong-Hing K. Crossed femoral stretching test: a case report. Spine 1996;21:1584–1586.

48. Kummel BM. Nonorganic signs of significance in low back pain. Spine 1996;21:1077–1081.

49. Lauder TD. Physical examination signs, clinical symptoms, and their relationship to electrodiagnostic findings and the presence of radiculopathy. Phys Med Rehabil Clin N Am 2002;13:451–467.

50. Lindblom K, Hultqvist G. Absorption of protruded disc tissue. J Bone Joint Surg Am 1950;32:557–560.

51. Loebl WY. Measurement of spinal posture and range of spinal movement. Ann Phys Med 1967;9: 103–110.

52. Macrae IF, Wright V. Measurements of back movement. Ann Rheum Dis 1969;28:584–589.

53. Magee DJ. Orthopedic Physical Asessement. Philadelphia: WB Saunders, 1992.

54. Main CJ, Waddell G. Spine update. Behavioral responses to examination: a reappraisal of the interpretation of "nonorganic signs." Spine 1998;23:2376–2371.

55. Mayer TG, Tencer AF, et al. Use of noninvasive techniques for quantification of spinal range of motion in normal subjects and chronic low back dysfunction patients. Spine 1984;9:588–595.

56. McCombe PF, Fairbank JCt, Cockersole BC, Pynsent PB. 1989 Volvo Award in Clinical Sciences. Reproducibility of physical signs in low-back. Spine 1989;14:908–918.

57. McGill SM. Low Back Disorders: Evidence-based Prevention and Rehabilitation. Champaign, IL: Human Kinetics, 2002.

58. McGregor AH, McCarthy ID, Hughes SP. Motion characteristics of the lumbar spine in the normal population. Spine 1995;20:2421–2428.

59. Mellin G. Correlations of spinal mobility with degree of chronic low back pain after correction for age and arthometric factors. Spine 1987;12:464–468.

60. Mellin G. Measurement of thoracolumbar posture and mobility with a Myrin inclinometer. Spine 1986; 11:759–762.

61. Mellin G. Method and instrument for noninvasive measurements of thoracolumbar rotation. Spine 1987; 12:28–31.

62. Merrit J, McLean T, Erickson R. Measurement of trunk flexibility in normal subjects: reproducibility of three clinical methods. Mayo Clin Pro 1986;61:192–197.

63. Miller SA, Mayer T, Cox R, Gatchel RJ. Reliability problems associated with the modified Schober technique for true lumbar flexion measurement. Spine 1992;17:345–348.
64. Moll JMH, Wright V. Normal range of spinal mobility: an objective clinical study. Ann Rheum Dis 1971;30:381–386.
65. Mooney V. Physical measurement of the lumbar spine. Phys Med Rehabil Clin N Am 1998;9:391–410.
66. Nadler SF, Campagnolo DI, Tomaio AC, Stitik TP. High lumbar disc: diagnostic and treatment dilemma. Am J Med Rehabil 1998;77:538–544.
67. Nadler SF, et al. The crossed femoral nerve stretch test to improve diagnostic sensitivity for the high lumbar radiculopathy: two case reports. Arch Phys Med Rehabil 2001;82:522–523.
68. Nattrass CL, Nitschke JE, Disler PB, Chou MJ, Ooi KT. Lumbar spine range of motion as a measure of physical and functional impairment: an investigation of validity. Clin Rehabil 1999;13(3):211–218.
69. Ng JK, Kippers V, Richardson CA, Parnianpour M. Range of motion and lordosis of the lumbar spine: reliability of measurement and normative values. Spine 2001;26:53–60.
70. O'Keeffe ST, Smith T, Valacio R, et al. A comparison of two techniques for ankle jerk assessment in elderly subjects. Lancet 1994;344:1619–1620.
71. Ohlen C, et al. Measurement of spinal configuration and mobility with Debrunner's Kyphometer. Spine 1989;14:580–583.
72. Penning L, Wilmink JT. Biomechanics of lumbosacral dural sac: a study of flexion–extension myelography. Spine 1981;6:398–408.
73. Pearcy MJ, Tibrewal SB. Axial rotation and lateral bending in the normal lumbar spine measured by three-dimensional radiography. Spine 1984;9:582.
74. Pearcy MJ, Portek J, Shepherd J. Three dimensional x-ray analysis of normal measurement in the lumbar spine. Spine 1984;9:294.
75. Porchet F, Frankhauser H, de Tribolet N. Extreme lateral lumbar disc herniation: a clinical presentation of 178 patients. Acta Neurochir (Wien) 1994;127:203–209.
76. Portek I, Pearcy MJ, Reader GP, et al. Correlation between radiographic and clinical measurements of lumbar spine movement. Br J Rheumatol 1983;22:197–205.
77. Reynolds PM. Measurement of spinal mobility: a comparison of three methods. Rheumatol Rehabil 1975;14(3):180–185.
78. Saur PMM, Ensink F-Bm, et al. lumbar range of motion: reliability and validity of the inclinometer technique in the clinical measurement of trunk flexibility. Spine 1996;21:1332–1338.
79. Schober P. The lumbar vertebral column and backaches. Much Med Wschr 1937;84:336.
80. Shiqing X, Quanzhi Z, Dehao F. Significance of the straight leg raising test in the diagnosis and clinical evaluation of lower lumbar intervertebral disc protrusion. J Bone Joint Surg 1987;69A:517–522.
81. Spangfort, E. Lasègue's sign in patients with lumbar disc herniation. Acta Orthop Scand 1971;42:459–460.
82. Spengler DM, Ouellette AE, Battie M, Zeh J. Elective discectomy for herniation of lumbar disc. J Bone Joint Surg 1990;72A:230–237.
83. Stankovic R, Johnell O, Maly P, Willner S. Use of lumbar extension, slump test, physical and neurological examination in the evaluation of patients with suspected herniated nucleus pulposus: a prospective clinical study. Man Ther 1999;4(1):25–32.
84. Sullivan MS, Dickinson CE, Troup JD. The influence of age and gender on lumbar spine sagittal plane range of motion: a study of 1126 healthy subjects. Spine 1994;19:682–686.
85. Supik LF, Broom MJ. Sciatic tension signs and lumbar disc herniation. Spine 1994;19:1066–1069.
86. Thomas M, et al. Surgical treatment of low backache and sciatica. Lancet 1983;2:1437–1439.
87. Thomas E, Silman AJ, Papageorgiou AC, Macfarlane GJ, Croft PR. Association between measures of spinal mobility and low back pain: an analysis of new attenders in primary care. Spine 1998;23:343–347.
88. Van Adrichmem JAM, Van der Krost JK. Assessment of the flexibility of the lumbar spine: a pilot study in children and adolescents. Scand J Rheumatol 1973;2:87–91.
89. Victor M, Ropper AH, Adams RD. Adams & Victor's Principles of Neurology, 7th edn. New York: McGraw-Hill Professional, 2001.
90. Viitanen JV, Kokko ML, Heikkila S, Kautiainen H. Assessment of thoracolumbar rotation in ankylosing spondylitis: a simple tape method. Clin Rheumatol 1999;18:152–157.
91. Vucetic N, Svensson O. Physical signs in lumbar disc hernia. Clin Orthop 1996;(333):192–201.
92. Waddell G, McCulloch JA, Kummel E, Venner RM. Nonorganic physical signs in low-back pain. Spine 1980;5:117–125.

93. Waddel G, et al. Normality and reliability in the clinical assessment of backache. Br Med J (Clin Res) 1982;284:1519–1523.

94. Waddell G, et al. Objective clinical evaluation of physical impairment in chronic low back pain. Spine 1992;17:617–628.

95. Wassermann S. Ueber ein neues Schenkelnersymptom nebstr Bemerkungen zur Diagnostik der Schenkelnerverkrankungen. Dtsch Z Nervenbeilk 1918/19;43:140–143.

96. White AA, Panjabi MM. Clinical Biomechanics of the Spine. Philadelphia: JB Lippincott, 1978.

97. Williams R, Binkley R, et al. Reliability of the modified-modified Schober and double inclinometer methods for measuring lumbar flexion extension. Phys Ther 1993;73;26–37.

98. Woodhall B, Hayes G. The well leg raising test of Fajerstajn in the diagnosis of ruptured lumbar intervertebral disc. J Bone Joint Surg 1950;32A:786–792.

Chapter 7

Physical Examination of the Sacroiliac Joint

JENNIFER SOLOMON, MD • SCOTT F. NADLER, DO •
HEIDI PRATHER, DO

Introduction

Evaluating and treating the patient with sacroiliac joint (SIJ) pain can be difficult. There is no gold standard for diagnosis by physical exam, and diagnosis often becomes one of exclusion. Complicating the clinical picture are the biomechanics of the SIJ and its interactions with the surrounding hip, pubic symphysis, and spine, which are complex. Researchers are still producing new information on force and load transmission across the pelvis. Clinicians need to keep the SIJ within the differential diagnosis of low back pain with radiculopathy, and so perform the standard physical assessment including provocative maneuvers and motion testing.

Anatomy and Biomechanics

The joints of the pelvis are intrinsically stable, and proper functioning is essential for normal biomechanics about the pelvis. High forces and repetitive loads can lead to ligamentous, muscle, and bone injuries or overuse syndromes. The pelvis also adapts to injuries of the spine and the lower extremities, which may lead to maladaptive syndromes.[51] SIJ dysfunction occurs when there is an alteration of the structural or positional relationship of the sacrum on the ilium. This dysfunction commonly originates through asymmetrical force transmission as well as degenerative changes.[51] Despite these well-known biomechanical changes it is still unclear whether altered motion at the SIJ is the source of pain.

227

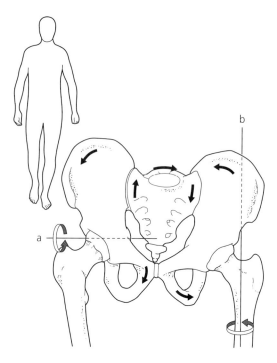

Figure 7–1. Biomechanics of the sacroiliac joints during walking: (a) rotation of the iliac bone at the non-weight-bearing side around a frontal horizontal axis; (b) rotation of the iliac bone at the weight-bearing side around a vertical axis. Adapted with permission from Ombregt L, Bisschop P, Ter Veer HJ, Van de Velde. Applied anatomy of the sacroiliac joint. In Ombregt L, Bisschop P, Ter Veer HJ, Van de Velde (eds), A System of Orthopedic Medicine. London: WB Saunders, 1995, p. 694.

The pelvis serves as the central base through which forces are transmitted both directly and indirectly (Figure 7–1). Inherently, the joints of the pelvis are stable; however, repetitive or high-velocity loads can lead to injury. In addition, adaptive or compensatory patterns may occur in the pelvis as a result of spine and lower-extremity injury or asymmetrical force transmission with resultant SIJ dysfunction. The natural degenerative changes that take place must be recognized as well.

Most research has focused on direct force transmission and motion about the SIJ, with an understanding that some motion at the SIJ may occur indirectly. Bodyweight and postural changes may create or inhibit motion at the SIJ, while the majority of indirect motion occurs secondary to the muscle groups surrounding the joint. These include the gluteals, hamstrings, hip external rotators, iliopsoas, abdominals, latissimus dorsi, quadratus lumborum, and erector spinae (Figure 7–2). Restriction of any of these muscle groups may subsequently alter mechanics about the SIJ. Acquired hyper- or hypomobility about the SIJ results in altered load transmission, which may impact on the other components of the lower-extremity kinetic chain. Studies have shown various ranges of motion about the SIJ, but most agree that approximately 4 degrees of rotation and 1.6 mm of translation occurs.[69,70] The amount of joint motion decreases with age. Women develop degenerative changes that restrict motion at age fifty while men develop them around age forty.[69,70] At the present time, the clinical impact of age-related degeneration about the SIJ is unclear.

Figure 7–2. Musculature about the sacroiliac joints: 1, psoas; 2, iliacus; 3, gluteus; 4, erector spinae; 5, sacroiliac joint. Adapted with permission from Ombregt L, Bisschop P, Ter Veer HJ, Van de Velde. Applied anatomy of the sacroiliac joint. In Ombregt L, Bisschop P, Ter Veer HJ, Van de Velde (eds), A System of Orthopedic Medicine. London: WB Saunders, 1995, p. 690.

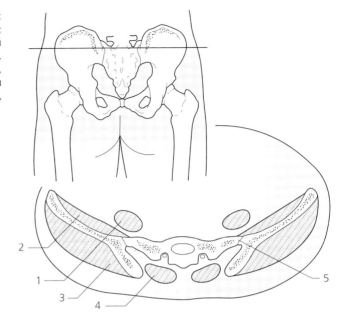

Motion/Biomechanics

Sacroiliac joint biomechanics are complex and as mentioned above may be affected by or indirectly affect motion at the spine, ilium, pubic symphysis, and hip. In 1878, Meyer described movement about two axes with respect to motion between the sacrum and innominates.[24,41] In 1955, Weisel demonstrated by radiographic assessment a constant movement of the SIJ in living subjects when changing from supine to standing.[71,72] He noticed a ventral shift of the sacral prominence of about 5.5 mm, with the axis of movement found to lie about 10 cm below the sacral prominence with a variability of about 5 cm.[69,70] Axes of motion of the sacrum on the ilium include sacral flexion, extension, rotation, lateral flexion, and torsion. Sacral flexion and extension occur at the second sacral segment, rotation occurs on a vertical axis, and lateral flexion occurs on an anteroposterior axis. Torsional motion is located from the superior end of the articular surface of the right side to the inferior end of the articular surface on the left side, and vice versa. In addition to isolated sacral mechanics, there exists motion of the innominates (ilium) on the sacrum – termed "nutation" and "counternutation" (Figure 7–3). Iliosacral motion occurs in anteroposterior and superoinferior planes.[69,70]

In light of the complex biomechanics surrounding SIJ motion, the interpretation of physical exam maneuvers can be difficult. This is further complicated by anatomical variation which makes identifying bony landmarks for measuring joint movement difficult. Colachis et al.[8] embedded pins into the iliac spines of medical students

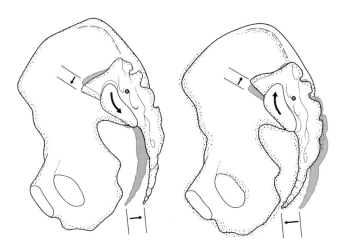

Figure 7–3. Nutation (*left*) and counternutation (*right*) of the sacroiliac joint. Adapted with permission from Ombregt L, Bisschop P, Ter Veer HJ, Van de Velde. Applied anatomy of the sacroiliac joint. In Ombregt L, Bisschop P, Ter Veer HJ, Van de Velde (eds), A System of Orthopedic Medicine. London: WB Saunders, 1995, p. 692.

and movement was measured in sitting, standing, trunk flexion, and extension. Movement varied significantly between individuals, with differences of 5 mm recorded between iliac spines. Frigerio[18] demonstrated movement in cadavers and living subjects using radiographic techniques. In living specimens, it was observed that movement between the sacrum and iliac crests varied up to 26 mm with torsional and flexion motions.

Several studies have used invasive techniques to analyze motion (or lack of motion) of the SIJ. Sturesson[65] used roentgen stereophotogrammetric analysis (RSA) where tantalum balls were implanted into the pelvis and then radiographically localized to measure SIJ motion in 34 patients with pain. Patients with bilateral symptoms had more rotation than patients with unilateral symptoms. Jacob[27] utilized surgically implanted Kirshner wires to measure SIJ motion in patients with and without SIJ pain. Twenty-three asymptomatic patients had less rotation and translation than the one patient with bilateral pain. These two studies suggest that asymmetrical motion could play a factor in SIJ pain; however, the studies were limited in sample size.

Epidemiology

Sacroiliac joint dysfunction is in the differential diagnosis of lumbosacral radicular pain; it has a prevalence between 15% and 30% and an unknown incidence.[15,23,55] Bernard and Kirkaldy-Willis[5] reported that of 1293 patients with low back pain, SIJ dysfunction was thought to be the pain source in 22.5% based on history and physical exam. The extensive neural circuitry from the lumbosacral region accounts for the difficulty in differentiating SIJ dysfunction from that of other surrounding structures. The SIJ can be affected in rheumatologic disorders such as seronegative spondyloarthropathies including reactive arthritis, psoriasis, juvenile chronic arthritis, ulcerative colitis, and Crohn's disease. It can also be affected by autoimmune and infectious diseases, malignancy with and without metastasis. Radiographic changes about the SIJ have been well documented in ankylosing spondylitis (AS), including joint space narrowing, subchondral sclerosis, and osteophytosis.[9,19,29,49] In the 1950s, Romanus and Yden[53] and Newton[46] described how physical exam maneuvers – including palpation of the anterior superior iliac spine, forced adduction of the flexed thigh, and lateral compression of the pelvis – were sometimes positive in early AS and might precede radiological changes. However these authors did not cite their reproducibility, specificity, or sensitivity. These studies set the stage for further evaluation of SIJ pathology and the clinical significance of provocative examination maneuvers.

Diagnosis

The validity of mobility studies is difficult to ascertain, and there is no gold standard for reference. In-vivo studies or the use of three-dimensional recording systems have been used; however, the conclusions are mixed.[64] The gold standard for mobility tests needs to be further delineated since reliability is not well established and a significant percentage of asymptomatic individuals may have positive tests.[64,65] Gemmell and Jacobson,[21] Miraeu et al.,[44] and Dreyfuss et al.[14] have shown positive provocative maneuvers in 26%, 33%, and 16% of asymptomatic populations.

Symptoms

The most common presenting symptom in patients with SIJ is pain or tenderness over the region of the posterior superior iliac spine.[10,16,17] Radiation may occur into the buttock, groin posterior proximal thigh, and rarely below the knee.[23] The presentation of SIJ dysfunction is similar to other forms of low back pain making clinical diagnosis more challenging.[37] Pain is often worse with long periods of sitting or standing, and stepping up on the affected leg. Pain or clicking with transitional activities such as getting up from a chair or in and out of a car may also be noted.[51] Studies have shown pain referral patterns, after injecting the SI joint, that extend to the medial or lateral buttocks, the greater trochanter, and the superior lateral thigh.[35,37,56–58] The area of maximal pain has been defined from the medial buttock extending approximately 10 cm caudally and 3 cm laterally from the PSIS (Figure 7–4).[16,17]

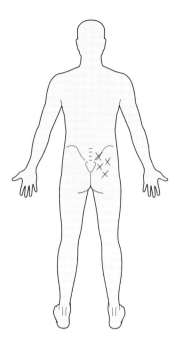

Figure 7–4. Typical pain location for sacroiliac joint dysfunction. Adapted with permission from George SZ, Delitto A. Management of the athlete with low back pain. Clin Sports Med 2002;21(1):112.

Tests for Sacroiliac Joint Pathology

A thorough musculoskeletal examination of the low back, pelvis, hips, and the remainder of the lower extremities should be performed to determine the origin of the dysfunction. The exam should include a full neurologic evaluation to rule out a neurologic source of pain, as SIJ dysfunction does not produce objective sensory, motor, or reflex changes. The examiner should be aware that SIJ dysfunction may coexist with other conditions, including primary conditions involving the hip, pelvic floor, or spine. In general, tests for SIJ dysfunction are divided into tests of motion or provocation.

Motion Tests

Standing Flexion Test

The standing flexion test was initially described by Henry Fryette in 1918, although he did not specifically call it a standing flexion test. Mitchell et al.[45] described the standing flexion test as follows (Figure 7–5):

> This test is performed with the patient standing, facing away from the examiner, with his feet approximately 12 inches apart so that the patient's feet are parallel and approximately acetabular distance apart. The examiner then places his thumbs on the

Figure 7–5. A,B: Standing flexion test. Reproduced with permission from Geraci MC, Alleva JT, McAdam FB. The physical examination of the spine and its functional kinetic chain. In Cole AJ, Herring SA (eds), The Low Back Pain Handbook: a Guide for the Practicing Clinician, 2nd edn. Philadelphia: Hanley & Belfus, 2003, p. 86.

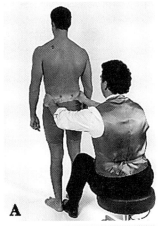

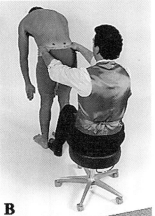

inferior aspect of each PSIS. The patient is asked to bend forward with both knees extended. The extent of the cephalad movement of each PSIS is monitored. Normally, the PSIS should move equally. If one PSIS moves superiorly and anteriorly to the other, this is the side of restriction and hypomobility.

This test only indicates asymmetry in motion or loss of lumbopelvic rhythm. A standing flexion test can be positive with an ipsilateral tight quadratus lumborum, contralateral tight hamstrings, sacroiliac joint arthritis, or hip joint restriction.[12]

There are varied suggestions for the distance the feet should be apart.[68] Bourdillon et al.[4] stated that the heels should be spaced about 6 inches or 15 cm, while others have suggested a lesser spacing. Schwarzer et al.[55] found no association between this test and those patients who had a positive fluoroscopically guided injection of lidocaine into the SIJ. This result is not surprising since altered motion is not always synonymous with pain.

Potter and Rothstein[50] found a 44% inter-examiner reliability for this test. Vincent-Smith and Gibbons[68] reported an inter-examiner reliability of 42% and a κ coefficient of 0.052, demonstrating poor reliability. The intra-examiner reliability was demonstrated to have a mean percentage agreement of 68% with a κ coefficient of 0.46, indicating moderate reliability. Levangie[34] assessed the association between innominate torsion and four clinical tests of the SIJ, including the standing forward flexion test in 150 patients with low back pain and 138 without. This study found the standing flexion test to have a sensitivity of 17%, specificity of 79%, a positive predictive value of 61%, and negative predictive value of 35%.

Dreyfuss et al.[13] determined the incidence of false-positive screening tests for SIJ dysfunction. Subjects who were asymptomatic had no back pain for the past 6 months. The control group consisted of subjects with active low back pain, but SIJ was not the confirmed source of the subject's pain. This study found this test to have a high false-positive rate in asymptomatic adults. For all 101 subjects, the incidence of false-positives on either side for the standing flexion test was 13%. At best, it appears that this test is useful in assessing symmetry of motion.

Seated Flexion Test

This is a test of the sacroiliac mobility that is used to differentiate sacroiliac from iliosacral dysfunction. Mitchell et al.[45] described the seated flexion as follows (Figure 7–6):

> This test is performed with the patient seated; both feet are flat on the floor facing away from the examiner and are firmly supported. The lower extremities should be abducted slightly to allow the patient's shoulders to descend between them. The examiner stands or sits behind the patient with the eyes at the level of the iliac crests and then the examiner should place his thumbs on each PSIS. The patient should be instructed to forward flex until his/her hands touch the floor as the examiner maintains contact with the PSISs. The test is positive if one PSIS moves unequally cephalad with respect to the other PSIS. The side with the greatest cephalad excursion implies articular restriction and hypomobility. While the patient is seated, the innominates are fixed in place, thus isolating out iliac motion.

A seated flexion test may be positive for reasons other than SIJ pain including a tight ipsilateral quadratus lumborum.[60–62]

Beal[1] reported poor inter-examiner reliability of this test (no-value given in the article). Potter and Rothstein[50] examined the inter-examiner reliability of the 13 tests including the seated flexion test for SIJ dysfunction and reported a 50% inter-examiner reliability. Dreyfuss et al.[13] concluded that this test has a low specificity as a result of the false-positive rate of 13.3%. Levangie[34] determined the sensitivity to be 9%, the specificity to be 93%, the positive predictive value to be 78%, and the negative

Figure 7–6. A,B: Seated flexion test. Reproduced with permission from Geraci MC, Alleva JT, McAdam FB. The physical examination of the spine and its functional kinetic chain. In Cole AJ, Herring SA (eds), The Low Back Pain Handbook: a Guide for the Practicing Clinician, 2nd edn. Philadelphia: Hanley & Belfus, 2003, p. 87.

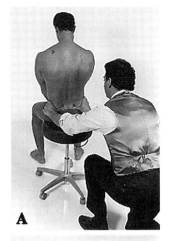

A

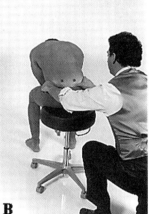

B

predictive value to be 28%. There is great disparity in the studies of reliability, specificity, and sensitivity, supporting the need for further study.

Gillet Test (One-leg Stork Test)

The Gillet test was described by Gillet and Liekens in 1981 to be a sensitive procedure to detect so-called partial iliosacral and SIJ dysfunction.[22] It is performed as follows (Figure 7–7)[43]:

> This test is performed with the patient standing, facing away from the examiner, with his feet approximately 12 inches apart. Once each PSIS is localized by the examiner's thumbs, the patient is asked to stand on one leg while flexing the contralateral hip and flexing his knee to his chest.

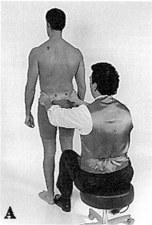

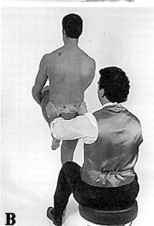

Figure 7–7. A,B: Gillet test. Reproduced with permission from Geraci MC, Alleva JT, McAdam FB. The physical examination of the spine and its functional kinetic chain. In Cole AJ, Herring SA (eds), The Low Back Pain Handbook: a Guide for the Practicing Clinician, 2nd edn. Philadelphia: Hanley & Belfus, 2003, p. 86.

Another method, the modified Gillet–Liekens test, has been described throughout the literature[21,50]:

> The examiner places one thumb directly under one PSIS and the other thumb at the S2 tubercle. The patient then stands on one leg and flexes the other hip toward the chest. The test is positive if the PSIS on the side of hip flexion fails to move posterior and inferior with respect to the other PSIS.

There are mixed results regarding inter-tester reliability of this test. Three studies found high inter-examiner reliability for this maneuver. Wiles et al.[73] evaluated 46 young asymptomatic patients and found an inter-rater reliability of 78%. Herzog[26] evaluated 11 patients examined by 10 chiropractors and determined the inter-examiner reliability to be between 54% and 78%. Carmichael et al.[6] looked at 53 healthy college students, and determined the inter-examiner reliability for the Gillet test to be 85%, and intra-examiner reliability to be 89.2%. Carmichael modified the original Gillet test by raising the leg as high as possible without bending the patients' knees. However, this study is difficult to apply to the general clinical population.

Several studies in the literature question outright the utility of the Gillet test.[6,67] Potter and Rothstein[50] found a 46% inter-examiner reliability among eight therapists who evaluated 17 patients with lateral buttock pain. Meijne et al.[43] found the intra-examiner to have a κ coefficient of 0.03–0.08 in all subjects (poor correlation), and an agreement of 70–83%. The inter-examiner reliability had a κ coefficient of –0.05 to 0.00, and 76–77% agreement. The authors concluded that this test has a very low level of reliability.

Dreyfuss et al.[3] found this test to have nearly 20% false-positive value, with females having more false-positives (26%) than males (12.5%). In a follow-up study, Dreyfuss et al.[14] evaluated 85 patients with SIJ-mediated low back pain. Patients were diagnosed with SIJ dysfunction based on a 90% reduction in pain after fluoroscopically guided injection of lidocaine and steroid. Twelve clinical examinations were evaluated on patients with pain reduction after fluoroscopy. The Gillet test was performed on 45 patients and was found to have a sensitivity of 43%, and specificity 68%. The inter-examiner reliability was found to be poor with a κ coefficient of 0.22 and agreement 45% of the time.

Levangie[34] assessed the association between innominate torsion and several physical examination tests including the Gillet test. This study looked at 150 patients with low back pain and compared them to 138 patients without low back pain. The Gillet test was found to have a sensitivity of 8%, a specificity of 93%, positive predictive value of 67%, and negative predictive value of 35%.

Sturesson et al.[64,65] studied the Gillet test with an invasive radiostereometric method looking at 22 patients with a positive Gillet test and presumptive SIJ dysfunction. No significant difference was noted between the left and right SIJ utilizing the Gillet test, and it was concluded that this test was of no value.

McCombe et al.[38] examined the reproducibility between observers of physical exam maneuvers in patients with low back pain. A total of 88 patients were examined, and the inter-examiner reliability for the Gillet test was found to have a poor κ coefficient of 0.16–0.09.

Maigne[36] concluded that there was no statistically significant association between this manual test and those patients who responded to fluoroscopically guided anesthetic injections.

Sturesson et al.[64,65] additionally evaluated the standing flexion test by using radiostereometric analysis. Only very small movements were registered in the sacroiliac joints and the authors indicated that the standing flexion test could not be supported as a diagnostic test for SIJ motion.

On a practical note, despite controversy regarding its ability to detect motion abnormalities, the Gillet's test can assess standing tolerance and balance.

Provocative Tests

Compression Test (Midline Sacral Thrust)

The history and description of the compression test are limited in the literature. However, the value of the compression test was debated in 1927 by F. J. Gaenslen, though the test was not fully described. In 1957, Newton[46] illustrated the SI compression test as performed in the supine position as follows (Figure 7–8):

> The examiner places both hands on the patient's ASIS and exerts a medial force bilaterally to implement the test. The compression test is more frequently performed with the patient in the sidelying position. The examiner stands behind the patient with their elbows locked in extension and palms interlocked over the anterolateral or upper part of the patient's iliac crest. The examiner exerts a medial or downward force towards the floor.

This test is reported to stretch the posterior ligaments and capsule dorsally over the reference and compresses the anterior part of the joint.[38] The test is considered positive if pain is elicited in the SIJ, or gluteal region.

Laslett and Williams[30,31] found good inter-examiner reliability utilizing seven pain provocation tests for SIJ dysfunction in 51 patients with low back pain. The inter-examiner agreement was over 90% with a κ coefficient of 0.73 (good reliability). However, the majority of published studies indicate significant variability of the inter-examiner reliability for this test. Potter and Rothstein[50] found a 70% inter-tester

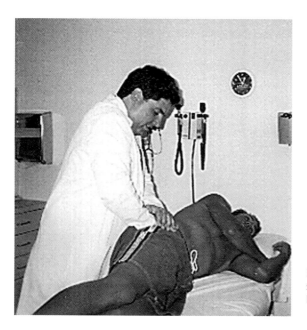

Figure 7–8. Compression test. Reproduced with permission from Nadler S, Stitik T. Occupational low back pain: history and physical examination. Occup Med State Art Rev 1998;13(1):77.

reproducibility, while Strender[63] noted a poor κ coefficient (0.26) for this test. However, neither of these studies addressed sensitivity or specificity, controls were not evaluated, and subjects did not have validated SIJ pathology.

With regard to the validity of SIJ tests, van der Wurff[66,67] calculated the sensitivity of the compression test to be 19% based upon a study done by Rantanen and Airaksinen,[52] 0% based upon a study by Blower,[6] and 7% based upon a study by Russell et al.[54] The specificity was calculated from Blower's study to be 100% specific, and 90% specific based on Russell et al.'s study.

Gapping Test (Distraction)

The history and description of the gapping (distraction) test are also limited in the literature (Figure 7–9). In 1957, Newton[46] described the SI gapping test as follows:

> The gapping test, also known as the distraction test, is performed with the patient in a supine position. The examiner places the heel of both hands at the same time on each ASIS, pressing downward and laterally.

This procedure is reported to stretch the anterior ligaments and capsule ventrally and compresses the posterior part of the joint.[38] If lumbar pain is elicited, support is placed at the low back to rule out lumbar involvement. The test is positive if pain is described in the gluteal or posterior crural areas.

Potter and Rothstein[50] and Laslett[30,31] showed over 94% and 88% inter-examiner agreement, respectively, when the gapping test was used to diagnose SIJ dysfunction. Laslett demonstrated a κ coefficient of 0.69 (good reliability), while a κ coefficient of 0.36 (poor reliability) was previously demonstrated by McCombe (1989).[38] It was concluded in the latter study that the gapping test was unreliable in the evaluation of SIJ dysfunction. The sensitivity for the gapping test has been documented to range only between 11% and 21%, whereas the specificity ranges from 90% to 100%.[3,52,54,66,67]

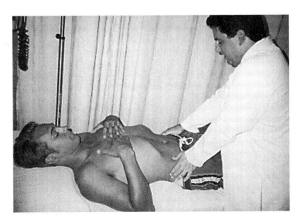

Figure 7–9. Gapping test. Reproduced with permission from Nadler S, Stitik T. Occupational low back pain: history and physical examination. Occup Med State Art Rev 1998;13(1):77.

Maigne[36] found no statistically significant association between the gapping test and those patients who had 75% or greater pain relief from fluoroscopically guided SIJ injections with lidocaine and steroid.

Patrick (FABERE) Test

In 1917, Hugh Patrick described this test originally for patients with hip arthritis.[48] This examination maneuver later became known as the FABERE sign, an acronym for *f*lexion, *ab*duction, *e*xternal *r*otation, and *e*xtension (Figure 7–10). It is described as follows:

> With the patient supine on a level surface, the thigh is flexed and the ankle is placed above the patella of the opposite extended leg. With the knee depressed and the ankle maintaining its position above the opposite knee, the patient will complain of pain before the knee reaches the level obtained in normal persons.

Kenna[28] described the Patrick test for use in those with hip or SIJ dysfunction as follows:

> The patient lies supine on the table and the foot of the involved side is externally placed on the opposite knee. The hip joint is now flexed, externally rotated and abducted. This position stresses the hip joint so that the inguinal pain on that side is a pointer to a defect in the hip joint or surrounding soft tissue. The range of motion for the hip joint in this position can be taken to the end point by pressing the knee downwards and simultaneously pressing on the region of the ASIS of the opposite side. This stresses the hip point as well as the SIJ on that side. If low back pain is reproduced the cause is likely to be due to a disorder of the SIJ.

Strender et al.[63] examined 71 patients with low back pain and evaluated the inter-examiner reliability of clinical tests used in the physical exam of patients with low back pain. Patrick's test was found unreliable in this study (κ 0.50 with 95% agreement).

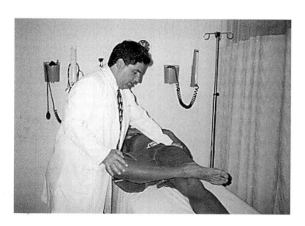

Figure 7–10. FABERE test. Reproduced with permission from Nadler S, Stitik T. Occupational low back pain: history and physical examination. Occup Med State Art Rev 1998;13(1):77.

Deursen et al.[11] also found this test to be unreliable (κ 0.38). Dreyfuss[13,14] found this test to be reliable with 85% agreement and a κ coefficient of 0.62. The sensitivity was found to be 69%, and a specificity of 16% was demonstrated.

Van der Wuff[66,67] determined the sensitivity to be low (57%) in a review of data from Rantanen and Airaksinen.[52] Broadhurst and Bond[5] reported 77% sensitivity and 100% specificity in their study of Patrick's sign correlated with double-blinded fluoroscopic SIJ joint block.

Gaenslen's Test

In 1929, F. J. Gaenslen described a diagnostic maneuver to differentiate between lumbosacral and sacroiliac lesions (Figure 7–11).[20] He described the following:

> The patient lies supine, flexes the ipsilateral knee and hip with the thigh crowded against the abdomen with the aid of both the patient's hands clasped about the

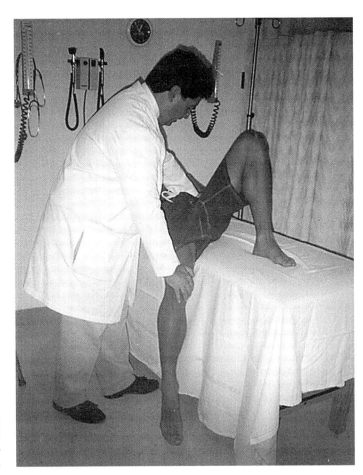

Figure 7–11. Gaenslen's test. Reproduced with permission from Nadler S, Stitik T. Occupational low back pain: history and physical examination. Occup Med State Art Rev 1998;13(1):76.

flexed knee. This brings the lumbar spine firmly in contact with the table and fixes both the pelvis and lumbar spine. The patient is then brought well to the side of the table, and the opposite thigh is slowly hyperextended with gradually increasing force by pressure of the examiner's hand on the top of the knee. With the opposite hand, the examiner assists the patient in fixing the lumbar spine and pelvis by pressure over the patient's clasped hands. The hyperextension of the hip exerts a rotating force on the corresponding half of the pelvis in the sagittal plane through the transverse axis of the sacroiliac joint. The rotating force causes abnormal mobility accompanied by pain, either local or referred on the side of the lesion.

This test can also be performed with the patient in side-lying position. The upper leg (test leg) is hyperextended at the hip. The examiner stabilizes the pelvis while extending the hip of the uppermost leg. This results in anterior rotation of the innominate and sacroiliac joint on the test side. Pain indicates SI joint pathology, but may also be caused by an L2–L4 nerve root lesion.[10,25]

Dreyfuss et al.[13,14] determined that this test was 68% sensitive, 35% specific, with a κ coefficient of 0.61 and 82% agreement. Others have challenged the discriminative information provided by the Gaenslen's test in the evaluation of a patient with low back pain.[54] Overall, there is limited research pertaining to the Gaenslen's maneuver in order to make strong conclusions.

Shear Test (Cranial Shear Test or Midline Sacral Thrust)

Mennell[39,40] and Laslett[30,31] described this test, but the original description could not be found. It has been described by Mennell as follows (Figure 7–12):

This test consists of the patient lying in the prone position and the examiner applies a pressure to the sacrum near the coccygeal end, directed cranially. The ilium is held

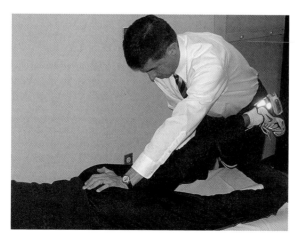

Figure 7–12. Shear test.

immobile through the hip joint as the examiner applies counter pressure against legs in the form of traction force – directed caudad. The test is considered positive if the maneuver aggravates the patient's typical pain.

Laslett found over 80% inter-tester reliability for the shear test, and no other studies have specifically evaluated the reliability of this test. With regard to sensitivity and specificity, Leboeuf et al.[56] examined 68 patients and found this test to have a specificity of 20% with a false-positive rate of 41% when comparing symptomatic with asymptomatic subjects. However, none of these patients was clearly defined as having SIJ complaints.

Dreyfuss et al.[13,14] further questioned the utility of this test, as there was no correlation among subjects who had a positive shear test with those who had a positive diagnostic fluoroscopically guided injection. They found this test to have a specificity of 40% and a sensitivity of 51%, with a κ coefficient of 0.30.

Broadhurst and Bond[5] performed a double-blinded trial to determine the sensitivity and specificity of pain provocative tests for SI joint dysfunction. They felt that Dreyfuss's pain reduction scale of 90% was too aggressive. Forty patients were subsequently randomized in a double-blind study to be injected fluoroscopically with either lidocaine or normal saline. None of the patients who received normal saline had any pain suppression. Positive pain relief was determined by 70% pain reduction, versus the 90% used by Dreyfuss. These authors found the shear test to be 100% specific and 80% sensitive. Even compared to the Dreyfuss criteria of 90% pain reduction, these authors still found 100% specificity and 70% sensitivity.

Other Tests

Palpation

O'Haire et al.[47] tested the inter- and intra-examiner reliability of ten senior osteopathic students using static palpation on ten asymptomatic subjects. Four assessments including the palpation of the posterior superior iliac spine (PSIS), sacral sulcus (SS), and the sacral inferior lateral angle (SILA) were performed on every subject by all examiners. Intra-examiner reliability ranged between κ = 0.21 (poor) to 0.33 (poor to fair) for palpation of the SILA, κ = 0.33 (poor to fair) for palpation of the PSIS, and κ = 0.24 (poor) for the SS. Inter-examiner reliability was poor for all palpation measurements, with κs ranging from 0.04 to 0.08.

Potter and Rothstein[50] determined that palpation in standing of iliac crest and PSIS levels had an inter-examiner reliability of only 35% for each assessment individually. The poor reliability of clinical tests involving palpation may be partially explained by error in landmark location.

Dreyfuss et al.[13,14] found sacral sulcus tenderness to be 90% sensitive and 15% specific when comparing the results to a diagnostic SIJ block. Inter-examiner reliability demonstrated a κ coefficient of 0.41 (fair).

Fortin Finger Test

Fortin described this test in 1991, as a simple diagnostic aid to clinicians to consider SIJ dysfunction:[16,17]

> The subject is asked to point to the region of pain with one finger. Positive sign was if the patient can localize the pain with one finger, the area pointed to was immediately inferomedial to the PSIS within 1 cm, and the patient consistently pointed to the same area over at least two trials.

Fortin and Falco[17] used provocation-positive sacroiliac joint injections to identify patients with sacroiliac joint dysfunction. Sixteen subjects were chosen from 54 consecutive patients by using the Fortin finger test. All 16 patients subsequently had provocation-positive joint injections validating sacroiliac joint abnormalities. A subset of 10 individuals underwent additional evaluation to exclude the possibility of confounding discogenic or posterior joint pains. All 10 patients had no indication of either discogenic or zygapophyseal joint pain generators. These results prompted the authors to conclude that a positive finding of the Fortin finger test successfully identified patients with sacroiliac joint dysfunction. This study did not determine interexaminer reliability, sensitivity, specificity, or positive predictive value of this test. A larger study is necessary to determine the clinical value of the test.

Combined Tests

Cibulka et al.[7] examined the sensitivity, specificity, and positive and negative predictive values of four commonly used tests of sacroiliac joint tests: (1) the standing flexion test, (2) sitting PSIS palpation, (3) the supine long sitting test, and (4) prone knee flexion tests. SIJ dysfunction was considered positive if at least three of the four tests were positive. Two hundred and nineteen patients with and without low back and SIJ-mediated pain were examined. The combination of these tests yielded a sensitivity of 0.82, specificity of 0.88, and positive predictive value of 0.86, and negative predictive value of 0.84. However, individual test results were not documented, so no conclusions can be made about their isolated validity.

Laslett and Williams[30,31] examined the inter-tester reliability of seven pain provocative tests commonly used to diagnose SIJ pathology: (1) distraction, (2) compression, (3) posterior shear, (4) pelvic rotation, (5) pelvic torsion, (6) sacral thrust, and (7) cranial shear test. Fifty-one patients with low pain, with or without radiation into the

Table 7–1. INTER-TESTER RELIABILITY OF SIJ TESTS

SI Test	κ Coefficient	Agreement (%)
Distraction	0.69	88.2
Compression	0.73	88.2
Sacral thrust	0.52	78.0
Thigh thrust	0.88	94.1
Pelvic torsion right	0.75	88.2
Pelvic torsion left	0.72	88.2
Cranial shear	0.61	84.3

Reproduced with permission from Laslett M, Williams M. The reliability of selected pain provocation tests for sacroiliac joint pathology. Spine 1994;19:1243–1249.

lower limb, were assessed by two examiners. Inter-tester reliability was determined for each test; however, combinations of these tests were not reported (Table 7–1).

Slipman et al.[59] determined the clinical validity of provocative SIJ maneuvers in making the diagnosis of SIJ dysfunction. Consecutive patients who described low back pain, including the region of the sacral sulcus, had a positive Patrick's test, ipsilateral sacral sulcus tenderness on palpation, and response to anesthetic SIJ block. The positive predictive value of provocative SIJ maneuvers in determining the presence of SIJ dysfunction was determined to be 60%. However, the negative predictive value was not reported. The authors felt that these results do not support the use of provocative SIJ maneuvers to confirm a diagnosis of SIJ dysfunction. Rather, these physical examination techniques can, at best, enter SIJ dysfunction into the differential diagnosis (Table 7–2).

Table 7–2. SACROILIAC JOINT TESTS IN THE LITERATURE

Test	First Author	κ Coefficient	Agreement	Sensitivity	Specificity
Grapping	Potter[50]		94%[a]		
	Laslett[31]	0.69	91%[a]		
	McCombe[38]	0.36			
	Russel[54]		11%	90%	
	Rantanen[52]			15%	
	Wurff[66,67]		11–21%	90–100%	
Compression	Potter[50]		76%[a]		
	Laslett[31]	0.77[a]	91%[a]		
	McCombe[38]	0.16			
	Rantanen[52]			19%	

Continued

Table 7–2. SACROILIAC JOINT TESTS IN THE LITERATURE—*cont'd*

Test	First Author	κ Coefficient	Agreement	Sensitivity	Specificity
	Russel[54]			7%	90%
	Strender[63]	0.26[a]			
	Blower[3]				100%
Gaenslen	Laslett[31]	0.72	63%		
	Dreyfuss[14]	0.61[a]	82%[a]	68%	35%
	Russel[54]			21%	72%
Patrick's	Dreyfuss[14]	0.62[a]	85%[a]	69%	16%
	Deursen[11]	0.38			
	Rantanen[52]			57%	
	Broadhurst[5]			77%	100%
	Strender[63]	0.50[a]	95%[a]		
Gillet	Meyne[42]	0.08	90%		
	Carmichael[6]	0.02	85%[a]		
			89.2[b]		
	Potter[50]		47%[a]		
	Dreyfuss[14]	0.22[a]	45%[a]	43%	68%
	Wiles[73]		78%[a]		
	Herzog[26]		54–78%[a]		
	Meijne[43]	0.03–0.08[b]	70–83%[b]		
		−0.05–0.00[a]	76–77%[a]		
	Levangie[34]			8%	93%
	McCombe[38]	0.16–0.09[a]			
Sitting flexion test	Potter[50]		50%[a]		
	Levangie[34]			9%	93%
Standing flexion test	Potter[50]		44%[a]		
	Vincent-Smith[68]	0.052[a]	42%[a]		
		0.46[b]			
			68%[b]		
	Levangie[34]			17%	79%
Shear test	Laslett[31]		80%[a]		
	Leboeuf[32]			20%	
	Dreyfuss[14]	0.30[a]		40%	51%
	Broadhurst[5]			70%	100%
Palpation	O'Haire[47]	0.21–0.33[b]			
		0.40–0.08[a]			
	Dreyfuss[14]			90%	15%
Fortin	Fortin[17]	NA	NA	NA	NA
Combined tests	Cibulka[7]			82%	88%

[a]Inter-examiner. [b]Intra-examiner. NA, not available.

Conclusion

Evaluation of the patient with sacroiliac joint pain can be difficult. The biomechanics of the SIJ are complex and there is no gold standard for diagnosis, which is often one of exclusion. The SIJ can be a source of pain with referral into the extremity and therefore needs to be included in the differential diagnosis of lumbar radiculopathy. As such, the standard physical assessment should include appropriate provocative maneuvers and motion testing. Sacroiliac motion testing via the standing or seated flexion tests along with the Gillet test are commonly performed, but clinicians must be aware that altered motion is not always synonymous with pain. In addition, there is great disparity in the studies of reliability, specificity, and sensitivity for all tests of the SIJ, supporting the need for further study.

REFERENCES

1. Beal MC. The sacroiliac problem: review of anatomy, mechanics, and diagnosis. J Am Osteopath Assoc 1982;81:667–679.
2. Bernard TN, Kirkaldy-Willis WH. Recognizing specific characteristics of nonspecific low back pain. Clin Orthop 1987;(217):266–280.
3. Blower PW, Griffin AJ. Clinical sacroiliac tests in ankylosing spondylitis and other causes of low back pain: two studies. Ann Rheum Dis 1984;43(2):192–195.
4. Bourdillon JF. Detailed examination. In Spinal Manipulation, 4th edn. London: William Heinemann Medical Books, 1987, pp. 58–72.
5. Broadhurst NA, Bond MJ. Pain provocation tests for the assessment of sacroiliac joint dysfunction. J Spinal Dis 1998;11:341–345.
6. Carmichael JP. Inter- and intra-examiner reliability of palpation for sacroiliac joint dysfunction. J Manip Physiol Ther 1987;10(4):164–171.
7. Cibulka MT, Koldehoff R. Clinical usefulness of a cluster of sacroiliac joint tests in patients with and without low back pain. J Orthop Sports Phys Ther 1999;29(2):83–89; discussion 90–92.
8. Colachis SC, Worden RE, Bechtol CO, Strohm BR. Movement of the sacroiliac joint in the adultmale: a preliminary report. Arch Phys Med Rehab 1963;44:490–499.
9. Crenshaw AH, Hamilton JF. Rheumatoid spondylitis. South Med J 1952;45:1055.
10. Daum WJ. The sacroiliac joint an under appreciated pain generator. Am J Orthop 1995;24:475–478.
11. Deursen van LLJM, Patijn J, Ockhuysen AL, et al. The value of some clinical tests of the sacroiliac joint. J Manual Med 1990;5:96–99.
12. DiGiovanna EL, Schiowitz S. An Osteopathic Approach to Diagnosis and Treatment. Philadelphia: JB Lippincott, 1991.
13. Dreyfuss P, Dreyer S, Griffin J, Hoffman J, Walsh N. Positive sacroiliac screening tests in asymptomatic adults. Spine 1994;19:1138–1143.
14. Dreyfuss P, Michaelsen M, Pauza K, McLarty J, Bogduk N. The value of medical history and physical examination in diagnosing sacroiliac joint pain. Spine 1996;21:2594–2602.
15. Ebraheim NA, Pananilam TG, Waldrop JT, Yeasting RA. Anatomic consideration in the anterior approach to the sacroiliac joint. Spine 1994;19:721–725.
16. Fortin JD, Dwyer AP, West S, Pier J. Sacroiliac joint: pain referral maps upon applying a new injection arthrography technique. 1: Asymptomatic volunteers. Spine 1994;19:1475–1482.
17. Fortin JD, Falco FJ. The Fortin finger test: an indicator of sacroiliac pain. Am J Orthop 1997;26:477–480.
18. Frigerio NA, Stowe RS, Howe JW. Movement of the sacroiliac joint. Clin Orthop Rel Res 1974;100:370. Communications: 1981;155:293–297.
19. Forestier J. Quoted in Romanus R, Yden S: Pelvo-Spondylitis Ossificans. Munksgaard, Copenhagen, 1955.

20. Gaenslen FJ. Sacro-iliac arthrodesis. JAMA 1927;89:2031–2035.
21. Gemmel HA, Johnson BH. Incidence of sacroiliac joint dysfunction and low back pain in fit college students. J Manip Physiol Ther 1990;13(2):63–67.
22. Gillet H, Liekens M. Belgian Chiropractic Research Notes, 11th edn. Huntington Beach, CA: Motion Palpation Institute, 1981.
23. Greenman PE. Clinical aspects of sacroiliac function in walking. J Man Med 1990;5(3):125–130.
24. Grieve GP. The sacro-iliac joint. Physiotherapy 1976;62(12);384–400.
25. Gross J, Fetto J, Rosen E. Musculoskeletal Examination. Cambridge, MA: Blackwell Science, 1996.
26. Herzog W, Read LJ, Conway PJ, Shaw LD, McEwen MC. Reliability of motion palpation procedures to detect sacroiliac joint fixations. J Manip Physiol Ther 1989;12(2):86–92.
27. Jacob HAC, Kissling RO. The mobility of the sacroiliac joints in healthy volunteers between 20 and 50 years of age. Clin Biomech 1995;10:352–361.
28. Kenna C, Murtagh J. Patrick or FABERE test to test hip and sacroiliac joint disorders. Aust Fam Physician 1989;18(4):375.
29. Knutsson F. Changes in the sacro-iliac joints in morbus bechterew and osteitis condensans. Acta Radiologica 1950;33:557.
30. Laslett M. The value of the physical examination in diagnosis of painful sacroiliac joint pathologies.Spine 1998;23:962–964.
31. Laslett M, Williams M. The reliability of selected pain provocation tests for sacroiliac joint pathology. Spine 1994;19:1243–1249.
32. Leboeuf C. The sensitivity and specificity of seven lumbo-pelvic orthopedic tests and the arm–fossa test. J Manip Physiol Ther 1990;13(3):138–143.
33. Lee D. The Pelvic Girdle. Edinburgh: Churchill Livingstone, 1989.
34. Levangie PK. Four clinical tests of sacroiliac joint dysfunction: the association of test results with innominate torsion among patients with and without low back pain. Phys Ther 1999;79:1043–1057.
35. Magee DJ. Orthopedic Physical Assessment. Philadelphia: WB Saunders, 1992.
36. Maigne JY, Aivaliklis A, Pfefer F. Results of sacroiliac joint double block and value of sacroiliac pain provocation tests in 54 patients with low back pain. Spine 1996;21:1889–1892.
37. Malanga GA, Nadler SF. Nonoperative treatment of low back pain. Mayo Clin Proc 1999;74:1135–1148.
38. McCombe PF, Fairbank JCt, Cockersole BC, Pynsent PB. Volvo Award in Clinical Sciences. Reproducibility of physical signs in low-back. Spine 1989;14:908–918.
39. Mennell J. Joint Pain: Diagnosis and Treatment using Manipulative Techniques. Boston: Little, Brown, 1964.
40. Mennell J. The science and art of joint manipulation. In The Spinal Column, Vol. II. Philadelphia: Blakiston Co., 1952.
41. Meyer GH. Der Mechanismus der Symphysis sacro-iliaca. Arch F Anat U Physiologie (Leipzig) 1878;I(1).
42. Meyne W, Neerbos K, Aufdemkampe G, van der Wur P. Intra- and inter-examiner reliability of the Gillet test. J Manip Physiol Ther 1999;1:4–10.
43. Meijne W, van Neerbos K, Aufdemkampe G, van der Wurff P. Intraexaminer and interexaminer reliability of the Gillet test. J Manip Physiol Ther 1999;22(1):4–9.
44. Mierau DR, Cassidy JD, Hamin T, Milne RA. Sacroiliac joint dysfunction and low back pain in school aged children. J Manip Physiol Ther 1984;7(2):81–84.
45. Mitchell FL, Morgan PS, Pruzzo NA. An Evaluation and Treatment Manual of Osteopathic Muscle Energy Techniques. Valley Park, MO: Mitchell, Moran & Pruzzo Associates, 1979.
46. Newton DRL. Discussion on the clinical and radiological aspect. Proc R Soc Med 1957;50:850–853.
47. O'Haire C, Gibbons P. Inter-examiner and intra-examiner agreement for assessing sacroiliac anatomical landmarks using palpation and observation: pilot study. Man Ther 2000;5(1):3–20.
48. Patrick HT. Brachial neuritis and sciatica. JAMA 1917;LXIX:2176–2179.
49. Polley HF, Slocumb CH. Rheumatoid spondylitis: a study of 1035 cases. Ann Int Med 1947;26:240.
50. Potter NA, Rothstein JM. Intertester reliability for selected clinical tests of the sacroiliac joint. Phys Ther 1985;65:1671–1675.
51. Prather H. Pelvis and sacral dysfunction in sports and exercise. Phys Med Rehabil Clin North Am 2000;11:805–836, viii.
52. Rantanen P, Airaksinen O. Poor agreement between so-called sacroiliac joint tests in ankylosing spondylitis patients. J Manip Med 1989;4:62–64.
53. Romanus R, Yden S. Pelvo-spondylitis Ossificans. Copenhagen: Munksgaard, 1955, pp. 18–23.

54. Russel AS, Maksymowych W, LeClercq S. Clinical examination of the sacroiliac joints: a prospective study. Arthritis Rheum 1981;24:1575–1577.

55. Schwarzer AC, Aprill CN, Bogduk N. The sacroiliac joint in chronic low back pain. Spine 1995;20:31–37.

56. Simons DG, Travell JG. Myofascial origins of low back pain. 1: Principles of diagnosis and treatment. Postgrad Med 1983;73(2):66, 68–70, 73 passim.

57. Simons DG, Travell JG. Myofascial origins of low back pain. 2: Torso muscles. Postgrad Med 1983;73(2):81–92.

58. Simons DG, Travell JG. Myofascial origins of low back pain. 3: Pelvic and lower extremity muscles. Postgrad Med 1983;73(2):99–105, 108.

59. Slipman CW, Sterenfeld EB, Chou LH, Herzog R, Vresilovic E. The predictive value of provocative sacroiliac joint stress maneuvers in the diagnosis of sacroiliac joint syndrome. Arch Phys Med Rehabil 1998;79: 288–292.

60. Solonen KA, Rokkanen P. Changes in the hip joint caused by asymmetry of the lower limbs: an experimental study on bipedal rats. Ann Chir Gynaecol Fenn 1967;56:189–192.

61. Solonen KA. Perforation of the anterior annulus fibrosus during operation for prolapsed disc. Ann Chir Gynaecol Fenn 1975;64:385–387.

62. Solonen KA. The sacroiliac joint in the light of anatomical, roentgenological, and clinical studies. Acta Othrop Scand 1957;27(suppl.):1–115.

63. Strender LE, Sjoblom A, Sundell K, Ludwig R, Taube A. Interexaminer reliability in physical examination of patients with low back pain. Spine 1997;22:814–820.

64. Sturesson B, Selvik G, Uden A. Movements of the sacroiliac joints: a roentgen stereophotogrammetric analysis. Spine 1989;14:162–165.

65. Sturesson B, Uden A, Vleeming A. A radiostereometric analysis of movements of the sacroiliac joints during the standing hip flexion test. Spine 2000;25:364–368.

66. Van der Wurff P, Hagmeijer RH, Meyne W. Clinical tests of the sacroiliac joint – a systemic methodological review. 1: Reliability. Manip Ther 2000;5(1):30–36.

67. Van der Wurff P, Meyne W, Hagmeijer RH. Clinical tests of the sacroiliac joint. Manip Ther 2000; 5(2):89–96.

68. Vincent-Smith B, Gibbons P. Inter-examiner and intra-examiner reliability of the standing flexion test. Manip Ther 1999;4(2):87–93.

69. Vleeming A, et al. The sacro-iliac joint: anatomical, biomechanical and radiological aspects. J Man Med 1990;5(3):100–102.

70. Vleeming A, et al. Mobility in the sacroiliac joints in the elderly: a kinematic and radiological study. Clin Biomech 1992;7(3):170–176.

71. Weisel H. Movements of the sacro-iliac joint. Acta Anat 1955;23:80–91.

72. Weisel H. Ligaments of sacro-iliac joint examined with particular reference to their function. Acta Anat 1954;20:201–213.

73. Wiles MR. Reproducibility and inter-examiner correlation of motion palpation findings of the sacroiliac joints. J Can Chiropr Assoc 1980;24(2):56–69.

Chapter 8

Physical Examination of the Hip

BRIAN J. KRABAK, MD • SCOTT J. JARMAIN, MD •
HEIDI PRATHER, DO

Introduction

The hip joint is one of the more stable joints of the body. The stability stems from the intimacy of the head of the femur within the acetabulum like a ball in a socket. Thus, the most severe injuries are often traumatic in nature. In general, injuries to the hip joint result in difficulty with ambulation. However, pain in the hip region may be referred from other areas such as the sacroiliac joint or lumbar spine. Therefore, careful examination of the hip and the surrounding regions is essential.

Inspection, Palpation, and Range of Motion

The initial examination should occur with the individual standing. The examiner should document any soft tissue or bony contour abnormalities, edema, skin discoloration, or scars. In addition, the examiner should note the alignment of the lower extremities; excess external rotation at the ankle is potentially indicative of femoral retroversion, while excess internal rotation – "toeing in" – is potentially indicative of femoral anteversion. Similarly, the individual should be examined while supine to further assess any obvious asymmetries of the anterior superior iliac spine, femoral or tibial height, which may result in shortening of one leg.

A general assessment of the patient's gait in both the sagittal and frontal planes is essential. Abnormal gait patterns – such as hip hiking, circumduction, or excess trunk extension – may be evidence of muscle weakness, leg length discrepancy, or pain. Any of these findings should prompt a more focused examination. In addition, the examiner will get a sense of the patient's overall posture and balance while ambulating.

Single-leg balance activities may support the presence of a "Trendelenburg sign" indicative of gluteus medius weakness, or the compensated variant in which the upper torso is shifted over the involved extremity.

During palpation of the hip area, the examiner should notice any areas of tenderness or warmth which may indicate underlying infection or inflammation. Anteriorly, the examiner can palpate the anterior superior iliac spine, traversing over the iliac crest and inferiorly toward the greater trochanter. The anterior soft tissue structures in the femoral triangle, including the inguinal ligament to the pelvic tubercles, iliopsoas, sartorius and adductor longus muscles, lymph nodes, and femoral artery are easily palpated. Laterally, the greater trochanter and iliac crest should be assessed along with the tensor fascia lata and gluteus medius and minimus. Tenderness over the trochanteric bursa overlying the greater trochanter may be indicative of bursitis, a common source of lateral hip pain. Posteriorly, the examiner can palpate the posterior superior iliac spine, at the base of the sacrum, and inferiorly, the ischial tuberosities where the hamstrings originate. Palpable soft tissue structures include the proximal hamstrings, piriformis, and gluteal muscles.[37]

Range of motion of the hip is generally assessed with the patient supine, with the exception of hip extension which is measured in the prone position. Internal and external rotation may be tested in either the supine or prone positions. Stabilization of the pelvis is important when assessing range of motion of the hip. There can be a wide range of what is considered "normal," so of greater importance is assessment for asymmetry from one side to the other.[37]

Tests for Muscle Tightness or Pathology of the Lumbopelvic Region

A variety of tests have been devised to assess for muscle tightness or pathology in the lumbopelvic region (Table 8–1). Some of the most common include the Thomas test (hip flexors), the Ely test (rectus femoris), the Ober test (iliotibial band), the piriformis test, popliteal angle measurement, and the Trendelenburg sign.

Thomas Test

In 1876, Hugh Owens Thomas described a novel method of diagnosing inflammation of the hip joint. He proposed that the Thomas test could help differentiate "morbus coxae," or inflammatory disease of the hip, from "abscesses, sciatica, or hysterical simulation" of hip joint pain. He described the test as follows:[54]

> Having undressed the patient and laid him on his back upon a table or other hard plane surface, the surgeon takes the sound limb and flexes it, so that the sound knee joint is in contact with the chest. Thus he makes certain that the spine and back of

Table 8–1. HIP TESTS

Test	Description	Reliability/Validity Tests	Comments
Thomas test	The patient lies supine while the examiner checks for excessive lordosis. The examiner flexes one of the patient's hips, bringing the knee to the chest to flatten out the lumbar spine, and the patient holds the flexed hip against the chest. If there is no flexion contracture, the hip being tested (the straight leg) remains on the examining table. If a contracture is present, the patient's leg rises off the table. The angle of contracture can be measured.	Lack of studies to provide definitive reliability and validity of the Thomas test. Thurston 1982[55] 5–20 degree variability in measuring the hip flexion deformity Bartlett 1985[2] Rater comparison error of 3 degrees (CI: 1.1–2.6 degrees) Harvey 1998[27] Intraclass coefficient reliability: 0.91	Rater reliability of two experienced therapists performing the Thomas test in 15 healthy children. Utilized a modified Thomas test to measure the flexibility of 113 elite athletes.
Ely test	The patient lies prone while the examiner passively flexes the patient's knee. Upon flexion of the knee, the patient's hip on the same side spontaneously flexes, indicating that the rectus femoris muscle is tight on that side and that the test is positive. The two sides should be tested and compared.	There are no studies to be found that investigated the specificity, sensitivity, or reliability of the Ely's test.	
Rectus femoris contracture test	The patient lies supine with the knees bent over the end or edge of the examining table. The patient flexes one knee onto the chest. The angle of the test knee should remain at 90 degrees. A contracture may be present if the test knee extends slightly.	Harvey 1998[27] Intraclass coefficient reliability: 0.94	Utilized a modified Thomas test to measure the flexibility of 117 elite athletes.
Ober test	The patient lies on his side, with the thigh next to the table flexed to obliterate any lumbar lordosis. The upper	There are no studies to be found that investigated the specificity, sensitivity, or reliability of this test.	

Continued

Table 8–1. HIP TESTS—*cont'd*

Test	Description	Reliability/Validity Tests	Comments
	leg is flexed at a right angle at the knee. The examiner grasps the ankle lightly with one hand and steadies the patient's hip with the other. The upper leg is abducted widely and extended so that the thigh is in line with the body. If there is an abduction contracture, the leg will remain more or less passively abducted.		
Piriformis test	The patient is placed in the side-lying position with the non-test leg against the table. The patient flexes the test hip to 60 degrees with the knee flexed, while the examiner applies a downward pressure to the knee. Pain is elicited in the muscle if the piriformis is tight.	There are no studies to be found that investigated the specificity, sensitivity, or reliability of this test.	
Popliteal angle measurement	The popliteal angle is measured with the patient supine and the hip flexed 90 degrees. The examiner attempts to extend the knee until firm resistance is met while the hip is maintained at 90 degrees. The popliteal angle is the angle from the tibia to the femur when the patient is supine with the hip fully flexed and knee extended.	Amiel-Tison 1968[1] Sensitivity: 51% Specificity: 92%. Positive-predictive value: 12% Negative predictive value: 99%	Performed in newborns with neurologic disorders.
Trendelenburg test	The patient is observed standing on one limb. The test is felt to be positive if the pelvis on the opposite side drops. A positive Trendelenburg test is suggestive of a weak gluteus muscle or an unstable hip on the affected side.	Bird 2001[6] Sensitivity: 72.7% Specificity: 76.9% Intra-observer κ: 0.676 (95% CI: 0.270–1.08)	24 women underwent MRI for gluteus medius tear.

Table 8–1. HIP TESTS—*cont'd*

Test	Description	Reliability/Validity Tests	Comments
FABERE test Patrick's test	The patient is placed in the supine position and the examiner flexes, abducts, and externally rotates the hip being tested ending with the ankle resting on the contralateral knee. The examiner then stabilizes the pelvis by applying pressure to the contralateral ilium. Pressure is then applied dorsally to the knee to further external rotation at the hip. The test is considered positive if this positioning recreates the patient's groin pain.	There are no studies to be found that investigated the specificity, sensitivity, or reliability of this test.	
Stinchfield test	With the patient supine with the knee extended, the examiner resists the patient's hip flexion at 20–30 degrees. Reproduction of groin pain is considered a positive test indicating intra-articular hip dysfunction.	There are no studies to be found that investigated the specificity, sensitivity, or reliability of this test.	
Quadrant test and hip scouring test	With the patient supine, the examiner flexes and adducts the hip until resistance is felt. The hip movement from adduction to abduction should be in a circular arc while applying compression in the direction of the shaft of the femur. Any irregularity in motion, reproduction of pain, locking, crepitus, click, or apprehension is considered a positive test.	There are no studies to be found that investigated the specificity, sensitivity, or reliability of this test.	
Axial hip distraction	With the patient supine, the examiner abducts the hip 30 degrees and applies long-axis traction by holding the leg just above the ankle. Reproduction on pain symptoms may indicate an intra-articular process.	There are no studies to be found that investigated the specificity, sensitivity, or reliability of this test.	

Continued

Table 8–1. HIP TESTS—*cont'd*

Test	Description	Reliability/Validity Tests	Comments
Leg-length discrepancy	*Direct tape measurement method:* (a) anterior superior iliac spine (ASIS) to the lateral malleolus (MM) of the tibia. (TMM) (b) ASIS to the lateral malleolus (LM) (c) umbilicus or the xiphisternum to the medial malleolus	Nicholas 1955[47] Clarke 1972[10] Fisk 1975[15]	 Used radiographs to compare the TTM and iliac crest palpation method. Used radiographs to analyze the Bourdillon indirect method.
	Indirect methods: (a) iliac crest palpation method with the use of lift blocks (b) iliac crest palpation with book correction method	Woerman 1984[58] The indirect method was the most precise and accurate method for LLD assessment. Mann 1984[39] Inter-rater reliability: 0.70 Gogia 1986[22] Inter-rater reliability: 0.98 Intra-rater reliability: 0.98 Beattie 1987[22] Intra-rater reliability: 0.807 Inter-rater reliability: 0.668 Lampe 1996[35] Iliac crest palpation with lift blocks within −1.4 and +1.6 cm of the results of the radiographs. TMM had significantly less agreement (95% CI: −1.8 to +2.1; $p = 0.002$) Jonson 1997[32] Inter-rater reliability: 0.70 Intra-rater reliability: 0.87 Gross 1998[24] Intra-rater reliability: 0.84 Inter-rater reliability: 0.77	Comparison of the direct methods of ASIS to MM, ASIS to LM, U to MM, and X to MM, and the indirect method of iliac crest palpation. Indirect method of iliac crest palpation. Studied the TMM. Studied the TMM as measured by two therapists. Comparison TMM, iliac crest palpation with lift blocks and radiography. Iliac crest palpation with lift blocks in naval shipman. Indirect method of rigid lift with a pelvic leveling device on 32 subjects with an LLD.

Table 8–1. HIP TESTS—*cont'd*

Test	Description	Reliability/Validity Tests	Comments
		Handi 2001[26] Intra-rater reliability: 0.98 Inter-rater reliability: 0.91	Iliac crest palpation and book correction method.
Fulcrum test	The patient is seated with lower legs dangling. The examiner's arm is used as gentle pressure is applied to the dorsum of the knee with the opposite hand. The test is positive if gentle pressure on the knee produces increased discomfort in the thigh.	There are no studies to be found that investigated the specificity, sensitivity, or reliability of this test.	
Hop test	A positive test occurs when the patient experiences pain in the area of a suspected stress fracture with the performance of a one-legged hop.	There are no studies to be found that investigated the specificity, sensitivity, or reliability of this test.	

the pelvis are lying flat on the table; an assistant maintains the sound limb in this fixed position; the patient is then urged to extend, as far as he is able, the diseased limb, and this he will be able to do in a degree varying with the previous duration of the infection … . By noticing the amount of flexion, the surgeon will, with practice, soon be able to guess the previous duration of the disease.

Over time, the Thomas test became the common method of measurement for fixed flexion deformities of the hip. Below is a current description of the Thomas test:[37]

The patient lies supine while the examiner checks for excessive lordosis. The examiner flexes one of the patient's hips, brings the knee to the chest to flatten out the lumbar spine, and the patient holds the flexed hip against the chest. If there is no flexion contracture, the hip being tested (the straight leg) remains on the examining table. If a contracture is present, the patient's leg rises off the table. The angle of contracture can be measured.

Since Thomas' original description of his test, several modified versions and altogether different techniques have been proposed to increase the accuracy of the measurement of hip extension. In 1936, Cave and Roberts described two methods for measuring hip extension, one with the patient positioned prone with the thigh of the unmeasured leg flexed over the end of the table at an angle of 90 degrees, and the other with the patient supine and the unmeasured thigh flexed to stabilize the pelvis.[9]

However, the placement of the goniometer was not defined for either method and normal limits of motion were not given.

West[57] measured hip extension with the patient in a prone position to "stabilize the torso." The axis of the goniometer was centered over the greater trochanter, the reference arm placed along the midaxillary line of the torso, and the movable arm along the lateral midline of the femur. Normal limits of extension were not given.

Milch[43] argued against the methods of Thomas and Cave, claiming they were not dependable for clinical purposes. Milch referred to the lack of agreement as to the extent to which the opposite leg should be flexed to obliterate the lumbar curve and the poor reliability of the testing methods. According to Milch, the similar style of Thomas and Cave "merely determines the amount of hip extension possible at any given degree of pelvic flexion. Since this latter cannot be fixed as a standard of reference, the whole procedure loses its validity." As an alternative, Milch proposed utilization of the *pelvifemoral angle* to measure the extension of the femur on the pelvis. The pelvifemoral angle was defined as the angle made between a plane (Nelaton's line) laid through both anterior superior iliac spines and ischial tuberosities and the axis of the extended femur.[42] Any increase in the size of this angle beyond the normal 50 degrees was the measure of the limitation of hip extension. To rule out the possibility of variants, the angle of maximum extension of the unaffected hip should be ascertained. The difference between this angle and the corresponding angle on the involved side would establish the amount of flexion deformity.

Moore[44] reported a method similar to that of West with the patient in either a prone or a side-lying position. The reference arm of the goniometer is placed parallel to a line from the greater trochanter to the crest of the ilium and parallel to the long axis of the trunk. With the axis over the greater trochanter, the movable arm is placed along the lateral midline of the femur toward the lateral epicondyle. The neutral position of the hip, 0 degrees, was defined as that position of the hip with the patient lying prone. Motion backward from neutral was hip extension. The normal range of hip extension was reported to be 0–15 degrees.

Mundale[46] described a new method that he believed took into account the position of the innominate bone prior to measuring the angle at the hip joint. To establish the position of the innominate bone, he used the anterior and posterior superior iliac spines as fixed subcutaneous landmarks. He chose the summit of the greater trochanter, which he believed to be situated approximately at the level of the center of the acetabulum, to represent the axis of motion. He drew a perpendicular line from the trochanter to the line connecting the iliac spines. The angle between this line and the line connecting the trochanter to the lateral epicondyle of the femur is the angle to be measured.

Staheli[53] presented a new method of measuring hip flexion deformity that allegedly obliterated the lumbar lordosis. She termed the method the "prone hip extension test." In performing the prone hip extension test, the patient is placed in the prone position with both hips comfortably flexed over the end of the examining table. To assure patient comfort, the contralateral limb may be supported between the examiner's knees, rested on a stool, or simply left hanging from the table's edge. The examiner places one hand on the pelvis and gradually extends the thigh with the other hand. The precise point at which the pelvis begins to rise marks the end of the hip motion and the beginning of spine motion. At this point, the horizontal–thigh angle is estimated or measured as the degree of hip flexion contracture.

Thurston[55] proposed a method for improving accuracy of measurement of fixed flexion deformities of the hip. He proposed placing the patient prone and near the edge of the examination couch, thereby allowing the thigh on the affected side to flex to about 60 degrees over the side of the couch. The examiner steadies the pelvis with one hand, while using the other hand to lift the dependent leg until the pelvis begins to move. The angle between the thigh and the top surface of the couch at the point at which the pelvis begins to move is the angle of fixed flexion deformity.

Despite the multiple recommendations regarding the measurement of hip flexion deformities, little is known about the accuracy of the Thomas test, its modified versions, and the other described techniques. Thurston attempted to compare the accuracy of the Thomas test with his own measurement method.[55] He compared measurements using each method as determined by black and white photographs taken during the examination of ten patients. The variability in measuring the hip flexion deformity in the Thomas test ranged from 5 to 20 degrees, while the variability was only from 0.5 to 4.5 degrees for his proposed method. The author felt Thomas's test consistently gave greater angles, depending on the amount of flexion imposed on the contralateral hip by the examiner.

Bartlett et al.[2] measured and compared the rater reliability of two trained and experienced therapists in performing four positioning techniques to measure hip extension: Staheli's prone hip extension test, the Thomas test, the Mundale method, and Milch's pelvifemoral angle method. They examined 45 subjects (90 hips) consisting of 15 children with spastic diplegia, 15 children with meningomyelocele, and 15 healthy children. Among patients with meningomyelocele, the rater comparison error was approximately 10 degrees for all tests except the Mundale method, where it approached 14 degrees (based on the 95% confidence interval [CI] for the mean difference between raters: 5.5–10.1 degrees, 4.4–8.4 degrees, 8.4–13.5 degrees, and 4.2–9.3 degrees for each method, respectively). Among patients with spastic diplegia, the Mundale and pelvifemoral angle methods yielded rater errors of 9 degrees (95% CI: 4.6–9.5 degrees and 5.4–8.8 degrees, respectively), while the prone hip extension and Thomas tests yielded rater errors close to 12 degrees (95% CI: 7.6–11.5 degrees and 6.2–12.2 degrees, respectively). Among the healthy subjects, rater error was 3 degrees for the prone hip extension and Thomas tests (95% CI: 1.2–2.9 degrees and

1.1–2.6 degrees, respectively), but approximated 10 degrees for the Mundale and pelvifemoral angle methods (95% CI: 5.0–9.3 degrees and 5.7–9.8 degrees, respectively). The authors concluded that while no single measurement technique was superior in all cases, the Mundale technique should be avoided among patients with myelomeningocele due to difficulties associated with identifying bony landmarks in the presence of obesity and deformities. Among patients with spastic diplegia, using techniques other than the Thomas test can attain improved reliability. Finally, single-rater reliability appears to be superior to multiple-rater reliability, with fewer errors occurring when the same examiner is used to perform repeated measurements.

Harvey[27] described the "modified Thomas test" (Figure 8–1) and proposed its use in measuring the flexibility of the iliopsoas, quadriceps, and tensor fascia lata/iliotibial band in 117 elite athletes. Harvey performed the modified Thomas test in the following manner:

> For the modified Thomas test, the subject sat on the end of the plinth, rolled back onto the plinth, and held both knees to the chest. This ensured that the lumbar spine was flat on the plinth and the pelvis was in posterior rotation. The subject held the contralateral hip in maximal flexion with the arms, while the tested limb was lowered towards the floor.

Harvey measured the angle of the hip to determine the length of the iliopsoas. The reliability intraclass correlation coefficient for the two trials of this measurement was 0.91 (excellent). The mean angle of hip flexion was −11.9 degrees.

Eland et al.[13] described a modified version for measuring hip extension, the "iliacus test."[13] This test is very similar to the Thomas test, but was felt to achieve

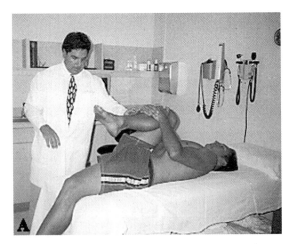
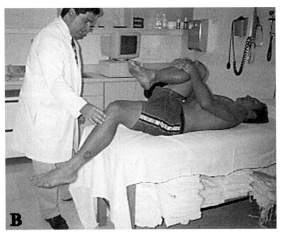

Figure 8–1. A: Normal modified Thomas test. **B**: Iliopsoas tightness demonstrated with modified Thomas test. Reproduced with permission from Nadler S, Stitik T: Occupational low back pain: history and physical examination. Occup Med 1998;13(1):72.

localization by stabilization of the innominate bone through palmar contact with the inferior surface of the anterior superior iliac spine. They performed the iliacus test to assess right hip extension as follows:

(1). The examiner instructs the subject to maintain the left hip and knee flexion with the left knee near the chest in the same comfortable position used for the Thomas test.

(2). The examiner then contacts the subject's right ASIS with his or her left palm. By using only enough pressure to maintain the position of the ASIS during extension of the right lower extremity, the examiner prevents anterior rotation of the right innominate bone ... and counterbalances the weight and leverage of the lower extremity and a downward force applied by the examiner at the knee.

(3). The examiner holds the right lower extremity until the subject lets the lower extremity relax and drop toward the floor, allowing the knee to bend. Gravity carries the lower extremity to its end point of hip extension, designated the *iliacus preangle measurement position*.

(4). Following passive maintenance of this gravity-dependent position for 3 to 5 seconds, the examiner carries the right thigh into further extension – but no further than the end of comfortable ROM as assessed by tissue-feel/end-range resistance defined by the examiner's contact with the knee. This end point is designated the *iliacus postangle measurement position*. The position of the innominate bone is maintained by continued contact with the ASIS. The subject continues to relax while the examiner maintains the palpable end point for another 3 to 5 seconds.

(5). Finally, the examiner returns the thigh to a neutral, supported position.

Eland and colleagues found a consistent difference in measurements of hip extension when comparing the results of the iliacus test and Thomas test ($p < 0.05$). The mean angle of the iliacus test (average post-angle: 17.0 degrees left, 16.5 degrees right) was significantly less ($p < 0.5$) than the means angle of the Thomas test (post-angle: 18.2 degrees left, 18.7 degrees right). Data analysis also showed a significant difference ($p < 0.001$) between the standard gravity-dependent end-point (pre-angle) and the examiner-induced knee pressure end-point (post-angle). The 95% CI values for the Thomas test were found to be the following: left pre-angle, 3.4–9.5; left post-angle, 15.7–20.8; right pre-angle, 7.5–13.0; right post-angle, 16.1–21.2. The 95% CI values for the iliacus test were found to be the following: left pre-angle, 1.7–7.0; left post-angle, 14.6–19.3; right pre-angle, 4.2–9.3; right post-angle, 14.5–18.5. When comparing sides, there was a significant difference ($p < 0.05$) in ROM for left (6.4 degrees) versus right (10.3 degrees) hip extension only for the standard (pre-angle/gravity-dependent end-point) Thomas test.

In summary, there is a lack of well-designed studies to evaluate the reliability, sensitivity, and specificity of the Thomas test and other hip extension flexibility measurement techniques.[2,13,55] Future studies are needed to better understand the accuracy and clinical utilization of these tests.

Ely Test or Rectus Femoris Contracture Test

Although the original description of Ely test could not be found, several sources have described the use of Ely's test to identify tightness of the rectus femoris muscle (Figure 8–2).[37] In Ely's test, the patient lies prone while the examiner passively flexes the patient's knee. Upon flexion of the knee, the patient's hip on the same side spontaneously flexes, indicating that the rectus femoris muscle is tight on that side and that the test is positive. The two sides should be tested and compared.

There are no studies to be found that have investigated the specificity, sensitivity, or reliability of the Ely test.

A different test used to identify tightness of the rectus femoris muscle is the rectus femoris contracture test. The test begins with the patient in a position similar to that used for the Thomas test. Magee describes the test in the following manner:[37]

> The patient lies supine with the knees bent over the end or edge of the examining table. The patient flexes one knee onto the chest and holds it. The angle of the test knee should remain at 90 degrees when the opposite knee is flexed to the chest. If it does not (i.e., the test knee extends slightly), a contracture is probably present. The examiner may attempt to passively flex the knee to see whether it will remain at 90 degrees of its own volition. The examiner should always palpate for muscle tightness when doing any contracture test. If there is no palpable tightness, the probable cause of restriction is tight joint structures (e.g., the capsule). The two sides should be tested and compared.

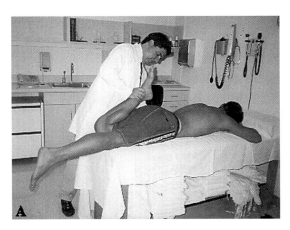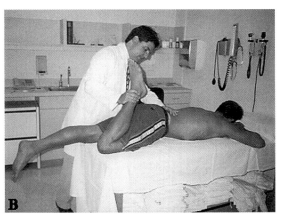

Figure 8–2. A: Normal Ely test. **B**: Rectus femoris tightness demonstrated with Ely test. Reproduced with permission from Nadler S, Stitik T: Occupational low back pain: history and physical examination. Occup Med 1998;13(1):71.

Harvey[27] measured the passive length of the quadriceps by determining the knee flexion angle of 117 elite athletes in the modified Thomas test position. The reliability intraclass correlation coefficient for the two trials was 0.94 (excellent). The mean angle of the knee was 52.5 degrees.

Ober Test

In 1936, Ober described the role of the iliotibial band and fascia lata as a factor in the causation of low back disabilities and sciatica.[48] Keenly observing that other surgeons were obtaining relief of sciatic pain when no bone pathology was visualized intraoperatively, Ober then surmised "that the relief of symptoms in these cases might be due to releasing the fascial pull exerted through the fascia lata and its attachments to the gluteus maximus muscle." He then described a method of identifying tightness of the tensor fascia lata and iliotibial band, or what he called the "abduction sign" (Figure 8–3). Ober performed this method in the following manner:[48]

> The patient lies on his side, with the thigh next to the table and flexed enough to obliterate any lumbar lordosis. The upper leg is flexed at a right angle at the knee. The examiner grasps the ankle lightly with one hand and steadies the patient's hip with the other. The upper leg is abducted widely and extended so that the thigh is in line with the body. If there is an abduction contracture, the leg will remain more or less passively abducted, depending upon the shortening of the iliotibial band. This band can be easily felt with the examining fingers between the crest of the ilium and the anterior aspect of the trochanter.

Despite the widespread use of this test, there are no studies that have measured the reliability, sensitivity, or specificity of the Ober test.

Piriformis Test

The purpose of the piriformis test is to help determine whether the piriformis muscle is playing a role in the etiology of sciatic pain. In his book *Anatomy of the Human Body*, Henry Gray was the first to describe anatomical variation of the sciatic nerve as related to the piriformis muscle, stating that "the muscle was frequently pierced by the

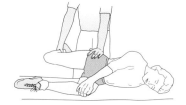

Figure 8–3. Ober test. Adapted with permission from Anderson B, Burke ER. Scientific, medical and practical aspects of stretching. In Delee JC, Drez D, Miller MD (eds), DeLee & Drez's Orthopaedic Sports Medicine: Principles and Practice, 2nd edn. Philadelphia: WB Saunders, 2003, p. 263.

common peroneal division of the sciatic nerve, which divides the muscle into two parts."[23] In 1928, Yeoman published the first reference to the piriformis muscle in relationship to sciatic pain.[59]

In 1934, Freiberg and Vinke reported that the sciatic nerve passed through the substance of the piriformis muscle in 10% of cadaver specimens.[16] Freiberg was the first to operatively target the piriformis muscle and surgically provide relief of associated sciatic pain.[17] Freiberg found that sciatic pain could be attributed to the piriformis muscle if Lasègue's sign[36] was positive and there was marked and constant tenderness at the sciatic notch and over the mesial part of the piriformis muscle. He proposed that forced internal rotation of the extended hip could reproduce the associated pain. This maneuver later became known as Freiberg's test.

In 1947, Robinson was the first to propose the term "piriformis syndrome."[51] The features of this syndrome included a history of trauma to the sacroiliac and gluteal region; pain in the region of the sacroiliac joint, greater sciatic notch and piriformis muscle extending down the leg exacerbated by walking; the presence of a palpable sausage-shaped mass over the piriformis muscle; a positive Lasègue's sign, and possibly gluteal atrophy.

Pace and Nagle[49] described a test to assist with the identification of piriformis syndrome (Figure 8–4). To perform what later became known as the Pace test, the patient remains seated at the edge of the table with legs hanging. The examiner places his/her hands on the lateral aspects of the patient's knees and asks the patient to push the hands apart by abducting and externally rotating the thighs against resistance. Faltering, pain, and weakness is noted on the affected side.

Solheim et al.[52] described the FAIR test to reproduce the pain in patients with piriformis syndrome. They noted that stretching of the piriformis muscle by combined *flexion/adduction/internal rotation* (FAIR) of the affected hip aggravated the pain in

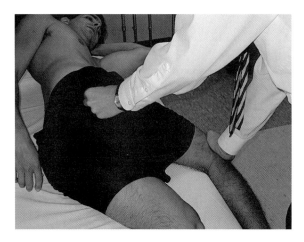

Figure 8–4. Piriformis test.

their patients. A positive Lasègue's sign was often present and subsequent diagnostic injection of local anesthetics in the piriformis muscle relieved the pain in their patients.

Currently, the piriformis test is performed by placing the patient in the side-lying position with the non-test leg against the table. The patient flexes the test hip to 60 degrees with the knee flexed, while the examiner applies a downward pressure to the knee. Pain is elicited in the muscle if the piriformis muscle is tight. Radiation of pain down the leg will occur if the substance of the piriformis muscle compromises the sciatic nerve.[37]

Benson and Schutzer[5] noted in 15 operative candidates for release of the piriformis that 14 had reproduction of their pain with the FAIR test.

In summary, several reports have defined the relationship of the piriformis muscle to the sciatic nerve in the development of piriformis syndrome. Over the years, few tests have been described to assess for piriformis syndrome, including the Freiberg, Pace, and FAIR tests. The reliability, sensitivity, and specificity of these clinical tests have not been studied.

Popliteal Angle Measurement

A variety of methods have been proposed to measure either the popliteal angle or popliteal fossa angle (hamstring flexibility/knee extension).[50] The proposed utility of this measurement has been in determining gestational age of neonates, helping to diagnose cerebral palsy, and assessing hamstring muscle tightness.[29] In 1966, Koenigsberger was the first to use the terminology "popliteal angle" when measuring the angle at the popliteal fossa to help determine gestational age of neonates, but he failed to state hip and contralateral limb position.[34]

In 1979, Bleck described the method of popliteal angle measurement which is most commonly used today (Figure 8–5).[7] According to Bleck:

> ... the popliteal angle is measured with the patient supine and the hip flexed 90 degrees. The examiner attempts to extend the knee until firm resistance is met while the hip is maintained at 90 degrees. The popliteal angle is the acute angle between the lower leg and an imaginary line extending up from the flexed femur.

While Bleck never stated the position of the opposite limb, Evans[14] had described a fairly similar method of assessing knee extensibility which allowed flexion of the opposite hip until lumbar lordosis was relieved. The accuracy of Bleck's method has not been studied.

Amiel-Tison[1] described the popliteal angle as the greatest angle from the tibia to the femur when the patient is supine with the hip fully flexed and knee extended. The sensitivity of Amiel-Tison's method was 51%, while the specificity was 92%. The positive-predictive value was determined to be 12% and the negative predictive value 99%.

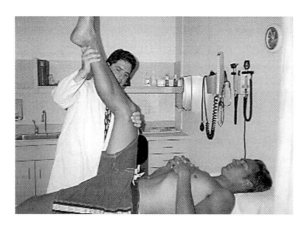

Figure 8–5. Popliteal angle measurement. Reproduced with permission from Nadler S, Stitik T. Occupational low back pain: history and physical examination. Occup Med State Art Rev 1998;13(1):72.

Trendelenburg Sign and Test

Friedrich Trendelenburg originally described the Trendelenburg sign in 1895 to assist with performing pelvic and lower abdominal procedures. As originally described, "if the right foot is put down ... the pelvis does not, like the upper part of the body, sink on the standing side, but sinks on the swinging side."[56]

More recently, the test has been described to assess the stability of hip adductors. The patient is observed standing on one limb. The test is felt to be positive if the pelvis on the opposite side drops (Figure 8–6). A positive Trendelenburg test is suggestive of a weak gluteus muscle or an unstable hip on the affected side.

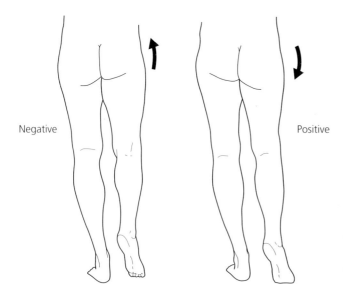

Negative

Positive

Figure 8–6. Trendelenburg's sign. Adapted with permission from Goldstein B, Chavez F. Applied anatomy of the lower extremities. Phys Med Rehabil State Art Rev 1996;10:601–630.

Few studies have evaluated the accuracy of the Trendelenburg sign (see Table 8–1). Bird et al.[6] used MRI images to study 24 women with clinical evidence of trochanteric bursitis to assess for the presence of Trendelenburg's sign, pain on resisted hip abduction, and pain on resisted hip internal rotation as predictors of a gluteus medius tear. Trendelenburg's sign was the most accurate in predicting a tendon tear, with a sensitivity of 72.7%, specificity of 76.9%, and calculated intra-observer κ of 0.676 (95% CI: 0.270–1.08).

Tests for Intra-articular or Periarticular Hip Joint Pathology

Patients with intra-articular hip pathology can present with a variety of complaints. These include posterior pelvic, groin, or thigh pain along with snapping at the groin or outer thigh. Functional complaints may include pain with sitting, standing or walking, and difficulty with transitional motions like getting in and out of a chair or car. Symptoms can be as a result of trauma such as a fall, but more commonly begin gradually and are related to incongruent weight-bearing or repetitive motion in the setting of muscle imbalance. The physical exam can be helpful in determining whether the symptom is related to hip joint pathology or from adjacent joint and myofascial structures such as the lumbar spine, sacroiliac joint, pelvic floor, or knee. Unfortunately, there are few studies showing validation of clinical examination tests (see Table 8–1).

FABERE Test

FABERE is the acronym that describes the positioning of the hip used during this test, which is *f*lexion, *ab*duction, *e*xternal *r*otation, and *e*xtension. This test is also known as the Patrick test and is often referred to as the FABERE Patrick test. A US neurologist and neuropsychiatrist who practiced in the late 1800s is credited for first describing the test, though the original description was not found. The purpose was to identify patients with hip arthritis through the application of compressive forces to the hip cartilage to induce pain.[31,37]

The patient is placed in the supine position and the examiner flexes, abducts, and externally rotates the hip being tested, ending with the ankle resting on the contralateral knee (Figure 8–7). The examiner then stabilizes the pelvis by applying pressure to the contralateral ilium. Pressure is then applied in a posterior direction to the knee causing further external rotation at the hip. The test is considered positive for hip joint pathology if this positioning recreates the patient's groin pain. This test also stresses the sacroiliac joint, pubic symphysis, adductors, lumbar spine, and inguinal ligament.

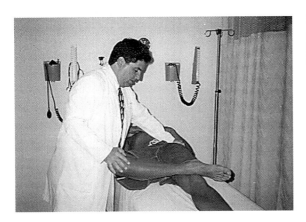

Figure 8–7. Patrick's (FABERE) test. Reproduced with permission from Nadler S, Stitik T. Occupational low back pain: history and physical examination. Occup Med State Art Rev 1998;13(1):76.

Therefore, if the test provokes pain, the examiner must ask the patient to specify the location of the pain to help determine the sight that is problematic. If the test reproduces posterior pelvic pain contralaterally, it is considered a positive test indicating that the sacroiliac joint is involved. A positive test that reproduces groin pain may indicate that there is a dysfunction within the hip joint, but does not specify the particular pathology.

The reliability, sensitivity, and specificity of this clinical test have not been studied.

Stinchfield's Test

The origin of Stinchfield's test is unknown, but it is named after Frank Stinchfield, an orthopedic surgeon whose academic career focused on hip joint arthroplasty.[41] The test description is as follows (Figure 8–8):[33]

> With the patient supine and the knee extended, the examiner resists the patient's hip flexion at 20–30 degrees. Reproduction of groin pain was considered a positive test indicating with intra-articular hip dysfunction.

The test is thought to increase intra-articular pressure, resulting in irritation of the articular sensory nerves.

Caution is indicated in interpreting a positive test result, as other extra-articular pathology may be provoked with this test. An example includes the iliopsoas muscle which may become contracted due to multiple factors, most commonly when guarding for a primary spine or hip joint disorder. This muscle may also activate in a shortened position due to primary dysfunction or adaptive changes involving the pelvis. Concentric activation of a contracted iliopsoas muscle may be painful during the Stinchfield's test secondary to muscular involvement alone. This test can be useful in

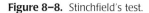

Figure 8–8. Stinchfield's test.

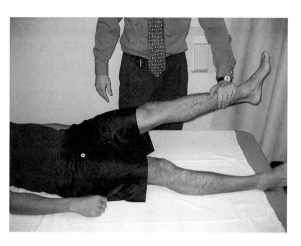

establishing a differential diagnosis, but a positive test does not specify the structure involved.

The reliability, sensitivity, and specificity of this clinical test have not been studied.

Quadrant Test and Hip Scouring Test

The hip quadrant test, also known as hip scouring, attempts to load as much of the acetabular surface area as possible (Figure 8–9). Maitland's description of the quadrant test emphasized the importance of determining whether joint loading reproduced symptoms or if irregularity of motion could be detected manually by the examiner.[38] The test assesses for pain, and restricted range of motion, while eliminating other structures including the iliopsoas muscle and hip joint capsule. This test should not be performed in patients with suspected fracture.[31] No validation of this test is available, but would likely be poor in that it is based on the patient's subjective report of pain and the perceived quality of motion.

The patient lies in a supine position and the examiner flexes and adducts the hip to end range where resistance is felt. The examiner then moves the hip into abduction while maintaining the flexed position. The motion from adduction to abduction should be in circular arc while applying compression in the direction of the shaft of the femur. The applied posterior compression in a circular motion is to load the surface area of the acetabulum. The four quadrants can be divided into the following arc of motion:

1. Flexion/abduction/external rotation to extension/abduction/external rotation
2. Flexion/adduction/external rotation to extension/adduction/external rotation
3. Flexion/abduction/internal rotation to extension/abduction/internal rotation
4. Flexion/adduction/internal rotation to extension/adduction/internal rotation

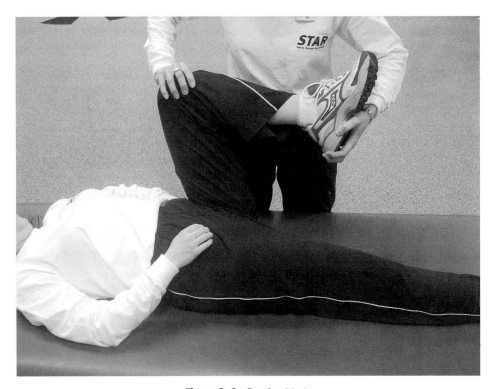

Figure 8–9. Quadrant test.

Any irregularity in motion, reproduction of pain, locking, crepitus, clicking, or apprehension is considered a positive test. A positive test may indicate intra-articular pathology but its sensitivity and specificity as well as its reliability have not been tested in order to validate its use.

Axial Hip Distraction

Axial hip distraction is also called a "caudal glide test" and may be useful in determining whether the patient's symptoms are related to compressive forces at the hip. No specific clinical studies utilizing the hip distraction technique have been identified, but distraction techniques are commonly used to unload any joint throughout the musculoskeletal system. Validation of this test is difficult, as it is dependent on the subjective report by the patient and the amount of force applied by the examiner.

The patient is in a supine position and the examiner abducts the hip 30 degrees and applies long-axis traction by holding the leg just above the ankle (Figure 8–10). If knee pathology is suspected or evident, the examiner should apply a shorter lever arm of traction by placing his/her hands around the thigh just proximal to the knee.

Figure 8–10. Axial hip distraction test.

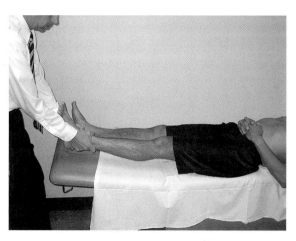

Relief of the patient's symptoms is reported to be a sign of an underlying intra-articular process. The examiner should also feel for giving way or telescoping as the traction is applied.[37]

No sensitivity, specificity, or reliability studies have been performed on this test.

Tests for Leg-length Discrepancy

Leg-length discrepancy (LLD) can be classified into two etiologic groups: structural (true) and functional (apparent or biomechanical). Structural LLDs are those in which an actual bony asymmetry exists somewhere between the head of the femur and the mortise of the ankle resulting in a true leg-length difference. Functional LLDs are those that occur as a physiologic response to altered mechanics along the kinetic chain anywhere from the foot to the lumbar spine, giving the appearance of a short leg when an asymmetry in the length of bones might not actually exist.[18,25,58]

A commonly used technique for the clinical assessment of LLD, and one that is purported to assess true anatomic differences, is the direct tape measurement method (TMM), measuring between the bony landmarks of the anterior superior iliac spine (ASIS) and the medial malleolus (MM) of the tibia (Figure 8–11).[58] The original description of this test's initial use has not been located. The German Society of Orthopaedics and Traumatology advocated a similar technique of direct tape measurement from the ASIS to the lateral malleolus (LM), claiming it is a more direct method and eliminates the contour of the thigh as a source of error.[12,45]

Measurement of functional LLD involves use of the umbilicus (U) or the xiphosternum (X) as the proximal reference point of direct tape measurement to the medial malleolus.[58] Whether this assessment should be performed in the weight-bearing

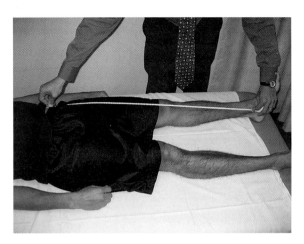

Figure 8–11. Leg length measurement from anterior superior iliac spine to the medial malleolus.

(standing) or supine position is controversial. Functional LLD assessment in the weight-bearing position may be of greater clinical value as it simulates the functional positioning of the patient and represents his or her posture in many activities of daily living (see Table 8–1).

In 1955, Nichols and Bailey determined the accuracy, or "observer error," of measuring leg-length differences by the TMM from the ASIS to MM.[47] They compared the results of measurements of leg-length differences of 50 patients by four doctors and determined that the "overall degree of accuracy of the measurement of leg lengths is such that differences of ½ inch (12.5 mm) or more may be accepted as diagnostically significant, but differences of less than ½ inch are not reliable unless based on the average of at least four measurements."

Gofton[21] described a useful way to estimate LLD. According to Gofton, three observations will be made in a standing patient if significant leg-length discrepancy exists:

1. The upper lateral thigh on the long side will protrude
2. Scoliosis will be apparent
3. The examiner's hands placed on top of the iliac crests will rest at different heights.

The examiner then places a lift under the foot of the presumed short side with correction of the observed imbalances. Gofton described the final step as the following:[21]

> The final step, and one which should not be omitted, is to place the same block under the presumed longer leg. The three observations originally made should now be exaggerated. Unless these simple checks confirm the initial observations the reliability of the estimated leg-length disparity is in doubt. The size of the block necessary to bring the pelvis to an appropriate level is an indication of the amount of disparity.

Gofton recognized that, with this method, obese or muscular subjects pose difficulties, because the hands of the examiner may not be able to palpate the top of the iliac crests and the scoliosis may be difficult to discern. Nevertheless, this method does include the feet, which the standard tape estimation does not, and allows the examiner to control apparent shortening more readily in the standing as opposed to the lying subject.

Bourdillon[8] listed four helpful methods to estimate LLD:

1. By comparing the levels of the posterior inferior iliac spines from behind with the patient standing
2. By comparing the levels of the posterior superior iliac spines from behind with the patient standing and fully flexed at the hip
3. By comparing the relative levels of the gluteal folds from behind with the patient erect
4. By comparing the levels of the iliac crests using the index fingers.

Bourdillon described a novel final step in which the examiner observes the patient in the sitting position:[8]

> With the patient in the sitting position, the effect of any leg-length discrepancy is eliminated. If, therefore, the right posterior inferior spine appears to be lower than the left in the standing position, but the two appear to be level with the patient sitting, this is additional evidence that the right leg is shorter than the left. If, with the patient sitting, the posterior inferior spine on the right side still appears lower than that on the left, the probable cause is a fixed torsion of the pelvis.

Clarke[10] described a radiographic method of measuring LLD and used it to study the accuracy of the direct tape measure method (TMM) using the ASIS and MM and the iliac crest palpation method without the use of lift blocks. Fifty patients were found to have an LLD with a degree of accuracy of 3 mm or less via the radiographic method. Using the TMM, both testers were within 5 mm of the x-ray result in only 20 of the 50 cases. If the 21 cases of 10 mm or more LLD are considered, in only 7 cases were both observers correct. Using the iliac crest palpation method, both testers were correct within 5 mm of the x-ray results in only 16 of the 50 cases. Of the 21 cases with LLD of 10 mm and more, only 9 were correctly assessed by both observers using iliac crest palpation.

Fisk[15] listed those variables that made clinical leg-length measurement unreliable: observer error, pelvic and sacroiliac joint asymmetry, and pelvic torsion. He found that when comparing radiographic to clinical examination results, the latter were inaccurate in 30% of cases. He concluded that the radiographic method of measuring LLD was more accurate than the clinical measurement methods.

Woerman and Binder-Macleod[58] tested and compared the results of five clinical methods of leg-length discrepancy assessment: the direct methods of ASIS to MM, ASIS to LM, U to MM, and X to MM, and the indirect method of iliac crest palpation with use of lift blocks for correction. The results were assessed against one another for their relative accuracy and precision compared to exact anatomic standards as determined by radiograph. The study made three statistical determinations:

1. Methods U and X were the most inaccurate and imprecise of all methods of direct LLD assessment tested.
2. Method LM proved to be a generally more accurate and precise tool in most test situations, especially after introduction and review of specific palpatory techniques.
3. The indirect method was the most precise and accurate method for LLD assessment of all methods tested, but tended to measure short to the actual.

Mann et al.[39] demonstrated an inter-rater reliability of roughly 70% in the determination of iliac crest heights by experienced physical therapists, compared to roughly 60% by inexperienced student therapists. Gogia and Braatz[22] demonstrated the strongest reliability of the TMM compared to radiographic assessment, with intra-examiner and inter-examiner reliability (intraclass correlation coefficient, ICC) of 0.98. No other studies have demonstrated such strong relationships. Beattie et al.[3] demonstrated intra-examiner reliability of 0.817, while inter-examiner reliability was 0.668. However, when the mean values of each therapist's two measurements were compared across observers, the ICC values increased to 0.910 for the total sample.

When comparing leg-length differences using the TMM (ASIS to MM) with those using a radiographic technique, Beattie et al. noted an ICC of 0.683 for all subjects.[4] When the means of the two values obtained by the tape measure method were compared with the radiographic measurements, the ICC for all subjects was 0.793.

Friberg et al.[19] reported that the indirect method of assessing LLD is an inaccurate and imprecise method, with a 7.5-mm mean difference compared to radiographs, and a 1.5-mm intra-examiner error. They also reported that the TMM (ASIS to MM) is equally as inaccurate with a mean difference in LLD measure of 8.6 mm compared to radiographs, and a 1.1-mm intra-examiner mean error. In contrast, Hoyle et al.[28] reported an inter-examiner reliability of 0.98 and an intra-examiner reliability ranging from 0.89 to 0.95 for the same measurements.

Lampe et al.[35] studied the agreement of LLD assessments using the TMM (ASIS to MM), iliac crest palpation with lift blocks, or "wooden boards," and radiography. They found that 95% of the measurements with lift blocks were within −1.4 and +1.6 cm of the results of the radiographs. The TMM had significantly less agreement (95% CI: −1.8 to +2.1; $p = 0.002$).

Jonson and Gross[32] used healthy naval shipmen to study the reliability of the method that employs lift blocks under the shorter limb and a pelvic leveling device at the iliac crests. The intra-examiner reliability ICC was 0.87, while the inter-examiner reliability was 0.70 ($N = 18$). The reliability ICC values for percentage discrepancy were 0.86 and 0.67, respectively. Intra-examiner and inter-examiner mean absolute differences for measuring total leg length were 0.43 and 0.75 cm, respectively. Gross et al.[24] used the indirect method of rigid lift with a pelvic leveling device and, when compared to radiographs, validity ranged from 0.55 to 0.76.

Hanada et al.[26] described the "iliac crest palpation and book correction" (ICPBC) method, performed by palpating the iliac crests and correcting identified differences with a book opened to the required number of pages. The measured thickness of the book correction is the LLD. By comparing the LLD using the ICPBC method and radiography in patients with simulated LLD that was induced, Hanada and colleagues determined the ICC for the intra-examiner and inter-examiner reliabilities to be 0.98 and 0.91, respectively. The ICCs for the construct and concurrent validities were 0.62 and 0.76, respectively. These authors concluded that the "ICPBC technique for measuring LLD is highly reliable and moderately valid."

In summary, most studies available have examined the indirect (rigid lift and pelvic observation) method or direct TMM. Because of conflicting results, there continues to be disagreement regarding the validity and reliability of both methods. The average of two measurements between the ASIS and MM may have acceptable validity and reliability when used as a screening tool and therefore is advocated. When accuracy is critical, radiographs or other imaging techniques should be considered.

Miscellaneous Tests

Fulcrum Test

In 1994, Johnson et al.[30] described the fulcrum test to assist in the diagnosis and management of stress fractures of the femoral shaft (see Table 8–1). Of note, this test was an outgrowth of historical data from four patients who reported aggravation of thigh discomfort when they sat on the edge of a desk or crossed their legs with the affected leg dangling in the air (Figure 8–12).[11,20] The fulcrum test was described in the following manner:[30]

> For this test the athlete is seated on the examination table with the lower legs dangling. The examiner's arm is used as a fulcrum under the thigh and is moved from distal to proximal thigh as gentle pressure is applied to the dorsum of the knee with the opposite hand. At the point of the fulcrum under the stress fracture, gentle pressure on the knee produced increased discomfort that was often described as a sharp pain and was accompanied with apprehension.

In their study, Johnson and colleagues prospectively followed 914 collegiate athletes over a two-year period. In that period, 34 stress fractures were sustained, seven of them (20.6%) involving the femoral shaft. The authors noted that for the

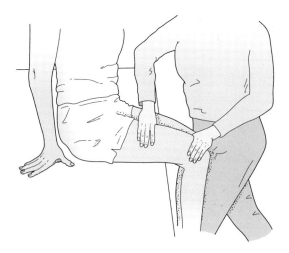

Figure 8–12. Fulcrum test utilizing the examination table as a fulcrum to increase force across the fracture site. Adapted with permission from Dugan S. Stress fractures. In Frontera WR, Silver JK (eds), Essentials of Physical Medicine and Rehabilitation. Philadelphia: Hanley & Belfus, 2002, p. 380.

seven patients with a femoral shaft stress fracture, the level at which the fulcrum test was positive corresponded to the site of the stress fracture in the femoral shaft as seen in a scintigram or radiograph. Only one false-positive was described in a patient with a quadriceps strain. In this patient the pain was less intense and there was no apprehension. One false-negative was described in a patient with a femoral neck stress fracture. The authors concluded that the fulcrum test is useful in diagnosing and managing femoral stress fractures. Future studies are needed to assess the reliability, sensitivity, and specificity of this test.

Hop Test

The hop test was originally described by Matheson et al.[40] to assess the likelihood of a stress fracture involving the lower extremity. Pain at the site of stress fracture reproduced by one-legged hopping indicated a positive hop test.

Clement et al.[11] studied 71 athletes with 74 stress injuries to the femur using a case-controlled design. During the clinical examination, when asked to hop on the affected limb, 70.3% of the patients had pain reproduced in the hip, groin, or anterior thigh. The authors concluded that the hop test was clinically useful in cases of suspected stress injury of the femur. These results should be used cautiously in that the true sensitivity, specificity, and reliability of this test have not been performed.

Conclusion

Evaluation of the hip requires a comprehensive understanding of the anatomy and biomechanics of the hip and related structures. The scientific evidence of the sensitivity, specificity and reliability of physical examination maneuvers of the hip is limited.

Therefore we must carefully utilize these tests in concert with historical information with an understanding of their usefulness in making specific diagnoses related to the hip.

REFERENCES

1. Amiel-Tison C. Neurologic evaluation of the maturity of newborn infants. Arch Dis Child 1968;43:89–93.
2. Bartlett MD, Wolf LS, Shurtleff DB, Staheli LT. Hip flexion contractures: a comparison of measurement methods. Arch Phys Med Rehabil 1985;66:620–625.
3. Beattie P, Rothstein JM, Kopriva LM. The clinical reliability of measuring the difference in leg lengths [abstract]. Phys Ther 1988;68:588.
4. Beattie P, Isaacson K, Riddle DL, Rothstein JM. Validity of derived measurements of leg-length differences obtained by use of a tape measure. Phys Ther 1990;70:150–157.
5. Benson ER, Schutzer SF. Posttraumatic piriformis syndrome: diagnosis and results of operative treatment. J Bone Joint Surg Am 1999;81:941–949.
6. Bird PA, Oakley SP, Shnier R, Kirkham BW. Prospective evaluation of magnetic resonance imaging and physical examination findings in patients with greater trochanteric pain syndrome. Arthritis Rheum 2001;44:2138–2145.
7. Bleck EE. Orthopedic Management of Cerebral Palsy, Vol. 2. Philadelphia: WB Saunders, 1979, pp. 29–33.
8. Bourdillon JF. Spinal Manipulation, 2nd edn. London: Heinemann, 1973.
9. Cave EF, Roberts SM. A method for measuring and recording joint function. J Bone Joint Surg 1936;18:455–465.
10. Clarke GR. Unequal leg length: an accurate method of detection and some clinical results. Rheum Phys Med 1972;11:385–390.
11. Clement DB, Ammann W, Taunton JE, et al. Exercise-induced stress injuries to the femur. Int J Sports Med 1993;14:347–352.
12. Eichler J. Methodological errors in documenting leg length and leg length discrepancies. In Hungerford DS (ed.), Progress in Orthopedic Surgery, Vol. 1. Berlin: Springer-Verlag, 1977, pp. 29–40.
13. Eland DC, Singleton TN, Conaster RR, et al. The "iliacus test": new information for the evaluation of hip extension dysfunction. J Am Osteopor Assoc 2002;102:130–142.
14. Evans EB. The knee in cerebral palsy. In Samilson RL (ed.), Orthopedic Aspects of Cerebral Palsy. London: SIMP/Heinemann; Philadelphia: JB Lippincott, 1975, pp. 173–194.
15. Fisk JW, Baigent ML. Clinical and radiological assessment of leg length. NZ Med J 1975;81:477–480.
16. Freiberg AH, Vinke TH. Sciatica and the sacro-iliac joint. J Bone Joint Surg 1934;16:126–136.
17. Freiberg AH. Sciatic pain and its relief by operations on the muscle and fascia. Arch Surg 1937;34:337–350.
18. Friberg O. Leg length asymmetry in stress fractures: a clinical and radiological study. J Sports Med 1982;22:485–488.
19. Friberg O, Nurminen M, Kouhonen K, Soininen E, Manttari T. Accuracy and precision of clinical estimation of leg length inequality and lumbar scoliosis: comparison of clinical and radiological measurements. Int Disability Stud 1988;10:49–53.
20. Fricker P, Masters S, Purdam C. Stress fractures of the femoral shaft: four case studies. Br J Sports Med 1986;20:14–16.
21. Gofton JP. Studies in osteoarthritis of the hip. IV: Biomechanics and clinical considerations. Can Med Assoc J 1971;104:1007–1011.
22. Gogia PP, Braatz JH. Validity and reliability of leg length measurements. J Orthop Sports Phys Ther 1986;8:185–188.
23. Gray H. Anatomy of the Human Body. Philadelphia: Lea & Febiger, 1924.
24. Gross MT, Burns CB, Chapman SW, et al. Reliability and validity of rigid lift and pelvic leveling device method in assessing functional leg length inequality. J Orthop Sports Phys Ther 1998;27:284–294.
25. Gurney B. Leg length discrepancy. Gait Posture 2002;15:195–206.
26. Hanada E, Kirby Lee, Mitchell M, Swuste JM. Measuring leg-length discrepancy by the "iliac crest palpation and book correction" method: reliability and validity. Arch Phys Med Rehabil 2001;82:938–942.
27. Harvey D. Assessment of the flexibility of elite athletes using the modified Thomas test. Br J Sports Med 1998;32:68–70.

28. Hoyle DA, Latour M, Bohannon RW. Intraexaminer, interexaminer, and interdevice comparability of leg length measurements obtained with measuring tape and metrecom. J Orthop Sports Phys Ther 1991;14:263–268.

29. Johnson A, Ashurst H. Is popliteal angle measurement useful in early identification of cerebral palsy? Devel Med Child Neurol 1989;31:457–465.

30. Johnson AW, Weiss CB, Wheeler DL. Stress fractures of the femoral shaft in athletes: more common than expected. A new clinical test. Am J Sports Med 1994;22:248–256.

31. Jones SL. Evaluation of the hip. In Fagerson TL (ed.), The Hip Handbook. Boston: Butterworth-Heinemann, 1998, pp. 97–159.

32. Jonson SR, Gross MT. Intraexaminer reliability, interexaminer reliability, and mean values for nine lower extremity skeletal measures in healthy naval midshipmen. J Orthop Sports Phys Ther 1997;25:253–263.

33. Khan NQ, Woolson ST. Referral patterns of hip pain in patients undergoing total hip replacement. Orthopedics 1998;21:123–126.

34. Koenigsberger MR. Judgement of fetal age. 1: Neurologic evaluation. Ped Clin N Am 1966;13:823–833.

35. Lampe HIH, Swierstra BA, Diepstraten FM. Measurement of limb length inequality: comparison of clinical methods with orthoradiography in 190 children. Acta Orthop Scand 1996;67:242–244.

36. Laègue C. Consideration sur la sciatique. Arch Gen de Med 1864;2:558.

37. Magee DM. Orthopedic Physical Assessment, 4th edn. Philadelphia: WB Saunders, 2002, pp. 606–640.

38. Maitland GD. The Peripheral Joints: Examination and Recording Guide. Adelaide: Virgo Press, 1973.

39. Mann M, Glasheen-Wray M, Nyberg R. Therapist agreement for palpation and observation of iliac crest heights. Phys Ther 1984;64:334–338.

40. Matheson GO, Clement DB, Mckenzie DC, et al. Stress fractures in athletes: a study of 320 cases. Am J Sports Med 1987;15:46–58.

41. McGrory BJ. Stinchfield resisted hip flexion test. Hosp Physician 1999;35(9);41–42.

42. Milch H. Nelaton's line. Med Record 1938;CXLVII, 229.

43. Milch H. Pelvifemoral angle: determination of hip-flexion deformity. J Bone Joint Surg 1942;24:148–153.

44. Moore ML. The measurement of joint motion. II: The technique of goniometry. Phys Ther Rev 1949;29:256–264.

45. Morscher E. Etiology and pathophysiology of leg length discrepancies. In Hungerford DS (ed.), Progress in Orthopedic Surgery, Vol. 1. Berlin: Springer-Verlag, 1977, pp. 9–19.

46. Mundale MO, Hislop HJ, Rabideau RJ, Kottke FJ. Evaluation of extension of hip. Arch Phys Med Rehabil 1956;37:75–80.

47. Nichols PJR, Bailey NTJ. The accuracy of measuring leg-length differences. Br Med J 1955;2:1247.

48. Ober FB. The role of the iliotibial band and fascia lata as a factor in the causation of low back disabilities and sciatica. J Bone Joint Surg 1936;18:105–110.

49. Pace JB, Nagle D. Piriformis syndrome. West J Med 1976;124:435–439.

50. Reade E, Hom L, Hallum, Lopopolo R. Changes in popliteal angle measurement in infants up to one year of age. Devel Med Child Neurol 1984;26:774–780.

51. Robinson DR. Pyriformis syndrome in relation to sciatic pain. Am J Surg 1947;73:355–358.

52. Solheim LF, Siewers P, Paus B. The piriformis muscle syndrome: sciatic nerve entrapment treated with section of the piriformis muscle. Acta Orthop Scand 1981;52:73–75.

53. Staheli LT. The prone hip extension test: a method of measuring hip flexion deformity. Clin Orthop 1977;123:12–15.

54. Thomas HO. Diseases of the Hip, Knee, and Ankle Joints and Their Deformities Treated by a New and Efficient Method, 3rd edn. Liverpool: T. Dobb & Co., 1876, pp. 17–19.

55. Thurston A. Assessment of fixed flexion deformity of the hip. Clin Orthop 1982;169:186–189.

56. Trendelenburg F. Trendelenburg's test 1895. Clin Orthop 1998;355:3–7.

57. West CC. Measurement of joint motion. Arch Phys Med 1945;26:414–425.

58. Woerman AL, Binder-Macleod SA. Leg length discrepancy assessment: accuracy and precision in five clinical methods of evaluation. J Orthop Sports Phys Ther 1984;5:230–239.

59. Yeoman W. Relation of arthritis of sacro-iliac joint to sciatica. Lancet 1928;ii:1119.

Chapter 9

Physical Examination of the Knee

STEPHEN ANDRUS, MD • GERARD A. MALANGA, MD •
MICHAEL STUART, MD

Introduction

The knee is particularly susceptible to traumatic injury because of its vulnerable location midway between the hip and the ankle, where it is exposed to the considerable forces transmitted from the ground through the knee to the hip. Thorough examination of all of the knee structures, including the ligaments and menisci, should be included in every knee evaluation. The examiner must rely on numerous physical exam maneuvers to evaluate these structures. It is crucial not only that these maneuvers are performed correctly, but also that the examiner is aware of the sensitivity and specificity of the various tests, as well as the limitations of the tests, in order to make the most accurate diagnosis possible.[58] In this chapter, we provide a review of the physical examination of the knee, followed by a literature-based review of the diagnostic accuracy of the major provocative tests used to diagnose knee injuries.

Inspection

Assessment of the knee should begin with an overall evaluation of lower-extremity alignment. Varus–valgus alignment of the lower extremity while weight-bearing with the knee in full extension should be noted. Normally, the tibia has a slight valgus angulation in comparison to the femur, and this angle is usually more pronounced in females. From the side, the knee should be fully extended when the patient is standing. Slight hyperextension of the knee is a normal finding, provided that it is present in both lower extremities. The position of the patella should be noted. When viewing the patella, the examiner should note whether the patella points straight ahead, tilts inward, outward, or is rotated in any way. Rotation and tilt may be caused by tight structures in the lower extremities that alter the position of the patella.

The skin around the knee joint should be inspected for any bruising, abrasions, lacerations, or surgical scars. External signs of injury can give a clue as to the mechanism of injury and internal structures damaged. Signs of swelling in the knee should be observed and may be suggested by the loss of the peripatellar groove on either side of the patella. Generalized swelling may be due to an effusion in the joint, whereas localized swelling may be due to an inflamed bursa or cyst.

The quadriceps muscle atrophies quickly when there is any type of knee joint pathology. Signs of muscular atrophy should, therefore, be observed and quantified with circumferential measurements that compare the affected and unaffected sides for differences in muscle girth.

Assessment of gait is an integral component of the comprehensive knee examination. In the normal gait cycle, the knee comes to full extension only at heel strike. During stance phase, slight flexion occurs, and it is the contraction of the quadriceps at this point that prevents giving way. At toe-off, the knee flexes to about 40 degrees and continues to flex through midswing to approximately 65 degrees. At this point, the quadriceps contract to begin acceleration of the leg, with the knee returning to full extension once again at heel strike. At heel strike, the hamstrings must contract in order to decelerate the leg. Abnormalities in gait pattern can occur from various causes. Weak hamstrings may not decelerate the knee properly and result in hyperextension at heel strike. Weakness in the quadriceps can cause a hard heel strike to occur, with excessive hip extension to force the knee into a hyperextended position to prevent buckling. Ligament injuries may result in a varus or valgus thrust, or even a buckling of the joint, depending on the extent of the ligament compromise. Finally, pain within the knee joint generally causes the patient to walk with an antalgic gait.[25]

Range of Motion

Active and passive range of motions of the knee should be measured. The neutral position (0 degrees) for the knee joint occurs when the femur and tibia are in a straight, fully extended position. Positive degrees of motion are measured for flexion, and negative degrees of motion are used to describe hyperextension of the knee. Normal values would be 135 degrees of flexion, and as much as 5–10 degrees of hyperextension. There can be a significant amount of normal variation, and it is therefore important to compare the involved and uninvolved sides.

As the examiner moves the knee through flexion and extension, the movements of the patella as it tracks along the femoral trochlea should be observed. The patella does not follow a straight path as the knee moves, but instead follows a curved pattern. The examiner should note whether the patella tilts laterally, tilts anteroposteriorly, or rotates during dynamic knee extension. The examiner should also observe for signs of quadriceps lag. This results from weakness of the quadriceps muscle and causes the patient to have difficulty in completing the last 10–15 degrees of knee extension. Although the majority of motion occurs with extension and flexion, the knee does possess the ability to rotate both internally and externally. Approximately 10 degrees of rotation in either direction is thought to represent a normal range, and significant increases in internal or external rotation may indicate ligament compromise.

Passive range of motion is assessed when the patient is not able to perform the full range of active movements. Flexion is tested with the patient lying prone. The leg is held just proximal to the ankle, and the knee is flexed. There are a number of causes for a decrease in range of motion at the knee. The most common cause is an effusion within the knee joint. A bucket-handle tear of the meniscus or loose body in the joint can act as a mechanical block, preventing full extension of the knee. Osteoarthritic changes can produce primarily a loss of full extension, as well as some loss of flexion. Significant ligamentous injuries can undermine the normal knee restraints, and allow abnormally increased ranges of motion to occur.

Palpation

The entire knee should be palpated in a sequential manner and compared with the uninjured side. The presence of an increase in temperature of the skin overlying the joint should be determined before other tests are performed. Palpation is the best way to determine the presence of swelling in and around the knee joint. A large joint effusion will be obvious to the examiner, whereas a small effusion can be identified by placing gentle thumb pressure over the lateral aspect of the patellofemoral joint and detecting a fluid wave with the index finger. In the ballottement test, one hand milks fluid from the suprapatellar pouch while the other hand presses down on the patella. The patella springing back indicates the presence of a larger effusion.

Localized tenderness is helpful in pinpointing the site of injury or pathology in the knee joint. A detailed knowledge of the bony and soft tissue surface anatomy is therefore of critical importance when trying to make a specific diagnosis in the knee. Palpation of the bony and soft tissue structures of the knee can be divided into four quadrants: anterior, medial, lateral, and posterior.

Medial Knee

Bony Structures

The bony structures of interest in the medial aspect of the knee include the medial tibial plateau, the tibial tubercle, medial femoral condyle, medial femoral epicondyle, and the adductor tubercle. The examiner's thumbs are placed on the anterior portion of the knee and pressed into the soft tissue depressions on each side of the infrapatellar tendon. Pushing a thumb slightly inferiorly into the soft tissue depression, the examiner palpates the distinct upper edge of the medial tibial plateau. The medial tibial plateau represents one site of attachment for the medial meniscus. Next, the infrapatellar tendon may be followed distally, to its insertion into the tibial tubercle. Moving the thumb upward from the starting position in the depressions on each side of the infrapatellar tendon, the medial femoral condyle will become palpable. The femoral condyle is more easily palpated if the knee is flexed to greater than 90 degrees. The adductor tubercle is located on the posterior medial aspect of the medial femoral condyle. It can be located by moving your thumbs posteriorly from the medial surface of the medial femoral condyle.[31]

Soft Tissue Structures

Palpation of the medial meniscus is performed along the medial joint line. The medial edge of the medial meniscus becomes more prominent when the tibia is internally rotated. Tears of the posteromedial portion of the medial meniscus are the most common, and are diagnosed clinically in part by the finding of tenderness at the posteromedial corner of the knee. The medial collateral ligament (MCL) is a broad ligament that spans from the medial femoral epicondyle to the tibia. The superficial MCL attaches to the medial femoral epicondyle proximally, and the medial aspect of the tibia distally, approximately 4 cm below the level of the joint line. The deep fibers of the MCL represent a thickening of the middle third of the joint capsule. The deep MCL has attachments to the underlying medial meniscus. The ligament should be palpated from origin to insertion for tenderness.

On the posteromedial side of the knee, the tendons of the sartorius, gracilis, and the semitendinosus muscles cross the knee joint, and insert into the lower portion of the medial tibial plateau. The pes anserine bursa lies at the common insertion of these muscles, and may become a source of pain when the bursa is inflamed (Figure 9–1).[25]

Lateral Knee

Bony Structures

The bony structures of interest in the lateral aspect of the knee include the lateral tibial plateau, lateral tubercle (Gerdy's tubercle), lateral femoral condyle, lateral femoral

Figure 9–1. The pes anserine bursa and medial knee structures. Adapted with permission from O'Donoghue DH. Treatment of Injuries to Athletes, 4th edn. Philadelphia: WB Saunders, 1984, p. 466.

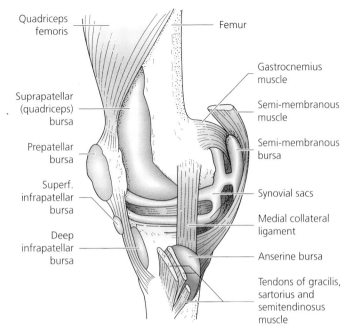

epicondyle, and the head of the fibula. Starting with your thumb in the soft tissue depression just lateral to the infrapatellar tendon, the edge of the lateral tibial plateau can be palpated inferiorly. The lateral tubercle is the large prominence of bone palpable just below the lateral tibial plateau. Moving upward and laterally from the starting point of the depression, the lateral femoral condyle becomes palpable. More of the lateral femoral condyle is palpable when the knee is flexed to greater than 90 degrees. The lateral femoral condyle lies just lateral to the femoral condyle. Finally, the fibular head is easily palpable along the lateral aspect of the knee, inferior to the joint line, at about the level of the tibial tubercle.[31]

Soft Tissue Structures

Palpation of the lateral meniscus is performed along the lateral joint line, with the knee in a slightly flexed position (Figure 9–2). The lateral meniscus is attached to the popliteus muscle, and not the lateral collateral ligament (LCL). The LCL is a palpable cord that runs between the lateral femoral condyle and the fibular head (Figure 9–3). Attaching posterior to the fibular head, and extending proximally, is the biceps femoris tendon. Additionally, the iliotibial band can be assessed for tenderness at its insertion point on Gerdy's tubercle of the tibia, and also as it crosses the lateral condyle of the femur. Complaints of "snapping" over the lateral femoral condyle are often associated with a tight iliotibial band. The common peroneal nerve can be palpated as it wraps around the fibula, and the nerve may be assessed for a positive Tinel's sign, indicative of nerve irritation or damage.[25]

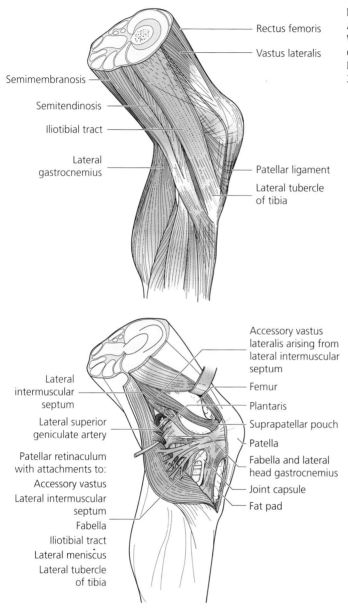

Figure 9–2. The lateral structures of the knee. Adapted with permission from Pagnani MJ, Warren RF, Arnoczky SP, Wickiewicz TL. Anatomy of the knee. In Nicholas J, Hershman E (eds), The Lower Extremity and Spine in Sports Medicine, 2nd edn. St Louis: Mosby, 1995, p. 607.

Anterior Knee

Bony Structures

The bony structures of interest in the anterior knee are the patella and the trochlear groove of the femur. The trochlear groove can be palpated by placing your thumbs over the medial and lateral joint lines and moving upward along the two femoral condyles. The depression of the trochlear groove is palpated in the midline, above the level of the patella.

Figure 9–3. Palpation of the lateral (fibular) collateral ligament (FCL). Adapted with permission from Zarins B, Fish DN. Knee ligament injury. In Nicholas J, Hershman E (eds), The Lower Extremity and Spine in Sports Medicine, 2nd edn. St Louis: Mosby, 1995, p. 854.

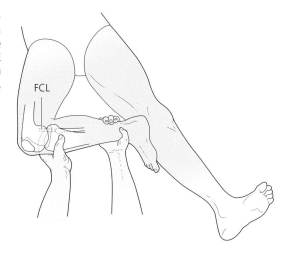

In flexion, the patella is fixed in the trochlear groove and therefore the undersurface of the patella is not easily palpated. In extension, the patella is more mobile, and palpation of the medial and lateral undersurfaces (facets) of the patella is possible in this position.[31]

Soft Tissue Structures

In the anterior aspect of the knee, an assessment of the tone and bulk of the quadriceps muscle should be made, as this is the main stabilizing muscle for the knee. Assessment of the vastus medialis is important when assessing the function of the patellofemoral joint. The prepatellar bursa overlies the anterior aspect of the patella (Figure 9–4). Thickening or swelling of the prepatellar bursa is commonly seen in people who frequently kneel. The patellar tendon is the continuation of the quadriceps tendon from the lower pole of the patella to the tibial tubercle. The superficial infrapatellar bursa lies between the skin and the patellar tendon, and is easily palpable on exam. The deep infrapatellar bursa lies beneath the patellar tendon.

Posterior Knee

The posterior fossa is bounded by the hamstring tendons proximally and the two heads of the gastrocnemius muscle distally. Passing through the posterior fossa is the tibial nerve, the popliteal artery, and the popliteal vein. Examination of the popliteal pulse is best performed with the knee in 90 degrees of flexion, so that the hamstring and calf muscles are relaxed. The popliteal artery is the deepest structure in the posterior fossa, and travels against the joint capsule. The posterior tibial nerve is the most superficial structure in the popliteal area, with the popliteal vein running directly beneath it. A cystic swelling within the fossa, called a Baker's cyst, can present as a

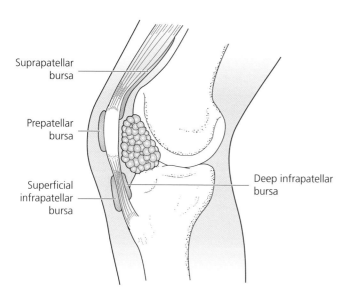

Suprapatellar bursa

Prepatellar bursa

Superficial infrapatellar bursa

Deep infrapatellar bursa

Figure 9–4. The bursa of the knee. Adapted with permission from Boland AL, Hulstyn MJ. Soft tissue injuries of the knee. In Nicholas J, Hershman E (eds), The Lower Extremity and Spine in Sports Medicine, 2nd edn. St Louis: Mosby, 1995, p. 909.

usually painless, mobile swelling on the medial side of the fossa. Many Baker's cysts directly communicate with the joint. The cyst is an enlargement of the normal gastrocnemius–semimembranosus bursa.

Neurovascular Testing

The quadriceps muscle is the primary extensor of the knee, and is innervated by the femoral nerve, with primarily L3 and L4 nerve root innervation. Manual testing of the quadriceps muscle can be performed with the patient in the sitting position. The patient should be asked to extend the knee actively. The examiner can use one hand to resist the extension of the leg, while the other hand can be used to palpate the tone and bulk of the muscle as it is contracting. The primary flexors of the knee are the hamstring muscles, which include the semimembranosus, semitendinosus, and biceps femoris. All of the hamstring muscles are innervated by the tibial portion of the sciatic nerve. The semimembranosus and semitendinosus receive the majority of their innervation from the L5 nerve root, while the biceps femoris receives most of its innervation from the S1 nerve root.

Manual testing of the hamstrings as a group can be performed by having the patient lie prone on the examination table. The patient is instructed to flex his/her knee while you resist this motion by holding the leg just proximal to the ankle joint. The patellar tendon reflex is a deep tendon reflex involving the L2, L3, and L4 neurologic levels, but for clinical application is primarily considered an L4 reflex. Sensation should also be assessed in the area of the knee and surrounding areas. Peripheral pulses should be tested in the femoral, popliteal, dorsalis pedis, and the posterior tibial arteries. The incidence of popliteal artery injury with knee dislocation is approximately 25%, so assessment of the vascular system is crucial, especially in acute knee injuries.[84]

Stability Testing

The ligaments of the knee joint are the primary structures responsible for maintaining stability of the joint (Figure 9–5). The knee should be checked for stability in the anteroposterior, medial–lateral, and rotatory directions. It is important to compare tests for stability with the normal contralateral knee, since there can be individual variation in the laxity of the ligaments tested. It can be helpful to evaluate the uninjured knee first, so that the patient has an understanding of what manipulations are going to be performed. In the acute situation, where the mechanism of injury is observed and the patient can be evaluated immediately before pain and secondary muscle spasm occur, the assessment of the ligaments can be much easier. Specific tests to assess the anterior cruciate ligament, posterior cruciate ligament, lateral collateral ligament, and medial collateral ligament will be described in the following sections, along with a literature review of the sensitivity and specificity of the individual tests.

Tests for the Anterior Cruciate Ligament

The anterior cruciate ligament (ACL) is one of the main stabilizers of the knee with injury often resulting in significant disability. Three of the most commonly applied tests are the anterior drawer, the Lachman test, and the pivot shift test (Table 9–1).

Anterior Drawer Test

Although the anterior drawer test has been widely used in the diagnoses of ACL ruptures, the origin of this maneuver remains obscure (Figure 9–6). According to Paessler,[70] as early as 1879, Paul Segund described the "abnormal anterior–posterior mobility" of the knee associated with ACL ruptures. George Noulis, who Paessler and Michell[70] credited with the earliest description of what we now call the Lachman test, also elucidated the drawer tests in large degrees of flexion. In a translation of Noulis' 1875 French thesis that appears in the textbook *Diagnostic Evaluation of the Knee* by Strobel and Stedtfeld,[79] Noulis describes the following test:

> [With] the patient's leg flexed, the thigh can be grasped with one hand at the lower leg with the other hand keeping the thumbs to the front and fingers to the back. If the lower leg is held in this grip and then moved backwards and forwards, it will be seen that the tibia can be moved directly backwards and forwards.

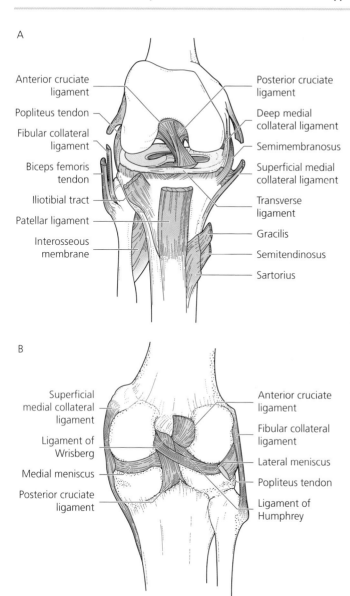

Figure 9–5. The ligaments of the knee. **A:** Anterior view. **B:** Posterior view. Adapted with permission from Scott WN (ed.). Ligament and Extensor Mechanism Injuries of the Knee. St Louis: Mosby, 1991.

Noulis observed a great deal of tibia displacement when both cruciate ligaments were severed. The assumption that a positive anterior drawer test indicates a tear of the ACL was not commonly accepted until much later.[35,71] Increased anterior tibial displacement as compared with the uninvolved side is now supported as indicative of a tear of the ACL.[47]

There remain some limitations of this test with sensitivities reported between 22.2% and 41% when performed in the alert patient and ranges of 79.6% to 91% when performed under anesthesia.[12,27,41,43,46,64] Differences in accuracy of the test are also

Table 9–1. ANTERIOR CRUCIATE LIGAMENT TESTS

Test	Description	Reliability/Validity Tests	Comments
Anterior drawer test	The subject is supine, hip flexed to 45 degrees and knee flexed to 90 degrees. The examiner sits on the subject's foot, with hands behind the proximal tibia and thumbs on the tibial plateau. Anterior force is applied to the proximal tibia. Hamstring tendons are palpated with index fingers to ensure relaxation. Increased tibial displacement compared with the opposite side is indicative of an ACL tear.	Harilainen 1987[27] Sensitivity: 41% Sensitivity (under anesthesia): 86%	350 acute knees evaluated, with 79 arthroscopically confirmed acute ACL injures. Prospective study.
		Katz 1986 and Fingeroth[43] Sensitivity: 22.2% (acute injuries) Sensitivity: 53.8% (chronic injuries) Specificity: >97% (acute + chronic)	*Testing performed only under anesthesia.* Retrospective study. Limited sample size: 9 acute ACL injuries and 12 chronic.
		Jonsson et al. 1982[41] Sensitivity: 33% (acute injuries) Sensitivity: 95% (chronic injuries)	107 patients, all with documented acute or chronic ACL ruptures. Specificity not assessed since only positive ACL ruptures included.
		Donaldson et al. 1985[12] Sensitivity: 70% (acute injuries) Sensitivity (under anesthesia): 91% Specificity: Not reported	Retrospective study. Study not designed to evaluate specificity since it was a review of only positive cases.
		Mitsou and Vallianatos 1988[64] Sensitivity: 40% (acute injuries) Sensitivity: 95.2% (chronic injuries) Specificity: Not reported	144 knees, with 60 acute injuries all assessed within 3 days of injury. In the group of 80 chronic injuries, the 4 false-negative drawer tests were associated with bucket-handle tears.
		Kim and Kim 1995[46] Sensitivity (under anesthesia): 79.6% Specificity: Not reported	*Testing performed only under anesthesia.* Retrospective study. All ACL injuries were chronic.
Lachman test	The patient lies supine. The knee is held between full extension and 15 degrees of flexion. The femur is stabilized with one hand while firm pressure is applied to the posterior aspect of the proximal tibia in an attempt to translate it anteriorly.	Torg et al. 1976[80] Sensitivity: 95% Specificity: Not reported	93 knees with combined tears of the ACL and median meniscus. All 5 false-negatives were associated with bucket-handle tears of the meniscus.
		Donaldson et al. 1985[12] Sensitivity: 99% Specificity: Not reported	Retrospective study. Study not designed to evaluate specificity since it was a review of only positive cases.

Continued

Table 9–1. ANTERIOR CRUCIATE LIGAMENT TESTS—*cont'd*

Test	Description	Reliability/Validity Tests	Comments
	The test is positive (indicating ACL rupture) when there is anterior translation of the tibia with "soft" end-point.	Katz and Fingeroth 1986[43] Sensitivity (under anesthesia): 84.6% Specificity (under anesthesia): 95%	*Testing performed only under anesthesia.* Retrospective study. Limited sample size: 9 acute ACL injuries and 12 chronic.
		Kim and Kim 1995[46] Sensitivity (under anesthesia): 98.6% Specificity: Not reported	*Testing performed only under anesthesia.* Retrospective review study. All ACL injuries were chronic.
		Mitsou and Vallianatos 1988[64] Sensitivity: 80% (acute injuries) Sensitivity: 98.8% (chronic injuries)	144 knees, with 60 acute injuries all assessed within 3 days of injury.
		Jonsson et al. 1982[41] Sensitivity: 87% (acute injuries) Sensitivity: 94% (chronic injuries)	107 patients, all with documented acute or chronic ACL ruptures. Specificity not assessed since only positive ACL ruptures included.
Pivot shift test	Leg picked up at the ankle. The knee is flexed by placing the heel of the hand behind the fibula. As the knee is extended, the tibia is supported on the lateral side with a slight valgus strain. A strong valgus force is placed on the knee by the upper hand. At approx. 30 degrees of flexion, the displaced tibia will suddenly reduce, indicating a positive pivot shift test.	Lucie et al. 1984[55] Sensitivity: 95% Specificity: 100%	50 knees tested. There was not an adequate sample size of intact ACLs to determine specificity.
		Katz and Fingeroth 1986[43] Sensitivity: 98.4% Specificity: >98%	*Testing performed only under anesthesia.* Retrospective study. Limited sample size: 9 acute ACL injuries and 12 chronic.
		Donaldson et al. 1985[12] Sensitivity: 35% Sensitivity (under anesthesia): 98% Specificity: Not reported	Retrospective study. Study not designed to evaluate specificity since it was a review of only positive cases.

Figure 9–6. Anterior drawer test. Adapted with permission from Micheo W, Amy E. Anterior cruciate ligament sprain. In Frontera WR, Silver JK (eds), Essentials of Physical Medicine and Rehabilitation. Philadelphia: Hanley & Belfus, 2002, p. 303.

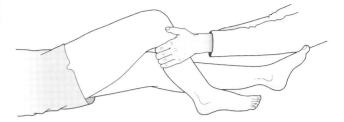

noted in those with acute versus chronic injury with the anterior drawer test present in 50–95% of chronic injuries.[47,71] Anterior drawer results may also be affected by the presence of concomitant injury, with 54% of those with no other injuries having a positive test, 67% of those with associated medial meniscal injuries, 82% in knees with associated lateral meniscal injuries, and 89% with associated medial collateral ligament injury demonstrated.[47] These figures suggest that the anterior drawer test becomes increasingly more sensitive as the secondary restraints of anterior stability are lost.

Falsely negative anterior drawer tests in instances of isolated ACL tears may occur secondary to protective spasm of the hamstring muscles and the anatomical configuration of the femoral condyle, while false-positive results may occur in the setting of posterior cruciate ligament (PCL) insufficiency.[64] In the presence of a PCL tear, sagging of the tibia may result in a false sense of its neutral position, resulting in a false sense of anterior movement when in fact the tibia is moving into its normal neutral position.

Overall, there is wide variation in the reported sensitivities of the anterior drawer test, with those performed under anesthesia having somewhat limited use in the clinical setting. The test's relatively low sensitivity for detecting ACL tears in the acute setting should serve to caution examiners not to rule out an acute ACL injury based solely on a negative anterior drawer. Conversely, the specificity of the test is quite high, and therefore a positive anterior drawer would strongly suggest the presence of ACL pathology.

Lachman Test

The Lachman test was described by Joseph Torg,[80] who trained under Dr Lachman at Temple University. Interestingly, Hans Paessler[70] traced descriptions of what we now call the Lachman as far back as 1875, when it was described in a thesis by George Noulis in Paris. Despite these very early descriptions, the test was not widely recognized or used until Torg's classic description of the Lachman test (Figure 9–7), which is given below:[80]

> The examination is performed with the patient lying supine on the table with involved extremity on the side of the examiner. With the patient's knee held between full extension and 15 degrees of flexion, the femur is stabilized with one hand while firm pressure is applied to the posterior aspect of the proximal tibia in an attempt to translate

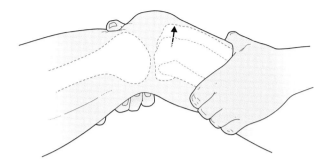

Figure 9–7. Lachman test. Adapted with permission from Ray JM. A proposed natural history of symptomatic anterior cruciate ligament injuries of the knee. Clin Sports Med 1988;7:699.

it anteriorly. A positive test indicating disruption of the anterior cruciate ligament is one in which there is proprioceptive and/or visual anterior translation of the tibia in relation to the femur with a characteristic 'mushy' or 'soft' end point. This is in contrast to a definite 'hard' end point elicited when the anterior cruciate ligament is intact.

There have been numerous studies looking at the sensitivity and specificity of the Lachman test, as well as studies comparing the accuracy of this test with the original anterior drawer. Torg originally reported that in 88 of 93 (95%) of individuals with combined lesions involving the anterior cruciate ligament and medial meniscus, the Lachman test was positive.[80] The false-negative tests were attributed to incarcerated bucket-handle tears blocking forward translation of the tibia. Donaldson et al.[12] noted a sensitivity of greater than 99% for this test and found it to be relatively unaffected by associated ligamentous or meniscal injuries. This was in contrast to the significant variability with anterior drawer when tested in those with injury to the secondary restraints of the knee. The sensitivity of the Lachman test has been reported to range between 80% and 100% with a specificity of 95%.[9,12,43,46,64,80] The Lachman test has therefore been found to be the most sensitive and specific test for diagnosis of ACL tears, especially in the setting of an acute injury.

There are certain limitations to the test. Draper and colleagues noted that the Lachman test is not easily performed when the patient has a large thigh girth and/or the examiner has small hands.[15,22,40] Various modifications of the Lachman have been proposed including "prone," "drop leg," and "stabilized" Lachman tests.[2,13,19,82] Few studies have been done comparing the sensitivity and specificity of these modified tests to the original.

Pivot Shift Test

The pivot shift is both a clinical phenomenon that gives rise to the complaint of giving way of the knee, and a physical sign that can be elicited upon examination of the injured knee (Figure 9–8).[22] Hey Groves in 1920 and Palmer in 1938 both published

Figure 9–8. Pivot shift test. Adapted with permission from Ray JM. A proposed natural history of symptomatic anterior cruciate ligament injuries of the knee. Clin Sports Med 1988;7:700.

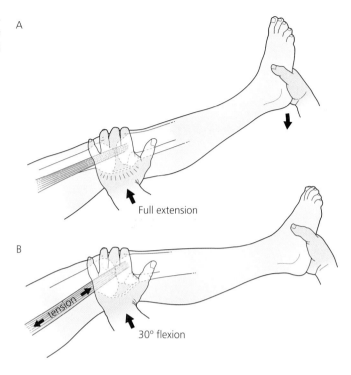

photographs demonstrating patients voluntarily producing what is called the pivot shift phenomenon.[29,71] The pivot shift phenomenon was characterized as an anterior subluxation of the lateral tibial plateau in relation to the femoral condyle when the knee approaches extension with reduction produced with knee flexion.[21,22,45,54,75] The pivot shift phenomenon is enhanced by the convexity of the tibial plateau in the sagittal plane.[48,51] The pivot shift test was initially described as follows:[22,56]

> The leg is picked up at the ankle with one of the examiner's hands, and if the patient is holding the leg in extension, the knee is flexed by placing the heel of the other hand behind the fibula over the lateral head of the gastrocnemius. As the knee is extended, the tibia is supported on the lateral side with a slight valgus strain applied to it. In fact, this subluxation can be slightly increased by subtly internally rotating the tibia, with the hand that is cradling the foot and ankle. A strong valgus force is placed on the knee by the upper hand. This impinges the subluxed tibial plateau against the lateral femoral condyle, jamming the two joint surfaces together, preventing easy reduction as the tibia is flexed on the femur. At approximately 30 degrees of flexion, and occasionally more, the displaced tibial plateau will suddenly reduce in a dramatic fashion. At this point, the patient will jump and exclaim, 'that's it!'

Several studies have been done to determine the diagnostic sensitivity and specificity of the pivot shift test in the diagnosis of ACL injuries. The reported sensitivity of pivot shift in the face of ACL injury ranges between 84% and 98% with a specificity of over

98% when performed under anesthesia, whereas in the alert patient values as low as 35% have been described.[12,43,55]

Many authors have recommended various modifications on the classic pivot shift test for producing the pivot shift phenomenon, including the addition of hip abduction, knee flexion, and external tibial rotation.[4,27,35,39,66]

As the specificity is high, the presence of the pivot shift will usually be indicative of an ACL tear. Additionally, the presence of a positive pivot shift test in a conscious patient may reflect an inability of the patient to protect the knee, which may suggest that these patients are less likely to succeed with non-operative treatment.

Tests for the Posterior Cruciate Ligament

Many authors have reported on the difficulties associated with the diagnosis of posterior cruciate ligament (PCL) injuries (Table 9–2).[7,53,72] Three commonly used tests for the diagnosis of PCL injuries are the posterior sag sign, the posterior drawer test, and the quadriceps active test.

Table 9–2. POSTERIOR CRUCIATE LIGAMENT TESTS

Test	Description	Reliability/Validity Tests	Comments
Posterior sag sign	Patient lies supine with the hip flexed to 45 degrees and the knee flexed to 90 degrees. In this position, the tibia "rocks back," or sags back, on the femur if the posterior cruciate ligament is torn. Normally, the medial tibial plateau extends 1 cm anteriorly beyond the femoral condyle when the knee is flexed 90 degrees. If this step off is lost, this step-off test is considered positive.	Rubenstein et al. 1994[72] Sensitivity: 79% Specificity: 100%	Double-blinded, randomized, controlled study. 39 subjects enrolled in study. (75 knees for analysis) Examiners all fellowship trained in sports medicine with at least 5 years' experience. Only included patients with chronic PCL tears.
Posterior drawer test	Subject is supine with the test hip flexed to 45 degrees, knee flexed to 90 degrees, and foot in neutral position. The examiner sits on the subject's foot with both hands behind the subject's proximal tibia and thumbs on the tibial plateau. A posterior force is applied to	Rubenstein et al. 1994[72] Sensitivity: 90% Specificity: 99% Loos et al. 1981[53] Sensitivity: 51% Specificity: Not reported	See above Compilation study from registry of knee surgeries in the US and Australia. 102 PCL injuries included. Multiple examiners at different sites, without

Table 9–2. POSTERIOR CRUCIATE LIGAMENT TESTS—*cont'd*

Test	Description	Reliability/Validity Tests	Comments
	the proximal tibia. Increased posterior tibial displacement as compared to the uninvolved side is indicative of a partial or complete tear of the PCL.		indication that study was randomized or controlled.
		Moore and Larson 1980[65] Sensitivity: 67% Specificity: Not reported	Retrospective study of 20 patients. All false-negatives were found to have both anterior and posterior cruciate injuries at surgery.
		Hughston et al. 1976[35,36] Sensitivity: 55.5% Specificity: Not reported	54 acute PCL tears studied over a 10 year period. Posterior drawer test was performed under anesthesia.
		Clendenin et al. 1980[6] Sensitivity: 100% Specificity: Not reported	Retrospective study of only 10 patients.
		Harilainen 1987[27] Sensitivity: 90% Specificity: Not reported	Prospective study which included only 9 patients with arthroscopically confirmed PCL tears.
Quadriceps active test	Subject is supine with knee flexed to 90 degrees in the drawer-test position. The foot is stabilized by the examiner, and the subject is asked to slide the foot gently down the table. Contraction of the quadriceps muscle in the PCL deficient knee results in an anterior shift of the tibia of 2 mm or more. The test is qualitative.	Daniel et al. 1988[7] Sensitivity: 98% Specificity: 100%	92 subjects included in study, 25 with no history of knee injury. Study was not blinded or randomized, as the examiners were told which knee was the index knee.
		Rubenstein et al. 1994[72] Sensitivity: 54% Specificity: 97%	Double-blinded, randomized, controlled study. 39 subjects enrolled in study. (75 knees for analysis) Examiners all fellowship trained in sports medicine with at least 5 years' experience. Only included patients with chronic PCL tears.

Posterior Sag Sign

Mayo Robson described this phenomenon in 1903, though it is unclear who coined the term posterior sag sign.[5,60] A detailed description of the test as it is performed today follows (Figure 9–9):

> The patient lies supine with the hip flexed to 45 degrees and the knee flexed to 90 degrees. In this position, the tibia 'rocks back,' or sags back, on the femur if the posterior cruciate ligament is torn. Normally, the medial tibial plateau extends 1 cm anteriorly beyond the femoral condyle when the knee is flexed 90 degrees. If this step off is lost, it is considered positive for a posterior cruciate tear.[28]

Few studies have been performed to establish the diagnostic sensitivity and specificity of the posterior sag sign in the diagnosis of PCL injuries. Rubenstein et al.,[72] in a blinded, randomized, controlled study to assess the accuracy of the clinical examination in the setting of posterior cruciate ligament injuries, reported a sensitivity of the posterior sag sign for detecting PCL injury of 79%, with a specificity of 100%. The overall sensitivity of the clinical exam for detecting PCL injury when all tests were utilized was 90%, with a specificity of 99%. In a non-randomized, unblinded, uncontrolled study, Stäubli and Jakob[77] evaluated the accuracy of the "gravity sign near extension" in which the knee is maintained in near extension. They reported that the gravity sign near extension was detectable in 20 of 24 PCL deficient knees, for a sensitivity of 83%.

Overall, the posterior sag sign is a useful test for diagnosing PCL injuries, with a relatively high sensitivity and very high specificity when used in isolation.

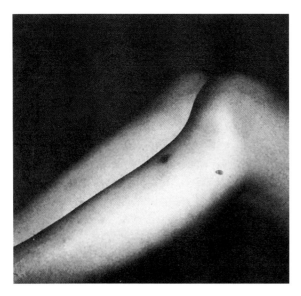

Figure 9–9. Posterior sag sign. Reproduced with permission from Zarins B, Fish DN. Knee ligament injury. In Nicholas J, Hershman E (eds), The Lower Extremity and Spine in Sports Medicine, 2nd edn. St Louis: Mosby, 1995, p. 857.

Posterior Drawer Test

George Noulis accurately described the opposing forces of the anterior and posterior cruciate ligaments in his 1876 thesis.[70,79] Paessler et al., in their historical review, give the following account of Noulis' description from the French text of his thesis:[70]

> When the leg was then moved forward and backward, it was found that the tibia will slide anteriorly and posteriorly. Noulis observed much movement of the tibia when both cruciates had been severed. When only the ACL was severed, movement of the tibia could be demonstrated when the knee was 'barely flexed.' However, when the posterior cruciate ligament had been divided, it took about 110 degrees of flexion to produce this movement of the tibia.

Paessler and colleagues clarify that Noulis's 110 degrees of flexion would translate into 70 degrees of flexion today since at that time they used 180 degrees as full extension. A more detailed and contemporary description of the posterior drawer test as it is commonly performed is seen below (Figure 9–10):[33]

> The subject is supine with the test hip flexed to 45 degrees, knee flexed to 90 degrees, and foot in neutral position. The examiner is sitting on the subject's foot with both hands behind the subject's proximal tibia and thumbs on the tibial plateau. Apply a posterior force to the proximal tibia. Increased posterior tibial displacement as compared to the uninvolved side is indicative of a partial or complete tear of the PCL.

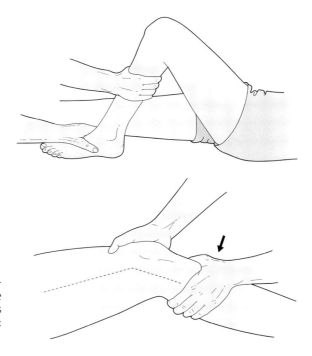

Figure 9–10. Posterior drawer test. Adapted with permission from Bienkowski P, Micheli LJ. Posterior cruciate ligament sprain. In Frontera WR, Silver JK (eds), Essentials of Physical Medicine and Rehabilitation. Philadelphia: Hanley & Belfus, 2003, p. 368.

Numerous studies in the literature report on the accuracy of the posterior drawer test for identifying injuries to the posterior cruciate ligament.[5,6,11,27,28,33–35,37,53,57,65,72,77] Many of these studies lack adequate sample sizes or have other flaws in their methodology, which makes interpretation of the results difficult. Rubenstein et al.[72] reported that the posterior drawer test was the most accurate test for identifying PCL injuries, with a sensitivity of 90% and a specificity of 99%. In general, when all of the clinical tests for PCL injuries were analyzed based on the grade of PCL tear, the examination sensitivity for grade I sprains was only 70% with a 99% specificity, whereas the sensitivity of grade II and III sprains was 97%, with 100% specificity. The study included only patients with chronic PCL tears, so the accuracy of the posterior drawer test in the setting of acute PCL injuries cannot be inferred.

Loos et al.[53] identified 102 PCL injuries in 13,316 knee operations performed in the US and Australia. In this study, the sensitivity of the posterior drawer test was 51%. The study was not designed to evaluate specificity, since only patients with surgically documented PCL injuries were included and no control group was reported.

Hughston[33] reported a sensitivity of 55.5% when the posterior drawer test was performed under anesthesia. The large number of false-negative results was explained by a lack of injury to the posteriorly situated arcuate complex. Studies of patients under anesthesia by Clendenin et al.[6] and Harilainen[27] noted positive posterior drawer test results in spite of intact posterior capsules.

In summary, the posterior drawer test has a high sensitivity and specificity with its accuracy increased when results are combined with other tests for posterior instability, such as the posterior sag sign.

Quadriceps Active Test

The quadriceps active test was described by Daniel et al.[7] Daniel's description of the test is given below (Figure 9–11):

> With the subject supine, the relaxed limb is supported with the knee flexed to 90 degrees in the drawer-test position. The subject should execute a gentle quadriceps contraction to shift the tibia without extending the knee. At this 90-degree angle, the patellar ligament in the normal knee is oriented slightly posterior and contraction of the quadriceps does not result in an anterior shift of the tibia although there may be a slight posterior shift. If the posterior cruciate ligament is ruptured, the tibia sags into posterior subluxation and the patellar ligament is then directed anteriorly. Contraction of the quadriceps muscle in the posterior cruciate-ligament deficient knee results in an anterior shift of the tibia of 2 mm or more. The test is qualitative.

In an unblinded, non-randomized study, Daniel reported a positive quadriceps active test in 41 of 42 knees that had a rupture of the PCL for a sensitivity of 98%. He reported a negative quadriceps active test result in all the normal knees and knees with

Figure 9–11. Quadriceps active test.

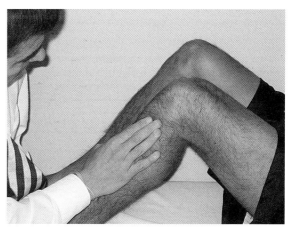

only ACL disruptions but intact PCLs, for a specificity of 100%. Rubenstein et al.[72] reported a sensitivity for the quadriceps active test of 54% and a specificity of 97%. This compares with findings of 79% sensitivity and 90% sensitivity for the posterior sag sign and posterior drawer test, respectively, with 99% or greater specificity for both tests.

Significantly different sensitivities for the quadriceps active test may be a reflection of study methodology and slightly different patient populations. The blinded, randomized, and controlled study by Rubenstein et al.[72] did not find the quadriceps active test to be as sensitive for detecting PCL disruption as other tests.

Tests for the Medial/Lateral Collateral Ligaments

The medial collateral ligament (MCL) is one of the most frequently injured ligaments in the knee. Valgus stress testing is the primary method used to diagnose MCL injury, but few studies have evaluated its accuracy or inter-examiner reliability. Injuries of the lateral collateral ligament (LCL) are rare, and there are even fewer studies evaluating the accuracy of the varus stress test in the diagnosis of this injury (Table 9–3).

Valgus and Varus Stress Tests

Although the originator of the valgus and varus stress tests for detecting ligament laxity is unclear, Palmer in 1938 described "abduction and adduction rocking" of the knee to determine the integrity of the collateral ligaments, an early reference to the valgus and varus stress tests used today. A description of Palmer's test from his 1938 paper is given below:[71]

In order to demonstrate lateral rocking, it is of the greatest importance that the patient be made to relax his muscles. In many cases this can be done if the extremity

Table 9–3. **MEDIAL AND LATERAL COLLATERAL LIGAMENT TESTS**

Test	Description	Reliability/Validity Tests	Comments
Valgus stress test	Patient supine on the exam table. Flex the knee to 30 degrees over the side of the table, place one hand about the lateral aspect of the knee and grasp the ankle with the other hand. Apply abduction (valgus) stress to the knee. The test must also be performed in full extension.	Harilainen 1987[27] Sensitivity: 86% Specificity: Not reported	72 patients studied with MCL tears confirmed on arthroscopy. Valgus stress testing was performed in 20 degrees of flexion, and testing in extension was not done. Clinical exam performed in the ER under unknown conditions, and no indication is given regarding the number of examiners or their training. There is also no documentation of the elapsed time between ER evaluation and arthroscopic evaluation.
		Garvin et al. 1993[23] Sensitivity: 96% Specificity: Not reported	Retrospective study of 23 patients who had undergone surgery for MCL tears. Non-standardized clinical examination of the MCL was used, sometimes under anesthesia, and sometimes performed prior to anesthesia.
		McClure et al. 1989[61] Inter-rater reliability in extension: 68% Inter-rater reliability in 30 deg. flexion: 56% Sensitivity: Not reported Specificity: Not reported	Physicians did not perform testing in this study, and the physical therapist's experience was varied. Standardized examination techniques between the examiners were not employed. Data variability of the clinical categories was insufficient to allow for accurate determination of reliability values.
Varus stress test	Patient supine on the exam table. Flex the knee to 30 degrees over the side of the table, place one hand about the medial aspect of the knee and grasp the ankle with the other hand. Apply adduction (varus) stress to the knee. The test must also be performed in full extension.	Harilainen 1987[27] Sensitivity: 25% Specificity: Not reported	Only 4 patients studied with LCL tears confirmed on arthroscopy. Varus stress testing was performed in 20 degrees of flexion, and testing in extension was not done. Clinical exam performed in the ER under unknown conditions, and no indication is given regarding the number of examiners or their training. There is also no documentation of the elapsed time between ER evaluation and arthroscopic evaluation.

is grasped so that it rests firmly and painlessly in the grip of the examiner. The best way is to hold the leg with the foot supported in the armpit with the calf resting against the forearm. The other hand supports the back of the knee. When it is felt that the muscles are relaxed, a surprise abduction movement is made. It is then felt how the articular surfaces snap apart and, when the muscles start to function as a reflex action, spring together again with a click which is clearly discernible to the hand supporting the back of the knee.

Modern varus and valgus testing is performed with slight abduction of the hip and 30 degrees of knee flexion (Figure 9–12). Hughston[35] concluded that a valgus stress test positive at 30 degrees and negative at 0 degrees indicates a tear limited to the medial-compartment ligaments (MCL ± posterior capsule), whereas a valgus stress test positive at 0 degrees indicates a tear of both the PCL and the medial-compartment ligaments. He did not find that the integrity of the ACL had any effect on the valgus stress test in extension. Marshall[59] noted that the valgus stress test in extension implicates one or both cruciates in addition to the MCL and posterior capsule.

Injuries resulting in straight lateral instability are rare. Hughston[36] reported on the operative findings of three patients with straight lateral instability demonstrated by positive varus stress testing in extension. Operation revealed a torn PCL, lateral capsule, arcuate ligaments, as well a torn ACL in two patients, among other findings. In his review of the subject, Marshall[59] reported that a positive varus stress test in flexion implicates the lateral collateral ligament (LCL), whereas a positive test in extension denotes a combined injury of the lateral collateral ligament, popliteus, and cruciate ligaments.

Little is known regarding the accuracy of valgus and varus stress testing. Harilainen[27] noted that, out of 72 patients with arthroscopically confirmed MCL tears,

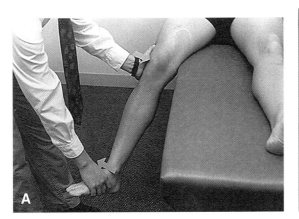
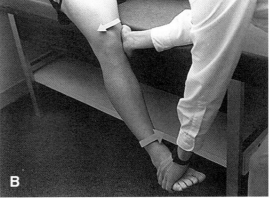

Figure 9–12. Varus and valgus stress testing for collateral ligament injury. Reproduced with permission from Mellion MB et al. (eds), The Team Physician's Handbook, 2nd edn. Philadelphia: Hanley & Belfus, 1996, pp. 558–559.

62 were diagnosed on clinical examination for a sensitivity of 86%. Out of four patients with a LCL tear confirmed on arthroscopy, one "instability" was diagnosed on clinical examination, for a sensitivity of 25%. The flawed design of this study significantly limits the overall clinical utility of the findings.

A few studies have been done comparing the clinical examination of collateral ligament injuries using varus/valgus stress testing with MRI imaging of the ligaments.[63,83] Yao et al.[83] reported that the agreement between MRI and the clinical grade of injury was modest with a 65% correct classification. Mirowitz et al.[63] reported a correlation coefficient between MR diagnosis and clinical diagnosis of 0.73 for MCL injuries. Garvin et al.[23] reported, in a retrospective study, that a tear of the MCL was predicted from the clinical examination in 22 of 23 patients, for a sensitivity of 96%. The retrospective design of the study with inclusion of only serious injuries, along with the non-standardized clinical exam primarily done under anesthesia, limits the clinical usefulness of this study.

McClure et al.[61] addressed the inter-examiner reliability of the valgus stress test. Tests were performed by three physical therapists on 50 patients with unilateral knee problems. Inter-examiner reliability was 0.6 with 68% agreement between examiners for the knee in extension and 0.16 with 56% agreement between examiners for the knee in 30 degrees of flexion.

In summary, there is a lack of well-designed studies that evaluate the sensitivity and specificity of the varus/valgus stress test, or the inter-examiner reliability of the test, in the diagnosis and grading of collateral ligament injuries.[61] Future studies would be clinically useful, but challenging to design as the majority of patients with collateral ligament injuries are currently managed without the need for surgery, and therefore the gold standard of arthroscopically identifying ligament injuries would be hard to justify.

Tests for Patellofemoral Disorders

Anterior knee pain is among the most common knee complaints that lead patients for evaluation by a physician. Two of the most common tests used in the evaluation of patellofemoral disorders are the patellar compression or "grinding" test and the patella apprehension test (Table 9–4).

Patellofemoral Grinding Test

The term "chondromalacia patellae" did not appear in published form until 1924.[16] Aleman is credited with using this term as early as 1917,[42] although the first mention of chondromalacia in the English language was in 1933 by Kulowski.[49] In 1936,

Table 9–4. PATELLOFEMORAL TESTS

Test	Description	Reliability/Validity Tests	Comments
Grinding test Compression test (for PFS)	The subject is supine with the knees extended. The examiner stands next to the involved side and places the web space of the thumb on the superior border of the patella. The subject is asked to contract the quadriceps muscle, while the examiner applies downward and inferior pressure on the patella. Pain with movement of the patella or an inability to complete the test is indicative of patellofemoral dysfunction.	No studies were found that document the sensitivity or specificity of the patellofemoral grinding test in the diagnosis of patellofemoral syndrome.	The diagnosis of PFS is based on clinical exam, including the patella compression test. The lack of another gold standard (such as arthroscopy) in the diagnosis of PFS makes any determination of sensitivity or specificity of specific clinical tests for this condition problematic.
Apprehension test (for patella dislocation)	Carried out by pressing on the medial aspect of the patella with the knee flexed 30 degrees with the quadriceps relaxed. It requires the thumbs of both hands pressing on the medial side of the patella to exert the laterally directed pressure. Often the finding is surprising to the patient and he becomes uncomfortable and apprehensive as the patella reaches the point of maximum passive displacement, with the result that he begins to resist and attempts to straighten the knee, thus pulling the affected patella back into a relatively normal position.	Sallay et al. 1996[73] Sensitivity: 39% Specificity: Not reported	19 patients underwent arthroscopic evaluation in this study, and all 19 exhibited gross lateral laxity of the patellofemoral articulation under anesthesia. This laxity was most prominent at 70–80 degrees of flexion.

Owre published the results of a clinical and pathological investigation of the patella.[69] The complete description of the patellofemoral grinding test by Owre is given below:

Pressure-pain over the patella is tested by clasping the patella with the thumb and index finger of each hand with the remaining fingers resting against the thigh and leg. While the patient lies with the leg relaxed and extended the patella is pressed against the medial and lateral femoral condyles. By moving the patella in an upward and downward direction the greater part of the surface cartilage may be examined in this manner. In some cases pain is elicited on the slightest pressure of the patella against the condyle, at other times considerable pressure must be exerted to obtain a positive response of an unpleasant sensation.

A positive test as indicated by pain was considered by Owre to be predictive of pathological changes to the retropatellar cartilage, or chondromalacia patella. In current use, a positive test may or may not be associated with the pathological diagnosis of chondromalacia patella as determined by direct arthroscopic visualization and probing. A more contemporary description of the test is as follows (Figure 9–13):[76]

> The subject is lying supine with the knees extended. The examiner stands next to the involved side and places the web space of the thumb on the superior border of the patella. The subject is asked to contract the quadriceps muscle, while the examiner applies downward and inferior pressure on the patella.

Pain with movement of the patella or an inability to complete the test is indicative of patellofemoral dysfunction.

There are no studies that document either the sensitivity or specificity of the patellofemoral grinding test in the diagnosis of patellofemoral syndrome. There are several studies over the last twenty years, however, that do show a generally poor correlation between retropatellar pain and articular cartilage damage.[1,8,10,38,44,52,81]

O'Shea[68] reported on the diagnostic accuracy of clinical examination of the knee in patients with arthroscopically documented knee pathology, including chondromalacia patella. He reported that only 11 of 29 patients were correctly diagnosed with having the pathological findings of chondromalacia patella based on the history, physical exam, and standard radiographs, for a sensitivity of 37%.

In summary, there is a poor correlation between the clinical history and exam and the diagnosis of chondromalacia patella. The explanation of the disparity between

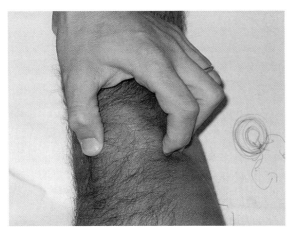

Figure 9–13. Patellofemoral grind test.

clinical signs and pathological findings is not easy, and reflects the continued question of what ultimately causes the pain in patients with patellofemoral syndrome.

Apprehension Test for Patellar Dislocation

This test was first described by Fairbank in 1935, and the test is often referred to as Fairbank's apprehension test. His description is:[18]

> While examining cases of suspected recurrent dislocation of the patella, I have been struck by the marked apprehension often displayed by the patient when the patella is pushed outwards in testing the stability of this bone. Not uncommonly, the patient will seize the examiner's hands to check the manipulation, which she finds uncomfortable and regards as distinctly dangerous. This sign, when present, I regard as strong evidence in favour of a diagnosis of slipping patella.

A more detailed and more recent description of the apprehension test for subluxation of the patella was given by Hughston. His description of the apprehension test is as follows (Figure 9–14):[32]

> This test is carried out by pressing on the medial side of the patella with the knee flexed about 30 degrees and with the quadriceps relaxed. It requires the thumbs of both hands pressing on the medial side of the patella to exert the laterally directed pressure. Accordingly the leg with muscles relaxed is allowed to project over the side of the examining table and is supported with the knee at 30 degrees of flexion by resting the leg on the thigh of the examiner who is sitting on a stool. In this position the examiner can almost dislocate the patella over the lateral femoral condyle. Often the finding is surprising to the patient and he becomes uncomfortable and apprehensive as the patella reaches the point of maximum passive displacement, with the result that he begins to resist and attempts to straighten the knee, thus pulling the affected patella back into a relatively normal position.

In their 1996 study, Sallay et al.[73] reported on the characteristic clinical and arthroscopically determined pathological findings associated with patellar dislocations. Only 39% of patients with a history of dislocation were noted to have a positive apprehension sign. In contrast, 83% exhibited a moderate to large effusion, and 70% of patients had significant tenderness over the posterior medial soft tissues. MRI imaging revealed a moderate to large effusion on all scans. Increased signal adjacent to the adductor tubercle was seen in 96%, tearing of the medial patellofemoral ligament (MPFL) was found in 87%, and increased signal was noted in the vastus medialis oblique (VMO) muscle in 78% of cases. Upon arthroscopic evaluation, gross lateral laxity of the patellofemoral articulation of all subjects was most prominent at 70–80 degrees of flexion. This degree of flexion is significantly higher than the 30 degrees classically recommended for the apprehension sign, and may explain the low sensitivity of this test in the diagnosis of patella dislocation.

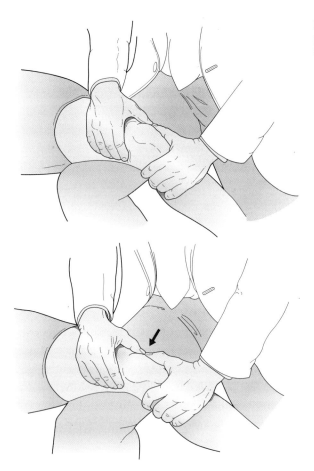

Figure 9–14. Patellar apprehension sign. Adapted with permission from Jacobson KE, Flandry FC. Diagnosis of anterior knee pain. Clin Sports Med 1989;8(2):183.

Tests for Meniscal Injuries

Meniscal tears occur commonly, but their clinical diagnosis is often difficult even for an experienced clinician (Table 9–5). Because the menisci are avascular and have no nerve supply on their inner two-thirds, an injury to the meniscus can result in little or no pain or swelling, which makes accurate diagnosis even more challenging. In 1803, William Hey described "internal derangement of the knee,"[30] and since that time there has been significant literature on the clinical diagnosis of meniscal tears.

Joint Line Tenderness

Joint line palpation is one of the most basic maneuvers, yet it often provides more useful information than the provocative maneuvers designed to detect meniscal tears. Flexion of the knee enhances palpation of the anterior half of each meniscus.

Table 9–5. TESTS FOR MENISCAL INJURIES

Test	Description	Reliability/Validity Tests	Comments
Joint line tenderness	The medial edge of the medial meniscus becomes more prominent with internal rotation of the tibia, allowing for easier palpation. Alternatively, external rotation allows improved palpation of the lateral meniscus.	Kurosaka et al. 1999[50] Sensitivity: 55% Specificity: 67%	Prospective blinded study of 160 patients with meniscal tears that were arthroscopically identified. Acute injuries were excluded.
		Fowler and Lubliner 1989[20] Sensitivity: 85% Specificity: 29.4%	Prospective study of 160 patients (161 knees) with meniscal tears that were arthroscopically identified.
		Anderson and Lipscomb 1986[3] Sensitivity: 77% Specificity: Not reported	Prospective evaluation of 100 patients by one examiner.
McMurray test	With patient lying flat, the knee is first fully flexed; the foot is held by grasping the heel. The leg is rotated on the thigh with the knee still in full flexion. By altering the position of flexion, the whole of the posterior segment of the cartilages can be examined from the middle to their posterior attachment. Bring the leg from its position of acute flexion to a right angle, while the foot is retained first in full IR and then in full ER. When the click occurs (in association with a torn meniscus) the patient is able to state that the sensation is the same as he experienced when the knee gave way previously.	Evans et al. 1993[17] Sensitivity: 16% Specificity: 98%	Prospective study of 104 patients. Interexaminer reliability between the two examiners of the study was only fair.
		Fowler and Lubliner 1989[20] Sensitivity: 29% Specificity: 95%	Prospective study of 160 patients (161 knees) with meniscal tears that were arthroscopically identified.
		Kurosaka et al. 1999[50] Sensitivity: 37% Specificity: 77%	Prospective blinded study of 160 patients with meniscal tears that were arthroscopically identified. Acute injuries were excluded.
		Anderson and Lipscomb 1986[3] Sensitivity: 58% Specificity: Not reported	Prospective evaluation of 100 patients by one examiner.
Apley grind test	The patient is prone. The surgeon grasps one foot in each hand, externally rotates as far as possible, then flexes both knees together to their limit. The feet are then rotated inward and knees extended.	Fowler and Lubliner 1989[20] Sensitivity: 16% Specificity: 80%	Prospective study of 160 patients (161 knees) with meniscal tears that were arthroscopically identified.
	The surgeon then applies his left knee to back of the patient's thigh. The foot is grasped in both hands, the knee is bent to a right angle, and powerful external rotation is applied.	Kurosaka et al. 1999[50] Sensitivity: 13% Specificity: 90%	Prospective blinded study of 160 patients with meniscal tears that were arthroscopically identified. Acute injuries were excluded.

Continued

Table 9–5. TESTS FOR MENISCAL INJURIES—*cont'd*

Test	Description	Reliability/Validity Tests	Comments
	Next, the patient's leg is strongly pulled up, with the femur being prevented from rising off the couch. In this position of distraction, external rotation is repeated. The surgeon leans over the patient and compresses the tibia downward. Again he rotates powerfully and if addition of compression had produced an increase of pain, this grinding test is positive and meniscal damage is diagnosed.		
Bounce home test	The test is performed with the patient supine with the patient's foot cupped in the examiner's hand. With the patient's knee completely flexed, the knee is passively allowed to extend. The knee should extend completely, or bounce home into extension with a sharp end-point. If extension is not complete or has a rubbery end feel, there is probably a torn meniscus or some other blockage present.	No studies were found that identified the accuracy of this specific test.	

The medial edge of the medial meniscus becomes more prominent with internal rotation of the tibia, allowing for easier palpation. Alternatively, external rotation allows improved palpation of the lateral meniscus.

The published literature notes a sensitivity for joint line tenderness of 55–85% with a specificity range of 29–67%.[20,50] Thus, joint line tenderness is likely to be present in those with meniscal tears. However, joint line tenderness alone is common to other diagnoses and is not pathognomonic for meniscal injury.

McMurray Test

The McMurray test is one of the primary clinical tests to evaluate for the presence of a meniscal tear (Figure 9–15). T. P. McMurray first described the test in 1940.[17,62] The original description of the test is as follows:[62]

> In carrying out the manipulation with patient lying flat, the knee is first fully flexed until the heel approaches the buttock; the foot is then held by grasping the heel and

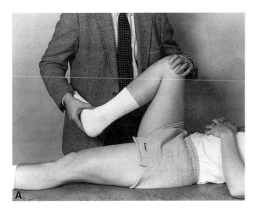
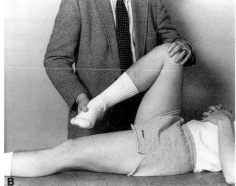

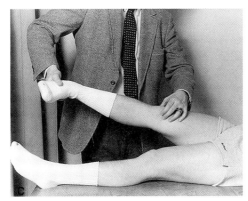

Figure 9–15. The McMurray test. Reproduced with permission from Mellion MB et al. (eds), The Team Physician's Handbook, 2nd edn. Philadelphia: Hanley & Belfus, 1996, p. 258.

using the forearm as a lever. The knee being now steadied by the surgeon's other hand, the leg is rotated on the thigh with the knee still in full flexion. During this movement the posterior section of the cartilage is rotated with the head of the tibia, and if the whole cartilage, or any fragment of the posterior section is loose, this movement produces an appreciable snap in the joint. By external rotation of the leg the internal cartilage is tested, and by internal rotation any abnormality of the posterior part of the external cartilage can be appreciated. By altering the position of flexion of the joint the whole of the posterior segment of the cartilages can be examined from the middle to their posterior attachment. Probably the simplest routine is to bring the leg from its position of acute flexion to a right angle, whilst the foot is retained first in full internal, and then in full external rotation. When the click occurs with a normal but lax cartilage, the patient experiences no pain or discomfort, but when produced by a broken cartilage, which has already given trouble, the patient is able to state that the sensation is the same as he experienced when the knee gave way previously.

Several studies have been performed to determine the clinical accuracy of the McMurray test in predicting meniscal pathology.[3,20,24,26,31,78] Four studies were found that evaluated the McMurray test as it was originally described without modification.

There appears to be a wide variation in the reported sensitivities (16–58%) and specificities (77–98%) of the McMurray test for detecting meniscal tears.[3,17,20,50]

Evans et al.[17] found a low agreement between examiners and the McMurray test was not found useful for diagnosing lateral meniscal tears.

Overall, these findings support a continued usefulness of the McMurray test in combination with other physical exam tests, and in patients with a history suggestive of meniscal involvement. The test should not be overly emphasized when negative, given its low diagnostic sensitivity.

Apley Grind Test

The Apley grind test was described by A. G. Apley in 1947.[24,26] The original description of the test is as follows (Figure 9–16):[26]

> For this examination the patient lies on his face. He should be on a couch not more than two feet high, or the tests become difficult, and he must be well over to the edge of the couch nearest the surgeon. To start the examination, the surgeon grasps one foot in each hand, externally rotates as far as possible, and then flexes both knees together to their limit. When this limit has been reached, he changes his grasp, rotates the feet inward, and extends the knees together again. The surgeon then applies his left knee to the back of the patient's thigh. It is important to observe that in this position his weight fixes one of the levers absolutely. The foot is grasped in both hands, the knee is bent to a right angle, and the powerful external rotation is applied. This test determines whether simple rotation produces pain. Next, without changing the position of the hands, the patient's leg is strongly pulled upward, while the surgeon's weight prevents the femur from rising off the couch. In this position of distraction, the powerful external rotation is repeated. Two things can be determined: (1) whether or not the maneuver produces pain and (2), still more important, whether the pain is greater than in rotation alone without the distraction. If the pain is greater, the distraction test is positive, and a rotation sprain may be diagnosed.

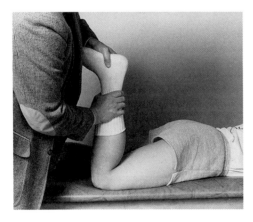

Figure 9–16. The Apley grind test. Reproduced with permission from Mellion MB et al. (eds), The Team Physician's Handbook, 2nd edn. Philadelphia: Hanley & Belfus, 1996, p. 259.

Then the surgeon leans well over the patient and, with his whole body weight, compresses the tibia downward onto the couch. Again he rotates powerfully, and if addition of compression had produced an increase of pain, this grinding test is positive, and meniscal damage is diagnosed.

In their report of five clinical signs for meniscal pathology, Fowler and Lubliner[20] prospectively evaluated the accuracy of the Apley grind test. They reported an overall sensitivity of 16% and a specificity of 80%. Kurosaka et al.[50] noted a sensitivity of 13%, a specificity of 90%, with an overall accuracy of 28% for the Apley grind. The results of these prospective studies demonstrate the limited predictive value of the Apley grind test for the diagnosis of meniscal injuries.

Bounce Home Test

This test is designed to evaluate a lack of full extension in the knee, which may indicate a torn meniscus, or other pathology such as a loose body or a joint effusion. The test is performed with the patient supine with the patient's foot cupped in the examiner's hand. With the patient's knee completely flexed, the knee is passively allowed to extend. The knee should extend completely, or bounce home into extension with a sharp end-point. If extension is not complete or has a rubbery end feel, there is probably a torn meniscus or some other blockage present.[57]

Oni[67] described a modification of the bounce home test, which he labeled the "knee jerk test," in which the knee is forcibly extended in one quick jerk and pain occurs in the region of tissue injury. Shybut and McGinty[74] described the forced hyperextension test of the knee which, in contrast to the bounce home test and the jerk test, involves forced hyperextension of an already extended knee.[74] A block to full extension indicates a positive test and may indicate a meniscal tear. Fowler and Lubliner, in their study on the predictive value of five clinical tests for meniscal pathology, reported a sensitivity of 44% and a specificity of 95% for the forced hyperextension of the knee test.[20]

Conclusion

The importance of a properly performed physical examination of the knee cannot be overemphasized. In the same light, understanding the diagnostic accuracy and the limitations of the various tests for knee pathology need to be understood. With this knowledge, the thoughtful clinician is better able to plan both diagnostic and treatment strategies for the painful knee.

REFERENCES

1. Abernethy P, Wilson G, Logan P. Strength and power assessment: issues, controversies and challenges. Sports Med 1995;19:401–417.
2. Adler GG, Hoekman RA, Beach DM. Drop leg Lachman test: a new test of anterior knee laxity. Am J Sports Med 1995;23:320–323.
3. Anderson AF, Lipscomb AB. Clinical diagnosis of meniscal tears: description of a new manipulative test. Am J Sports Med 1986;14:291–293.
4. Bach BR, Warren RF, Wickiewicz TL. The pivot shift phenomenon: results and description of a modified clinical test for anterior cruciate ligament insufficiency. Am J Sports Med 1988;16:571–576.
5. Barton TM, Torg JS, Das M. Posterior cruciate ligament insufficiency: a review of the literature. Sports Med 1984;1:419–430.
6. Clendenin MB, DeLee JC, Heckman JD. Interstitial tears of the posterior cruciate ligament of the knee. Orthopedics 1980;3:764–772.
7. Daniel DM, Stone ML, Barnett P, Sachs R. Use of the quadriceps active test to diagnose posterior cruciate–ligament disruption and measure posterior laxity of the knee. J Bone Joint Surg Am 1988;70:386–391.
8. Darracott J, Vernon-Roberts B. The bony changes in chondromalacia patellae. Rheum Phys Med 1971; 11:175–179.
9. DeHaven KE. Arthroscopy in the diagnosis and management of the anterior cruciate ligament deficient knee. Clin Orthop 1983;172:52–56.
10. Dehaven KE, Dolan WA, Mayer PJ. Chondromalacia patellae in athletes: clinical presentation and conservative management. Am J Sports Med 1979;7:5–11.
11. De Lee JC. Ligamentous injury of the knee. In Stanitski CL, DeLee JC, Drez D (eds), Pediatric and Adolescent Sports Medicine. Philadelphia: WB Saunders, 1994.
12. Donaldson WF, Warren RF, Wickiewicz T. A comparison of acute anterior cruciate ligament examinations: initial versus examination under anesthesia. Am J Sports Med 1985;13:5–10.
13. Draper DO. A comparison of stress tests used to evaluate the anterior cruciate ligament. Phys Sports Med 1990;18:89–96.
14. Draper DO, Schulthies SS. A test for eliminating false positive anterior cruciate ligament injury diagnoses. J Athl Train 1993;28:355–357.
15. Draper DO, Schulthies SS. Examiner proficiency in performing the anterior drawer and Lachman tests. J Orthop Sports Phys Ther 1995;22:263–266.
16. Dugdale TW, Barnett PR. Historical background: patellofemoral pain in young people. Orthop Clin N Am 1986;17:211–219.
17. Evans PJ, Bell GD, Frank C. Prospective evaluation of the McMurray test. Am J Sports Med 1993; 21:604–608.
18. Fairbank HA. Internal derangement of the knee in children and adolescents. Proc R Soc Med 1936;427–432.
19. Feagin JA, Cooke TD. Prone examination for anterior cruciate ligament insufficiency. J Bone Joint Surg [Br] 1989;71:863.
20. Fowler PJ, Lubliner JA. The predictive value of five clinical signs in the evaluation of meniscal pathology. Arthroscopy 1989;5(3):184–186.
21. Galway HR, Beaupre A, MacIntosh DL. Pivot shift: a clinical sign of symptomatic anterior cruciate insufficiency. J Bone Joint Surg [Br] 1972;54B:763–764.
22. Galway HR, MacIntosh DL. The lateral pivot shift: a symptom and sign of anterior cruciate ligament insufficiency. Clin Orthop 1980;147:45–50.
23. Garvin GJ, Munk PL, Vellet AD. Tears of the medial collateral ligament: magnetic resonance imaging findings and associated injuries. Can Assoc Radiol J 1993;44(3):199–204.
24. Gillis L. Diagnosis in Orthopedics. Toronto: Butterworth, 1969.
25. Goodfelllow DB. The knee. In Marcus RE (ed.), Orthopaedics: Problems in Primary Care. Los Angeles: Practice Management Information Corp., 1991, pp. 141–159.
26. Gould JA, Dabies GJ. Orthopaedic and Sports Physical Therapy. Toronto: Mosby, 1985.
27. Harilainen A. Evaluation of knee instability in acute ligamentous injuries. Ann Chir Gynaecol 1987;76(5):269–273.
28. Hawkins RJ. Musculoskeletal Examination. St Louis: Mosby, 1993.
29. Hey Groves EW. The crucial ligaments of the knee joint: their function, rupture and the operative treatment of the same. Br J Surg 1920;7:505–515.

30. Hey W. Practical Observations in Surgery. Philadelphia: James Humphreys, 1805.

31. Hoppenfeld S. Physical Examination of the Spine and Extremities. Norwalk, CT: Appleton–Century–Crofts, 1976, pp. 171–196.

32. Hughston JC. Subluxation of the patella. J Bone Joint Surg Am 1968;50:1003–1026.

33. Hughston JC. The absent posterior drawer test in some acute posterior cruciate ligament tears of the knee. Am J Sports Med 1988;16:39–43.

34. Hughston JC. Extensor mechanism examination. In Fox JM, Del Pizzo W (eds), The Patellofemoral Joint. New York: McGraw-Hill, 1993.

35. Hughston JC, Andrews JR, Cross MJ, Moschi A. Classification of knee ligament instabilities. I: The medial compartment and cruciate ligaments. J Bone Joint Surg Am 1976;58A:159–172.

36. Hughston JC, Andrews JR, Cross MJ, Moschi A. Classification of knee ligament instabilities. II: The lateral compartment. J Bone Joint Surg Am 1976;58:173–179.

37. Hughston JC, Bowden JA, Andrews JR, Norwood LA. Acute tears of the posterior cruciate ligament: results of operative treatment. J Bone Joint Surg Am 1980;62:438–450.

38. Hvid I, Anderson LI. The quadriceps angle and its relation to femoral torsion. Acta Orthop Scan 1982;53:577–579.

39. Jakob RP, Staubli HU, Deland JT. Grading the pivot shift: objective tests with implications for treatment. J Bone Joint Surg [Br] 1987;69:294–299.

40. Johnson RJ. The anterior cruciate: a dilemma in sports medicine. Int J Sports Med 1982;3:71–79.

41. Jonsson T, Althoff B, Peterson L, Renstrom P. Clinical diagnosis of ruptures of the anterior drawer sign. Am J Sports Med 1982;10:100–102.

42. Karlson S. Chondromalacia patellae. Acta Chir Scand 1939;83:347–381.

43. Katz JW, Fingeroth RJ. The diagnostic accuracy of ruptures of the anterior cruciate ligament comparing the Lachman test, the anterior drawer sign, and the pivot shift test in acute and chronic knee injuries. Am J Sports Med 1986;14:88–91.

44. Kelly MA, Insall JN. Historical perspectives of chondromalacia patellae. Orthop Clin N Am 1992; 23:517–521.

45. Kennedy JC. Anterior subluxation of the lateral tibial plateau. In James SL (ed.), Late Reconstructions of Injured Ligaments of the Knee. New York: Springer-Verlag, 1978, pp. 94–98.

46. Kim SJ, Kim HK. Reliability of the anterior drawer test, the pivot shift test, and the Lachman test. Clin Orthop 1995;317:237–242.

47. Konin JG. Special Tests for Orthopedic Examination. Thorofare, NJ: Slack, 1997.

48. Kujala UM, Nelimarkka O, Koskinen SK. Relationship between the pivot shift and the configuration of the lateral tibial plateau. Arch Orthop Trauma Surg 1992;111:228–229.

49. Kulowski J. Chondromalacia of the patella; fissural cartilage degeneration; traumatic chondropathy: report of three cases. JAMA 1933;100:1837–1840.

50. Kurosaka M, Yagi M, Yoshiya S, Muratsu H, Mizuno K. Efficacy of the axially loaded pivot shift test for the diagnosis of a meniscal tear. Int Orthop 1999;23:271–274.

51. Larson RL. Physical examination in the diagnosis of rotatory instability. Clin Orthop 1983;172:38–44.

52. Leslie IJ, Bentley G. Arthroscopy in the diagnosis of chondromalacia patellae. Ann Rheum Dis 1978;37:540–547.

53. Loos WC, Fox JM, Blazina ME, Del Pizzo W, Friedman MJ. Acute posterior cruciate ligament injuries. Am J Sports Med 1981;9:86–92.

54. Losee RE, Johnson TR, Southwick WO. Anterior subluxation of the lateral tibial plateau: a diagnostic test and operative repair. J Bone Joint Surg Am 1978;60:1015–1030.

55. Lucie RS, Wiedel JD, Messner DG. The acute pivot shift: clinical correlation. Am J Sports Med 1984; 12:189–191.

56. MacIntosh DL, Galway HR. The lateral pivot shift: a symptomatic and clinic sign of anterior cruciate insufficiency. Read at the Annual Meeting of the American Orthopaedic Association, Tucker's Town, Bermuda, 1972.

57. Magee DJ. Orthopedic Physical Assessment, 3rd edn. Philadelphia: WB Saunders, 1997, pp. 506–598.

58. Malanga GA, Andrus SA, Nadler SF, McLean J. Physical examination of the knee: a review of the original test description and scientific utility of common orthopedic tests. Arch Phys Med Rehabil 2003;84:592–603.

59. Marshall JL, Rubin RM. Knee ligament injuries: a diagnostic and therapeutic approach. Orthop Clin N Am 1977;8:641–668.

60. Mayo Robson AW. Ruptured cruciate ligaments and their repair by operation. Ann Surg 1903;37:716–718.

61. McClure PW, Rothstein JM, Riddle DL. Intertester reliability of clinical judgments of medial knee ligament integrity. Phys Ther 1989;69:268–275.

62. McMurray TP. The semilunar cartilages. Br J Surg 1942;29:407–414.

63. Mirowitz SA, Shu HH. MR imaging evaluation of knee collateral ligaments and related injuries. Comparison of T1-weighted, T2-weighted, and fat-saturated T2-weighted sequences – correlation with clinical findings. J Magn Reson Imaging 1994;4:725–732.

64. Mitsou A, Vallianatos P. Clinical diagnosis of ruptures of the anterior cruciate ligament: a comparison between the Lachman test and the anterior drawer sign. Injury 1988;19:427–428.

65. Moore HA, Larson RL. Posterior cruciate ligament injuries: results of early surgical repair. Am J Sports Med 1980;8:68–78.

66. Noyes FR, Grood ES, Cummings JF, Wroble RR. An analysis of the pivot shift phenomenon: the knee motions and subluxations induced by different examiners. Am J Sports Med 1991;19:148–155.

67. Oni AO. The knee jerk test for diagnosis of torn meniscus [letter]. Clin Orthop 1985;193:309.

68. O'Shea KJ, Murphy KP, Heekin RD, Herzwurm PJ. The diagnostic accuracy of history, physical examination, and radiographs in the evaluation of traumatic knee disorders. Am J Sports Med 1996;24:164–167.

69. Owre A. Chondromalacia patellae. Acta Chir Scand 1936;77(suppl. 41):1–159.

70. Paessler HH, Michel D. How new is the Lachman test? Am J Sports Med 1992;20:95–98.

71. Palmer I. Injuries to the ligaments of the knee joint. Acta Chir Scand 1938;81(suppl. 53).

72. Rubinstein RA, Shelbourne KD, McCarroll JR, VanMeter CD, Rettig AC. The accuracy of the clinical examination in the setting of posterior cruciate ligament injuries. Am J Sports Med 1994;22:550–557.

73. Sallay PI, Poggi J, Speer KP, Garrett WE. Acute dislocation of the patella: a correlative pathoanatomic study. Am J Sports Med 1996;24:52–60.

74. Shybut GT, McGinty JB. The office evaluation of the knee. Orthop Clin N Am 1982;13:497–509.

75. Slocum DB. Late reconstruction of the knee. Presentation to American Academy Instructional Course. Cleveland, OH, 1975.

76. Solomon DH, Simel DL, Bates DW, Katz JN, Schaffer JL. Does this patient have a torn meniscus or ligament of the knee? Value of the physical examination. JAMA 2001;286:1610–1620.

77. Staubli HU, Jakob RP. Posterior instability of the knee near extension: a clinical and stress radiographic analysis of acute injuries of the posterior cruciate ligament. J Bone Joint Surg [Br] 1990;72:225–230.

78. Stratford PW, Binkley J. A review of the McMurray test: definition, interpretation, and clinical usefulness. J Orthop Sports Phys Ther 1995;22(3):116–120.

79. Strobel M, Stedtfeld HW, Feagin JA, Telger TC. Diagnostic Evaluation of the Knee. New York: Springer-Verlag, 1990.

80. Torg JS, Conrad W, Kalen V. Clinical diagnosis of anterior cruciate ligament instability in the athlete. Am J Sports Med 1976;4:84–93.

81. Tria AJ, Palumbo RC, Alicea JA. Conservative care for patellofemoral pain. Orthop Clin N Am 1992; 23:545–554.

82. Wroble RR, Lindenfeld TN. The stabilized Lachman test. Clin Orthop 1988;237:209–212.

83. Yao L, Dungan D, Seeger LL. MR imaging of tibial collateral ligament injury: comparison with clinical examination. Skeletal Radiol 1994;23:521–524.

84. Zarins B, Nemith VA. Acute knee injuries in athletes. Orthop Clin N Am 1985;16:285–302.

Chapter **10**

Physical Examination of the Foot and Ankle

GARRETT S. HYMAN, MD, MPH •
JENNIFER SOLOMON, MD • DIANE DAHM, MD

Introduction

This chapter provides a review of foot and ankle anatomy and examination followed by an evidence-based discussion of the major provocative tests employed to diagnose ankle and foot injuries. Epidemiologically, lateral ankle sprains are the most common sports injuries.[16,39] Among a series of 321 consecutive acute ankle sprains, Broström[8] described a prevalence of complete ligament rupture in 75% of cases. Of these, isolated rupture of the anterior talofibular ligament (ATFL) occurred in about 65% of cases, combined ATFL–CFL (calcaneofibular ligament) tears in about 20%, and isolated tibiofibular (syndesmosis) rupture in about 10%. Our goal here is to provide the clinician with an understanding of the science (or lack thereof) that guides our examination and its subsequent interpretation. The present body of research calls into question the utility of much of what we do in common clinical practice, including certain aspects of both the standard ankle and foot physical examination.

Anatomy and Physical Examination

Inspection

Assessment of the foot and ankle begins as the patient enters the examination room with observation of a patient's gait pattern, static standing posture, and wear on the sole of the shoes. Gait abnormalities may result from neuromuscular weakness, soft tissue contractures, lower-extremity malalignment, or pain. With the shoes and socks removed, the weight-bearing posture of the ankle and foot may reveal pes cavus or planus (e.g., high-set longitudinal arch or flat foot, respectively), calcaneus or equino-varus, and hindfoot varus or valgus deformities. Hallux valgus and hammertoes as well as skin and nail deformities may also be readily apparent.

The transverse and longitudinal arches should be grossly evaluated for accentuation or collapse. The longitudinal arch can be separated into lateral and medial portions. The lateral longitudinal arch is formed by the calcaneus, cuboid, fourth and fifth metatarsals, and bears the bodyweight in early stance. The medial longitudinal arch is formed by the calcaneus, talus, navicular, three cuneiforms, and three media metatarsals, and provides support of bodyweight in the mid and late stance phases of gait. There are three transverse arches: the tarsal arch formed by the cuneiforms medially and the cuboid laterally; the posterior metatarsal arch created by the metatarsal bases; and the flexible anterior metatarsal arch fashioned by the distal metatarsal bones.[10] Integrity of interosseous ligaments as well as the intrinsic and extrinsic foot muscles contributes to the maintenance of these biomechanically important curvatures of the foot.

Inspection of the patient's stance and gait is important. Normally, the foot pronates during early stance phase. The foot should not remain pronated during heel rise and lift off. Heel inversion should occur during heel rise (normal contribution of intrinsic and extrinsic foot muscles). The foot should contact the ground with the heel first, and the heel should begin to rise at 35% of the gait cycle. Early heel rise may occur due to tightness of the gastrocsoleus complex. Late heel rise may be secondary to weakness of the calf musculature.[28]

Particular attention must be given to careful skin inspection of dorsal, plantar, and interdigital regions of the neuropathic foot (e.g., diabetics with peripheral polyneuropathies) to examine for bruising, erythema, pressure sores, nail abnormalities, blisters, callus, and other signs of infection. Often, straightforward modifications to shoe wear or the use of custom-molded cushioned orthotics are all that is needed to remedy or prevent problems in the neuropathic ankle and foot.

Palpation

Bony Structures

The foot can be divided into sections: hindfoot, midfoot, and forefoot (Figure 10–1). The hindfoot consists of the talus and calcaneus. The midfoot comprises the navicular, cuboid, and cuneiforms. The metatarsals and phalanges make up the forefoot.

Proximally at the ankle, the medial malleolus of the tibia and the lateral malleolus of the fibula are prominent and should always be palpable. Note that the lateral malleolus of the fibula extends further distally than does the medial tibial malleolus, thereby limiting the eversion range of the ankle joint. When ankle injury is in question, one should palpate the tibial and fibular shafts several centimeters proximal

Figure 10–1. Anatomic zones of the foot. Adapted with permission from Starkey C, Ryan JL. Evaluation of Orthopedic and Athletic Injuries. Philadelphia: FA Davis, 2001, p. 48.

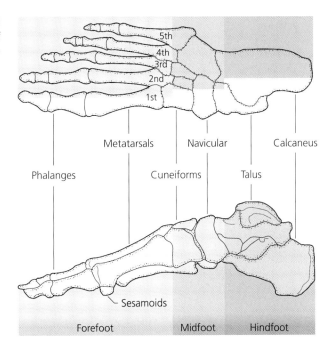

to the malleoli looking for gross deformity or tenderness and from the fibular head several centimeters distally because syndesmotic, medial, and lateral ankle injuries can all be associated with fractures of the proximal fibula (called a Maisonneuve fracture). This follows the general tenet of orthopedic physical examinations that one should always examine the joints above and below an injury.

At the proximal portion of the ankle mortise is the distal tibiofibular joint (or tibiofibular syndesmosis) and the tibiotalar articulation. Anteromedially, at the ankle just medial to the extensor hallucis longus tendon, one can palpate the head of the talus. Gentle lateral and medial rocking of the talocalcaneal joint by gripping the calcaneus in the opposite hand while pressing in this location will cause the talar head to slide under one's fingertips, making it more readily appreciated. Anterior and slightly distal to the lateral malleolus, a depression between the talus and calcaneus, termed the sinus tarsi, is accessible without difficulty. Several ligaments, origins of the extensor retinaculum, fat, and a nutrient vascular supply run through it. Tenderness and swelling at the sinus tarsi may be noted in severe ankle sprains. In addition, it is important to palpate the lateral process of the talus, because fractures here are commonly missed during evaluation of an "ankle sprain."

Moving distally to the hindfoot, several calcaneal prominences can be localized. The anterior process of the calcaneus should be palpated and any tenderness noted since fractures here are frequently overlooked. Posteriorly, the Achilles tendon inserts on the calcaneal tuberosity. Pain and swelling in this region may be related to tendonitis, enthesitis, superficial tendo-achilles ("pump bump"), or retrocalcaneal bursitis, and in the pediatric or adolescent, a calcaneal apophysitis (e.g., Sever's disease). Medially, the sustentaculum tali is the prominence just distal to the medial malleolus and functions as the insertion site for the calcaneal attachment of the deltoid and spring ligaments. Inferior and just distal to the lateral malleolus lies the peroneal trochlea, below which passes the peroneus longus tendon.

Other bony landmarks and structures of clinical importance include the navicular tuberosity medially and the styloid process of the fifth metatarsal laterally. The metatarsal shafts are appreciated on the dorsum of the foot and tenderness may be indicative of a fracture, while the metatarsal heads are accessible on the plantar sole. The presence of calluses and tenderness of the metatarsal heads suggests metatarsalgia, often seen in a pes cavus foot. Pain at the plantar aspect of the first metatarsophalangeal (MTP) joint may be seen with inflammation of that joint capsule (i.e., "turf toe") or injury to the two sesamoid bones that buttress the flexor hallucis longus tendon just proximal to the MTP joint (i.e., sesamoiditis).

Ligamentous and Articular Structures

The medial and lateral collateral ligaments of the ankle comprise the anterior talofibular ligament (ATFL), posterior talofibular ligament (PTFL), and calcaneofibular ligament (CFL) laterally (Figure 10–2), and the deltoid ligament complex medially (Figure 10–3). The ATFL, PTFL, and CFL should each be palpated from their origin on the lateral malleolus to their insertion points.

The ATFL is actually an extension of the anterior joint capsule, and is in the order of 20 mm long, 10 mm wide, and 2–5 mm thick. It originates from the anterior border of the lateral malleolus and inserts distally on the body of the talus just anterior to the

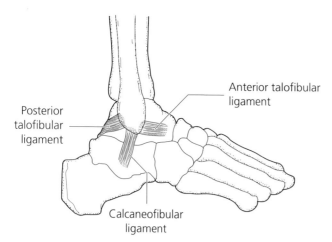

Figure 10–2. The lateral ankle ligaments. Adapted with permission from Starkey C, Ryan JL. Evaluation of Orthopedic and Athletic Injuries. Philadelphia: FA Davis, 2001, p. 89.

Figure 10–3. The deltoid ligament complex. Adapted with permission from Starkey C, Ryan JL. Evaluation of Orthopedic and Athletic Injuries. Philadelphia: FA Davis, 2001, p. 89.

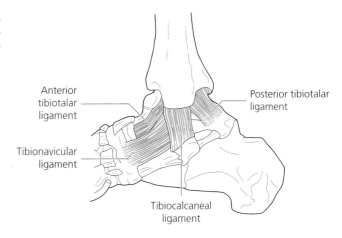

articular facet. Its fibers are oriented approximately 75 degrees to the floor. The ligament is most taut and positioned essentially in-line with the long axis of the tibia in the plantar flexed ankle.[9] It requires the least load to failure of any of the lateral ligaments.[2,42] Rupture of this ligament is associated with tearing the anterior joint capsule,[4] and bony avulsion of the fibular malleolus is also relatively common.[21,42]

The CFL is extracapsular, crosses both the tibiotalar and talocalcaneal joints, and measures on average 2 cm long, 5 mm wide, and 3 mm thick.[23] It is most taut with the ankle in neutral or slight dorsiflexion, when its fibers are positioned in-line with the long axis of the tibia.[9] The origin of this ligament, which is two and a half times stronger than the ATFL,[2,23] is from the distal pole of the fibular malleolus and the insertion is into a small posterolateral tubercle on the calcaneus. The peroneal tendons sheath passes under the lateral malleolus adjacent to the CFL. Broström[7] noted intraoperatively that the ruptures of the CFL were associated with tears of the medial wall of this tendon sheath. Rubin and Witten[38] found the CFL to be lax in weight-bearing, and this supports the fact that ankle stability during axial loading derives primarily from the tibiotalar and talocalcaneal joint articulations.[40,48]

The PTFL, like the ATFL, is confluent with the ankle joint capsule. It traverses from its origin on the posterior fibular malleolus to a lateral tubercle on the posterior talus. Its fibers are oriented nearly horizontal. The PTFL is the strongest of the lateral ligaments, and is taut only at the extremes of dorsiflexion with avulsion of the lateral malleolus occurring before PTFL disruption.[4,39,42]

The deltoid ligament courses from the medial malleolus dividing into four parts: the anterior and posterior tibiotalar ligaments, the tibiocalcaneal ligament, and the tibionavicular ligament. It has both superficial and deep portions and is stronger than any of the lateral ankle ligaments.

The distal tibiofibular syndesmosis is important since it is involved in many moderate-to-severe ankle sprains. There are four ligaments that make up the distal tibiofibular syndesmosis: the anterior tibiofibular, posterior tibiofibular, transverse tibiofibular, and interosseous ligaments. The anterior tibiofibular ligament is palpable at the anterolateral ankle, although its proximity to the anterior talofibular ligament may limit the specificity of diagnosing a syndesmotic versus lateral ankle sprain when palpation of this structure is painful.

Connecting the sustentaculum tali of the calcaneus to the navicular tuberosity is the plantar calcaneonavicular or spring ligament.

The talonavicular and calcaneocuboid joints, together termed the "transverse tarsal joint," are palpated in the midfoot. In the forefoot, the first metatarsophalangeal joint capsule is easily appreciated.

Spanning the sole of the foot from the calcaneus to the bases of the proximal phalanges is the plantar aponeurosis or plantar fascia, which is often tender at its medial calcaneal origin when inflamed.

Tendons

At the medial aspect of the ankle, behind the medial malleolus, pass three tendons along with the posterior tibial artery and nerve through the flexor retinaculum. A useful mnemonic for remembering these three tendons is "*Tom, Dick, and Harry*," which stands for the posterior *t*ibialis, the flexor *d*igitorum longus, and the flexor *h*allucis longus. Passing just anterior to the medial malleolus is the anterior tibialis tendon, which is recognized prominently during ankle dorsiflexion. The extensor hallucis longus tendon can also be palpated as it crosses the dorsomedial ankle and foot on its way to insertion at the great toe.

Posterior to the lateral malleolus pass the peroneus longus and brevis, while the peroneus tertius crosses the ankle anterior to the lateral malleolus just lateral to the extensor digitorum longus. Asking the patient to evert the ankle should allow one to distinguish the peroneus tertius from the extensor digitorum longus (Figure 10–4).

The pulses of the posterior tibial and dorsalis pedis arteries are both palpable in normal individuals. The posterior tibial pulsation can be found just posterior to the medial malleolus as it runs alongside the tendons of the posterior tibialis, flexor digitorum longus, and flexor hallucis longus contained by the flexor retinaculum. The pulse of the dorsalis pedis is readily appreciated in the interspace between the proximal aspect of the first and second metatarsals.

Joint Range of Motion and Biomechanics

The motions occurring at the ankle and foot are complex. Multiplanar joint movements and joint-to-joint interactions generate the motions we simplify in our clinical descriptions

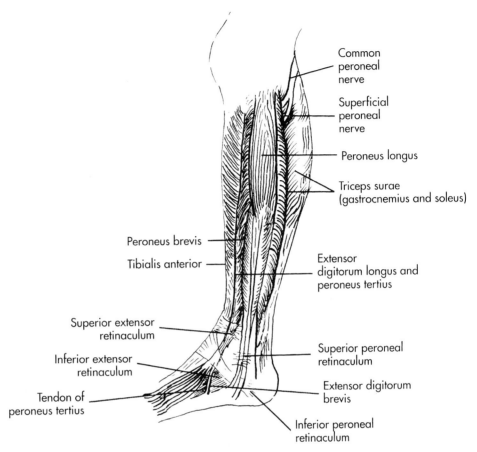

Figure 10–4. Lateral soft tissue anatomy. Reproduced with permission from Bachner EJ, Friedman MJ. Injuries to the leg. In Nicholas J, Hershman E (eds), The Lower Extremity and Spine in Sports Medicine, 2nd edn. St Louis: Mosby, 1995, p. 527.

(i.e., dorsiflexion, plantar flexion, inversion, eversion, pronation, supination). There is a lack of consistency in characterizing the movements of the ankle and foot. Tibiotalar, talocalcaneal, and transverse tarsal motions are complex, interdependent, and not confined to one plane.[29,43] For this reason, we will clarify our use of the following terms: *dorsiflexion* and *plantar flexion* refer to tibiotalar joint motion; *inversion* and *eversion* delineate talocalcaneal (subtalar) joint movement; *internal rotation* and *external rotation* of the ankle refer to combined tibiotalar and talocalcaneal motion; and *pronation* and *supination* are composite movements involving the midfoot and forefoot and are described further below.[43]

Movements of the lower extremity are influenced by each part of the kinetic chain, and this is particularly apparent when leg–ankle–foot interactions are considered.

During human locomotion, actions at the ankle and foot are coordinated with external and internal rotation of the tibia. The rotational forces, or torques, are transmitted distally through the tibiotalar (= talocrural), talocalcaneal (= subtalar), and transverse tarsal joints. "Kinematic coupling" produces the composite movements we term "pronation" and "supination."[43] Pronation is characterized by external rotation and abduction of the forefoot relative to the tibia combined with hindfoot eversion. Supination represents an internal rotation and adduction of the foot on the tibia combined with hindfoot inversion.[47]

Limitations of joint motion may be due to any combination of osseous, cartilaginous, ligamentous, musculotendinous, or fibrous restrictions. Ligamentous laxity is common, and may contribute to individual differences in the ankle range of motion of healthy subjects.[5,38] In a cohort of 18 healthy subjects who underwent a biomechanical analysis of ankle range of motion, Siegler et al.[45] found no significant side-to-side differences.

Tibiotalar Joint

Ankle plantar flexion and dorsiflexion are sagittal plane motions that occur primarily at the tibiotalar joint. Dorsiflexion involves cephalad tilting of the foot toward the tibial shaft, with a range of 20 degrees. Downward pointing of the foot occurs with plantar flexion, with the normal range of 50 degrees. Interestingly, Siegler et al.[43] showed *in vitro* that up to 20% of dorsiflexion or plantar flexion motion is generated at the subtalar joint.

Dorsiflexion is the position of stability for the tibiotalar joint. Rubin and Witten[38] noted that, in the dorsiflexed ankle, the broader anterior part of the talus is in firm contact with the malleoli and resists talar tilt. In dorsiflexion, the fibular malleolus is displaced 2–3 mm laterally. The main function of the lateral ankle ligaments is to stabilize the joint near its neutral position, while at extremes of range of motion bone-to-bone contact provides stability.[44] Furthermore, several researchers have demonstrated that the ankle articulation is inherently stable under loaded conditions.[25,32,40,48] Boardman et al.[3] added that the integrity of the anterolateral joint capsule also contributes significantly to ankle stability.

Talocalcaneal Joint

Hindfoot inversion and eversion occur primarily at the subtalar or talocalcaneal articulation. While some advocate that subtalar motion should be measured with the tibiotalar joint held in neutral dorsiflexion to ensure that the talus is firmly grasped in the mortise, others have noted good joint congruence throughout the range of talocalcaneal motion.[37] Inman[18] noted a large variability in subtalar motion, from 20 to

60 degrees, due to variation in subtalar axis and anatomy, kinematic coupling with the ankle joint, and maintenance of true subtalar neutral positioning. Siegler et al.[43] showed that, at extremes of motion besides subtalar motion, the tibiotalar joint also contributes to inversion and eversion.

Talocalcaneal motion is assessed with the patient sitting, holding the calcaneus in one hand and the forefoot in the other. The examiner subsequently can move the subtalar joint into inversion and eversion. There is usually twice as much inversion as eversion and a lack of subtalar motion may indicate abnormalities such as arthritis, peroneal spastic flat foot, or tarsal coalition. Excessive inversion may be noted after injury to the lateral ankle ligaments.[28]

Transverse Tarsal Joint (Chopart's Joint)

The talonavicular and calcaneocuboid articulations together comprise the transverse tarsal joint. Forefoot supination and pronation occur at this collective joint, and should be tested with the hindfoot maintained in subtalar neutral since motion at the transverse tarsal joint is affected by talocalcaneal inversion and eversion. As with the talocalcaneal joint, side-to-side comparison is helpful in determining unilateral restrictions. Decreased transverse tarsal motion may be seen in chronic tibialis posterior tendon insufficiency and arthrosis involving the transverse tarsal joint. Midfoot amputation at this level is commonly called a Chopart's amputation.

Tarsometatarsal Joint (Lisfranc's Joint)

The cuboid and three cuneiforms adjoin the five metatarsal bones to form the collective tarsometatarsal joint, or Lisfranc's joint. Tenderness at the interval between the first and second metatarsal bases may indicate rupture of Lisfranc's ligament. Foot amputation at this level is called a Lisfranc amputation.

Extrinsic Muscles of the Ankle and Foot

Plantar Flexion

The triceps surae or gastrocnemius–soleus complex contains the prime plantar flexors of the ankle (Figure 10–5). The gastrocnemius has medial and lateral heads originating from the medial and lateral femoral condyles, respectively. Their obliquely oriented fibers adjoin into a common Achilles tendon that is also shared by the soleus muscle and inserts into the calcaneal tuberosity. The posterior tibialis, peroneus longus, flexor digitorum longus, and flexor hallucis longus, and to a lesser extent the plantaris muscle, comprise the accessory plantar flexors of the ankle and foot.[37]

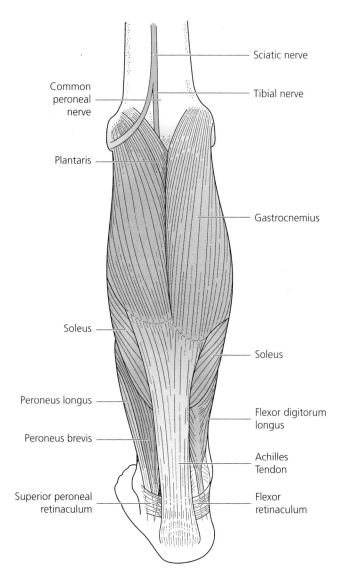

Figure 10–5. The posterior soft tissue anatomy. Adapted with permission from Bachner EJ, Friedman MJ. Injuries to the leg. In Nicholas J, Hershman E (eds), The Lower Extremity and Spine in Sports Medicine, 2nd edn. St Louis: Mosby, 1995, p. 526.

Sciatic nerve

Common peroneal nerve

Tibial nerve

Plantaris

Gastrocnemius

Soleus

Soleus

Peroneus longus

Flexor digitorum longus

Peroneus brevis

Achilles Tendon

Superior peroneal retinaculum

Flexor retinaculum

Dorsiflexion

The most important ankle dorsiflexors of the ankle and foot are the tibialis anterior and the extensor digitorum longus. The peroneus tertius and extensor hallucis longus serve as supplemental dorsiflexors.

Inversion and Supination

The main invertors are the tibialis anterior and tibialis posterior. These muscles contribute as well to forefoot supination. The flexor digitorum longus and flexor hallucis longus can serve as auxiliary forefoot supinators as well. The triceps surae produce calcaneal inversion.

Eversion and Pronation

The peroneus longus, peroneus brevis, and peroneus tertius act in concert to evert the forefoot. The lateral portion of the extensor digitorum longus can aid in this function.

Intrinsic Muscles of the Foot

Interphalangeal and Metatarsophalangeal Flexion

The flexor digitorum longus (FDL) and brevis (FDB), the flexor hallucis longus (FHL), and the quadratus plantae all serve as interphalangeal joint flexors. The metatarsophalangeal joints are flexed by the FDL, FDB, FHL, flexor hallucis brevis and flexor digiti minimi brevis, abductor hallucis and abductor digiti minimi, and all the lumbricals and interossei.

Metatarsophalangeal Extension

The lumbricals and interossei, extensor digitorum longus and brevis, and the extensor hallucis longus and brevis, all contribute to metatarsophalangeal extension.

Innervation of the Foot Muscles and Ankle Joint

The tibial nerve enters the ankle and foot region coursing behind the medial malleolus and subsequently dividing into medial and lateral plantar branches. The tibial nerve supplies the ankle plantar flexors, invertors, and extrinsic toe flexors in the leg, and then divides into the medial and lateral plantar branches that are analogous to the median and ulnar nerves in the hand. The medial plantar nerve innervates the abductor hallucis, flexor digitorum brevis, flexor hallucis brevis, and first two lumbricals, and provides cutaneous sensation to the medial three and a half digits. The lateral plantar nerve supplies the quadratus plantae, flexor digiti quinti brevis, abductor digiti quinti, the lateral three lumbricals, the interossei, and cutaneous sensation to the lateral plantar aspect of the foot.

While the peripheral nerves innervating the structures of the ankle and foot are not typically palpable, the examiner should be aware of interdigital neuromas (e.g., Morton's neuroma) (Figure 10–6), and nerve entrapments, including the controversial tarsal tunnel syndrome (entrapment of the tibial nerve as it crosses the ankle through the flexor retinaculum) as sources of foot pain (Figure 10–7). The examination for interdigital neuroma includes squeezing or compressing the metatarsals

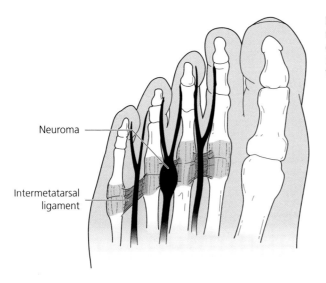

Figure 10–6. Morton's neuroma. Adapted with permission from Mann RA. Entrapment neuropathies of the foot. In DeLee JC, Drez D (eds), Orthopedic Sports Medicine Principles and Practice. Philadelphia: WB Saunders, 1994, p. 1838.

Neuroma

Intermetatarsal ligament

as well as looking for a "Mulder's click," demonstrated by compression of the distal metatarsals combined with translation in a superior/inferior direction.[34] A "click" is often felt or heard when a neuroma is present (this is due to the distal metatarsals contacting the thickened soft tissue mass which is the neuroma). A positive Tinel's sign at the tarsal tunnel supports a diagnosis of tarsal tunnel syndrome.

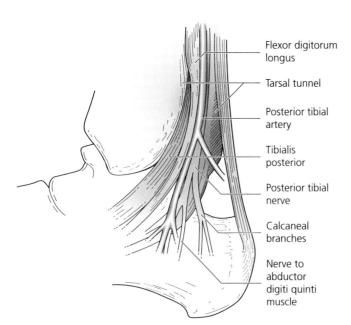

Flexor digitorum longus

Tarsal tunnel

Posterior tibial artery

Tibialis posterior

Posterior tibial nerve

Calcaneal branches

Nerve to abductor digiti quinti muscle

Figure 10–7. The tarsal tunnel. Adapted with permission from Mann RA. Entrapment neuropathies of the foot. In DeLee JC, Drez D (eds), Orthopedic Sports Medicine Principles and Practice. Philadelphia: WB Saunders, 1994, p. 1832.

Figure 10–8. The superficial peroneal nerve. Adapted with permission from Mann RA. Entrapment neuropathies of the foot. In DeLee JC, Drez D (eds), Orthopedic Sports Medicine Principles and Practice. Philadelphia: WB Saunders, 1994, p. 1837.

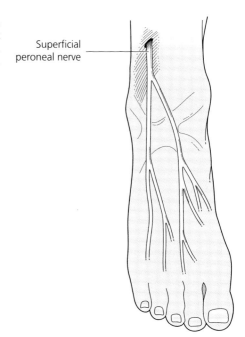

Superficial peroneal nerve

The common peroneal nerve divides behind the fibular head into deep and superficial portions. The deep peroneal nerve supplies the tibialis anterior, extrinsic toe extensors, and peroneus tertius, while its terminal branch brings cutaneous sensation to the interspace between the first and second toes. The superficial peroneal nerve supplies the peroneus longus and brevis, the prime ankle evertors, and then provides cutaneous sensation to the anterolateral lower leg and dorsum of the foot (Figure 10–8).

The sural nerve is formed from branches of the tibial and common peroneal nerves, and supplies sensation to the lateral dorsum and heel of the foot (Figure 10–9).

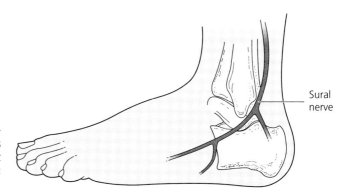

Sural nerve

Figure 10–9. The sural nerve. Adapted with permission from Mann RA. Entrapment neuropathies of the foot. In DeLee JC, Drez D (eds), Orthopedic Sports Medicine Principles and Practice. Philadelphia: WB Saunders, 1994, p. 1835.

The joint capsules and collateral ligaments of the ankle are richly innervated with pain and proprioceptive fibers.

Special Tests for the Ankle and Foot

Lateral Ankle Ligaments

Lateral ankle sprains are the most common lower-extremity injury. In a series of 321 consecutive acute ankle sprains, Broström[8] described 239 arthrographically proven acute lateral ligament ruptures. Thus, one or more lateral ligaments were completely ruptured in at least 75% of cases. Isolated ATFL rupture occurred in about 65% of cases, combined ATFL–CFL tear in about 20%, and isolated tibiofibular (syndesmosis) rupture in about 10%.

Anterior Drawer

In 1968, Landeros et al. described the maneuver as follows:[22]

> With the patient relaxed, the knee flexed and the ankle at right angles, the ankle is grasped on the tibial side by one hand, whose index finger is placed on the posteromedial part of the talus and whose middle finger lies on the posterior tibial malleolus. The heel of this hand braces the anterior distal leg. On pulling the heel forward with the other hand, relative anteroposterior motion between the 2 fingers (and thus between talus and tibia) is easily palpated and is also visible to both patient and examiner.

In 1976, Frost and Hanson devoted a short article to further describing the technique, noting several pearls. Excerpts are provided below[13]:

> The anterior and posterior muscles which actuate the ankle joint must be relaxed. … The ankle must be positioned at 90 degrees to the leg. … Place the heel of the right hand over the anterior ankle distal tibia just proximal to the ankle joint. Extend the fingers around the medial side of the tibia, and place the index finger on the posterior prominence of the astragalus (i.e., talus), the third finger on the posterior tibial malleolus on its medial aspect. These fingers serve as 'sensors' to detect any relative anteroposterior displacement of the talus on the tibia. Curve the left hand around the foot, the palm on the underside of the heel, the fingers curled around the posterior aspect of the tuber os calcis. … Pull forward on the heel with the left hand, and push posteriorly on the distal tibia with the right hand, thereby attempting to draw the talus anteriorly in the mortise.

A recent study by Tohyama et al.[55] showed that a relatively low anterior load (30 N) during the anterior drawer test was more sensitive than a higher load (60 N)

Figure 10–10. The anterior drawer test. Adapted with permission from Renstrom P, Kannus P. Injuries of the foot and ankle. In DeLee JC, Drez D (eds), Orthopedic Sports Medicine Principles and Practice. Philadelphia: WB Saunders, 1994, p. 1709.

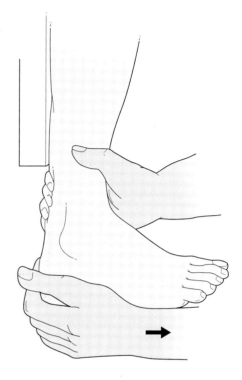

in distinguishing a significant difference between injured to normal anterior displacement. The greater anterior load tends to elicit a protective muscle contraction which may mask the anterior talar displacement.

Anterior drawer testing is performed to assess the integrity of the lateral ankle ligaments, and in particular the ATFL (Figure 10–10). Isolated ATFL tears constitute between one-third and two-thirds of all lateral ligament injuries, and tears are usually complete and involve the anterior joint capsule.[7,19]

The validity, sensitivity, and specificity of such manual stress testing as the anterior drawer maneuver has been studied, and the results are conflicting. Lindstrand[24] consecutively examined 100 skiers with acute ankle sprains with a modified anterior drawer maneuver, the results of which were compared with findings at surgery. Eighty of 100 persons had a positive drawer sign, nine of which were only observed under local anesthesia. Overall, the sensitivity of the anterior drawer sign was 95%, the specificity was 84.2%, the positive predictive value of the test was 96.25%, while the negative predictive value was 80%.

Funder et al.[15] examined 444 patients with acute lateral ankle sprains for direct and indirect ligament tenderness, manually elicited anterior drawer (at 30 degrees plantar flexion), and talar tilt (ankle flexion angle not specified) tests without local anesthesia, and swelling anterior and over the lateral malleolus. Findings were compared to arthrography as the gold standard. There were 209 arthrographically confirmed ligament ruptures. Of the 35 cases with a positive anterior drawer sign, 71% of these had arthrographically proven ligament tears. Of the 53 positive talar tilt tests, 68% of those had arthrographically demonstrated ligament rupture. Arthrography could not distinguish between or confirm which ligaments had ruptured. Swelling over the lateral malleolus ≥ 4 cm in diameter proved to be the single most valuable diagnostic sign; 70% with this sign had ligament rupture. If such swelling was present in conjunction with direct and indirect tenderness of the lateral ligaments, there was a 91% probability of ligament rupture.

Caution must be exercised in assessing the anterior drawer in those with ligamentous laxity as false-positive findings may be seen in up to 19% of uninjured ankles in those with such laxity.[19]

Van Dijk et al.[56] compared physical examination delayed 5 days after ankle sprain to arthrography and surgical findings in 160 consecutive patients. Of these 160 patients, 135 patients went on to have surgery, and of those 122 ligament tears were confirmed. The anterior drawer test was found to have a sensitivity of 80%, specificity of 74%, positive predictive value of 91%, and negative predictive value of 52%. The combination of pain on lateral ligament palpation, hematoma formation at the lateral ankle, and a positive anterior drawer test diagnosed a lateral ligament lesion correctly in 95% of cases.

Talar Tilt

The earliest English language description of the talar tilt test we could find was by Rubin and Witten (Figure 10–11):[38]

> By definition, talar tilt angle is the angle formed by the opposing articular surfaces of the tibia and talus when these surfaces are separated laterally by a supination force applied to the hind part of the foot.

In 1944, Bonnin[5] stated that 4–5% of ankles without a history of injury had a significant tilt up to 25 degrees. Rubin and Witten[38] reported that normal talar tilt could range from 0 to 23 degrees. Broström[8] described 239 cases of arthrographically confirmed lateral ligament rupture. He found that talar tilt instability was frequently seen in the contralateral uninjured ankle, and so he concurred with Rubin and Witten who asserted the talar tilt test is not a reliable indicator of ligament injury.[8,38]

Frost and Amendola[14] additionally found that talar tilt x-rays were not reliable in diagnosing lateral ligament injury. In the most methodologically sound studies reviewed, there still was a significant degree of variability in the values defining a normal talar tilt; they included 7 degrees, 10 degrees, 11 degrees, and 3 mm as the upper limits of normal utilizing both manual and mechanical devices to induce

Figure 10–11. The talar tilt test. Adapted with permission from Renstrom P, Kannus P. Injuries of the foot and ankle. In DeLee JC, Drez D (eds), Orthopedic Sports Medicine Principles and Practice. Philadelphia: WB Saunders, 1994, p. 1710.

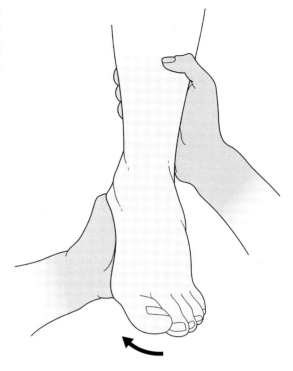

stress (Telos radiographic ankle stress apparatus, Telos Medical, Fallston, MD, USA). Overall, the literature does not support the use of either the talar tilt test, with or without radiography.

Information on the sensitivity, specificity, positive and negative predictive values of the talar tilt test is reported in Table 10–1.

Syndesmosis Injuries

The distal tibiofibular syndesmosis consists of four stabilizing ligaments, termed the anterior, posterior, transverse, and interosseous tibiofibular ligaments (Figure 10–12). Maisonneuve[27] first described how an external rotation of the talus in the ankle mortise could result in fractures at the ankle and proximal fibula and could be associated with damage to the tibiofibular ligaments. Sprains of the distal tibiofibular syndesmosis occur in between 1% and 11% of all ankle injuries and are thought to be the result of a strong external rotation force at the ankle.[6,17] Recovery times for syndesmotic ankle sprains may be extended, up to twice as long as for patients with complete lateral ligament injuries.[6,17,35,50] Syndesmosis ligament injury is difficult to detect utilizing x-ray and arthrography as minor disruption of the ligaments may be missed, especially

Table 10–1. ANKLE STABILITY

Test	Description	Reliability/Validity Tests	Comments
Anterior drawer test	In Landeros et al.[22]; and see this text.	Lindstrand 1976[24] Sensitivity: 95% Specificity: 84.2%	Findings at operation were gold standard.
	In Frost and Hanson[13]; and see this text.	van Dijk et al. 1996[56] Sensitivity: 80% Specificity: 74%	
Talar tilt	In Rubin and Witten[38]; and see this text.	NA	

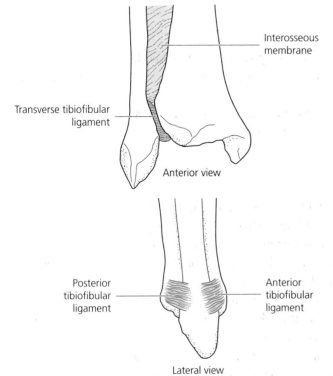

Interosseous membrane

Transverse tibiofibular ligament

Anterior view

Posterior tibiofibular ligament

Anterior tibiofibular ligament

Lateral view

Figure 10–12. The distal tibiofibular syndesmosis. Adapted with permission from Starkey C, Ryan JL. Evaluation of Orthopedic and Athletic Injuries. Philadelphia: FA Davis, 2001, p. 90.

in the acute setting.[1,33] Magnetic resonance imaging (MRI) is the most sensitive and is also quite specific in both acute and chronic settings, but its expense makes it impractical as a screening test. Delayed radiography several weeks following syndesmosis injury may reveal heterotopic ossification of the interosseous membrane in 50% or more of those with a partial rupture.[17,50]

Three well-described exam maneuvers are used to detect syndesmosis injury: the external rotation test (Figure 10–13), syndesmosis ligament palpation (Figure 10–14) and the squeeze test (Figure 10–15). There are no studies, however, that specifically validate these tests for syndesmotic injury (Table 10–2), and there is no information available on the true sensitivity or specificity of these tests. Utilizing combinations of tests may be a more sensitive and specific indicator of syndesmotic injury and additionally may ultimately be a better predictor of severity. Alonso et al.[1] noted that subjects with both positive external rotation and dorsiflexion-compression tests had significantly longer recovery time, suggesting more serious injury.

External Rotation or Kleiger's Test

Barnard Kleiger (1954) was the first to explain the external rotation, or Kleiger's test, to identify syndesmotic injury (see Figure 10–13). The original description of the test is as follows[20]:

Table 10–2. SYNDESMOSIS TESTS

Test	Description	Reliability/Validity Tests	Comments
External rotation or Kleiger's test	In Kleiger[20]; and see this text. In Boytim et al.[6]; and see this text.	NA	
Syndesmotic ligament palpation test	The palpation test involves palpation over the area of the anterior tibiofibular ligament and proximal to the anterior talofibular ligament, with a positive test result indicated by the report of tenderness in this area.	NA	
Syndesmosis squeeze test	The squeeze test is performed by manually compressing the fibula to the tibia above the mid point of the calf. A positive test produces pain over the area of the syndesmotic ligaments.[17]	NA	

Figure 10–13. The external rotation test. Copyright © 1990 by the American Orthopaedic Foot and Ankle Society (AOFAS), originally published in Foot and Ankle International, June 1990, Volume 10, Number 6, page 326 and reproduced here with permission.

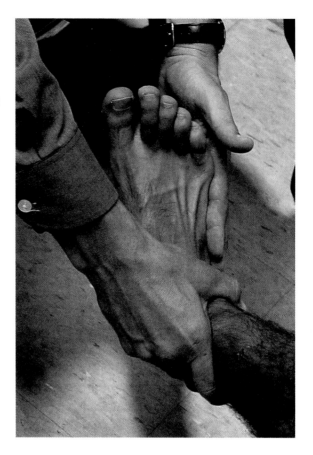

The diagnosis can occasionally be confirmed clinically when the talus can be felt to move laterally as the foot is rotated externally. This is possible only when swelling is slight and the talus can be felt with the examining finger. The diagnosis can best be established by taking roentgenograms with the ankle under external rotation stress.

Kleiger proceeded to outline suggestions for performing external rotation stress radiographs.

The physical examination maneuver has been explained further by Boytim et al.[6] The patient is seated with the knee flexed to 90 degrees and the foot relaxed. The examiner applies a small force on the foot, rotating it laterally. The patient will have pain anterolaterally when the test is positive. The examiner may also feel the talus displace from the medial malleolus, which would suggest a deltoid ligament tear. The rotation causes the talus to press against the lateral malleolus, resulting in tibiofibular joint widening of the syndesmosis ligaments.

Boytim et al.[6] analyzed the records of 15 professional football players with syndesmosis sprains and compared them to others with lateral ankle injuries. The diagnosis was made based upon tenderness over the anterior and/or posterior tibiofibular and interosseous ligaments, and increased pain on external rotation stress. Acute radiographs showed an avulsion of the posterior tibial tubercle in 2 of 13 players and no abnormalities of the mortise were seen. Follow-up radiographs 1 month later demonstrated calcification of the interosseous membrane in 6 of 8 players. The 15 players with syndesmosis sprains missed significantly more games and practices and required more physical therapy than those with lateral ankle sprains.

Alonso et al.[1] investigated the inter-rater reliability of various tests for syndesmotic injury. While the authors failed to describe the gold standard by which syndesmotic injury was identified, they concluded that the external rotation test has the best inter-rater reliability, with a κ coefficient of 0.75. The straightforward biomechanics involved in the external rotation test is likely to contribute to the high reliability of the test.

Stricker et al.[49] compared the findings of a standardized history and physical examination with radiography among 74 patients with acute ankle injuries in order to determine factors significantly associated with fractures and syndesmosis injuries. Two examiners performed the external rotation stress test, direct syndesmosis palpation, and mid-calf squeeze test for syndesmotic injuries, and they found that the external rotation stress was the only test that showed significant association with an abnormal mortise or fracture. The possibility of a fracture or abnormal mortise was 5.1 times greater in those with syndesmosis pain during the external rotation test.

Syndesmotic Ligament Palpation Test

The palpation test involves palpation over the area of the anterior tibiofibular ligament and proximal to the anterior talofibular ligament, with a positive test result indicated by the report of tenderness in this area (see Figure 10–14).[1,6]

The palpation test has been used frequently as a diagnostic tool for syndesmosis ligament damage. However, Alonso et al.[1] found this test to have only fair inter-rater reliability. We could find no study that examines the specificity, sensitivity, positive predictive value, or the negative predictive value of the palpation test. Alonso et al. explain that it is extremely difficult to precisely apply direct pressure accurately over the anterior tibiofibular ligament, and any injury in this area can cause pain limiting the specificity of the test. Variation in the area palpated can increase the rate of false positives. The anterior tibiofibular ligament is located close to the more commonly injured lateral ligaments, specifically the anterior talofibular ligament. A varying amount of pressure applied by each examiner can lead to different findings.

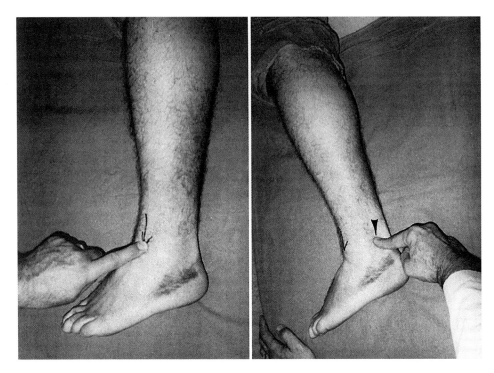

Figure 10–14. The syndesmosis ligament palpation test. **A:** Over anterior tibiofibular ligament. **B:** Over posterior tibiofibular ligament. Reproduced with permission from Turco VJ, Gallant GG. Occult trauma and unusual injuries in the foot. In Nicholas J, Hershman E (eds), The Lower Extremity and Spine in Sports Medicine, 2nd edn. St Louis: Mosby, p. 476.

Syndesmosis Squeeze Test

The squeeze test is performed by manually compressing the fibula to the tibia above the mid point of the calf (see Figure 10–15).[17,51] A positive test produces pain over the area of the syndesmotic ligaments.

Hopkinson et al.[17] retrospectively studied 1344 ankle sprains of West Point cadets to compare the duration of disability with the specific ligaments involved and the severity of ankle injury. The prevalence of syndesmosis injuries in this review was 1%. Fifteen cadets were diagnosed with syndesmosis sprain, and all had a positive squeeze test. Nine out of 10 ankles that underwent a second set of radiographs several weeks following the initial injury had calcification of the interosseous membrane.

Xenos et al.[57] performed an in-vitro study on 25 cadaver ankles administering a machine-applied external rotation torque to produce syndesmotic ligament injuries. The authors found that the degree of distal tibiofibular diastasis seen on x-ray during application of an external rotation torque correlates to the degree of syndesmosis injury.

Alonso et al.[1] found the squeeze test had moderate inter-rater reliability, with a κ coefficient of 0.50. The authors suggested that in order to obtain a

Figure 10–15. The syndesmosis squeeze test. Redrawn with permission from Hopkinson WJ, St Pierre P, Ryan JB, Wheeler JH. Syndemosis sprains of the ankle. Foot Ankle 1990;10(6), as it appeared in Canale ST. Ankle injuries. In Canale ST. Campbell's Operative Orthopaedics, 9th edn. St Louis: Mosby, 1998.

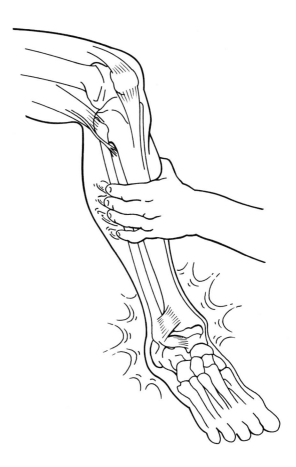

positive result the compressive forces must either be very large or the actual injury very severe.

Achilles Tendon Rupture

Achilles tendon rupture can occur in a relatively healthy tendon or in one that is scarred from repetitive trauma.[11] The most common mechanisms of Achilles rupture are pushing off with the weight-bearing forefoot while extending the knee, sudden unexpected dorsiflexion of the ankle, or violent dorsiflexion of the plantar flexed foot as in a fall from a height.[31,54] Disruption also can occur from a direct blow to the contracted tendon or from a laceration.

Thompson's Test (Simmonds–Thompson or Squeeze Test)

There is controversy over who to credit with first identifying the squeeze test (Figure 10–16). As described by Thompson and Doherty in 1962, it is performed in the following manner:[52]

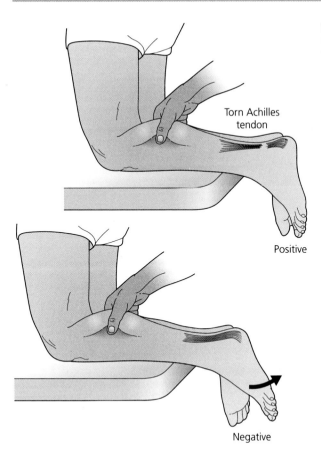

Figure 10–16. Thompson's test for Achilles tendon rupture. Reproduced with permission from The athletic heel. Foot Ankle Clin 1999:867.

The patient is placed in a prone position with his foot extending over the end of the table. The calf muscles are squeezed in the middle one-third below the place of the widest girth. Passive plantar movement of the foot is seen in a normal reaction. A positive reaction is seen when there is no plantar movement of the foot and indicates a rupture of the heel cord.

In 1957, Simmonds[46] first published a description of the calf squeeze test for rupture of the calcaneal tendon (Table 10–3). Five years later, Thompson[53] published his description of the test, and explained that he had observed the effects of this examination in 1955, two years prior to Simmonds. They both noted that when examining a patient with heel cord rupture, no motion of the foot occurred when squeezing the calf of the affected leg. However, when squeezing the calf of the unaffected leg, the foot responded by being passively plantar-flexed.

In 1962, Thompson and Doherty[52] noted (and Scott et al. later confirmed[53]) that plantar flexion of the foot with a squeeze of the calf requires an intact soleus musculotendinous unit. When performed on cadavers, if 90% of the soleus tendon

Table 10–3. ACHILLES TENDON RUPTURE TESTS

Test	Description	Reliability/Validity Tests	Comments
Thompson's test (Simmonds–Thompson or squeeze test)	Simmonds[46] published the first description of the calf squeeze test for rupture of the calcaneal tendon in 1957. In Thompson and Doherty in 1962[52]; and see this text.	Maffulli 1998[26] Sensitivity: 0.96 Specificity: 0.93	Positive in almost 100% of ruptures of Achilles tendon.
Matles test	In Matles[30]; and see this text.	Mafulli 1998[26] Sensitivity: 0.88 Specificity: 0.85	
O'Brien test	In O'Brien 1984[36]; and see this text.	Maffulli 1998[26,36] Sensitivity: 0.80 Specificity: ?	
Copeland's test	In Copeland[12]; and see this text.	Maffulli 1998[26] Sensitivity: 0.78 Specificity: ?	
Palpation test	In Maffulli[26]; and see this text.	Maffulli[26] Sensitivity: 0.73 Specificity: 0.89	

was cut, the foot responded less strongly. When the tendon was completely cut, the foot remained in neutral position on the squeeze test.

Maffulli[26] studied 174 patients with complete Achilles tendon tears using all four provocative tests described herein, with and without the influence of anesthesia. The calf squeeze test was found to have a sensitivity of 0.96, and a specificity of 0.93, and a positive predictive value of 0.98.

Matles Test

The Matles test was first described in 1975 by Arthur Matles as follows:[30]

> In the prone position, with the foot over the end of the table, the patient is asked to actively flex the knee through 90 degrees. The position of the foot is observed throughout the arc, and if the foot falls into neutral or the slightest position of dorsiflexion, the test is positive. In normal patients, the foot is held in plantar flexion.

The test cannot be used if the patient has an associated knee injury preventing knee flexion. Active flexion of the knee causes shortening of the Achilles tendon because the gastrocnemius is a two-joint muscle and crosses the knee.

The knee may be passively flexed as well, as when a patient is anesthetized. Whether the test is performed with active or passive knee flexion, the position of the ankle and foot is carefully observed during flexion of the knee. If the foot on the affected side falls into neutral or into dorsiflexion, an Achilles tendon tear is diagnosed. On the uninjured side, the foot remains in slight plantar flexion when the knee is 90 degrees. Mafulli[26] studied the Matles test and noted a sensitivity of 0.88 and a positive predictive value of 0.92. The specificity was 0.85.

O'Brien Test

The O'Brien test was described in 1984 by Tim O'Brien as follows:[36]

> The patient is in the prone position. Using aseptic technique, a 25-gauge needle was inserted at a right angle through the skin of the calf just medial to the midline at a point ten centimeters proximal to the superior border of the calcaneus. The needle was inserted gently through the skin until further resistance was felt, so that the needle's tip was just within the substance of the Achilles tendon but did not transfix it. The foot was then passively and alternately dorsiflexed and plantarflexed gently, and the movement of the hub of the needle was noted.
>
> Two distinct types of response may occur. One response is swiveling of the needle about its pivot point in the skin so that it points in the direction opposite to the movement of the foot. This indicates that the tendon is intact throughout its distal ten centimeters. The other possible response is the absence of swiveling or only a slight movement of the needle that corresponds to the movement of the skin (the needle moves slightly distally as the foot is dorsiflexed). Such an opposite motion or the lack of a swiveling is a positive test, indicating the loss of continuity of the Achilles tendon between its insertion and the position of the needle.

O'Brien notes that only the needle technique dynamically tests the integrity of the distal 10 cm of the Achilles tendon. Maffulli[26] noted the sensitivity of the O'Brien test to be 0.80 with a positive predictive value of 0.85. The O'Brien test was only performed under anesthesia due to its uncomfortable nature.[36]

Copeland's Test

Copeland described his novel test as follows:[12]

> The patient lies face down on the examination couch. The knee is flexed to 90 degrees and a sphygmomanometer cuff is applied around the bulk of the calf muscle. The cuff is inflated to approximately 100 mmHg with the ankle plantar flexed. The ankle is then passively dorsiflexed by pressure on the sole of the foot. If the Achilles tendon is intact, the column will be seen to rise to approximately 140 mmHg. If the tendon is disrupted, only a flicker of movement is seen in the Mercury column.

The sensitivity of the Copeland test was 0.78 with a positive predictive value of 0.92 in the study done by Maffulli.[26]

Palpation Test

As described by Maffulli: "The examiner gently palpates the course of the tendon. The gap is classified as present or absent."[26] The palpation test may be uncomfortable in the setting of acute injury, and calf swelling may diminish its accuracy. The palpation test was found to be the least sensitive at 0.73 in the study by Maffulli. The specificity was noted to be 0.89.

Summary

Maffulli[26] concluded that each of the four tests described above could diagnose a subcutaneous Achilles tendon tear with a high degree of certainty. These tests may also be used to correctly determine when the Achilles tendon is not torn. When two or more of these tests indicate a subcutaneous Achilles tendon tear, the diagnosis of tear is established. The sensitivity of the tests increased under anesthesia but the differences did not reach statistical significance. The sensitivity of the squeeze and Matles tests both approached 0.90, and were significantly more sensitive than the other maneuvers.

Conclusion

Injuries of the ankle and foot are commonly seen in clinical practice. Not only must the musculoskeletal medicine practitioner understand ankle and foot anatomy and biomechanics, but he or she should be knowledgeable of the routinely employed physical exam maneuvers. In this chapter, we have provided the original description of selected commonly employed special tests of the ankle and foot, and outlined the validity of these special tests as substantiated by the current literature. We found little evidence that supports the validity of these tests. The Achilles tendon squeeze test was the only maneuver shown to have greater than 90% sensitivity and specificity and positive and negative predictive value. The examiner should use caution, therefore, in interpreting these special orthopedic tests that are commonly used in physical examination of the ankle and foot.

REFERENCES

1. Alonso A, Khoury L, Adams R. Clinical test for ankle syndesmosis injury: reliability and prediction of return of function. J Orthop Sports Phys Ther 1998;27:276–284.
2. Attarian DE, McCrackin HJ, DeVito DP, et al. Biomechanical characteristics of human ankle ligaments. Foot Ankle 1985;6(2):54–58.

3. Boardman DL, Liu SH. Contribution of the anterolateral joint capsule to the mechanical stability of the ankle. Clin Orthop 1997;341:224–232.

4. Bonnin JG. Editorials and annotations: injury to the ligaments of the ankle. J Bone Joint Surg 1965;47B:609–611.

5. Bonnin JG. The hypermobile ankle. Proc R Soc Med 1944;37:282–286.

6. Boytim MJ, Fischer DA, Neumann L. Syndesmotic ankle sprains. Am J Sports Med 1991;19:294–298.

7. Broström L. Sprained ankles. I: Anatomic lesions in recent sprains. Acta Chir Scand 1964;128:483–495.

8. Broström L. Sprained ankles. III: Clinical observations in recent ligament ruptures. Acta Chir Scand 1965;130:560–569.

9. Bulucu C, Thomas KA, Halvorson TL, et al. Biomechanical evaluation of the anterior drawer test: the contribution of the lateral ankle ligaments. Foot Ankle 1991;11:389–393.

10. Cailliet R. Structural functional anatomy. In Cailliet R, Foot and Ankle Pain, 3rd edn. Philadelphia: FA Davis Co., 1997, pp. 1–46.

11. Cook J, Khan K, Purdam C. Achilles tendinopathy. Man Ther 2002;7(3):121–130.

12. Copeland SA. Rupture of the Achilles tendon: a new clinical test. Ann R Coll Surg Engl 1990;72:270–271.

13. Frost H, Hanson CA. Technique for testing the drawer sign in the ankle. Clin Orthop 1977;123:49–51.

14. Frost SC, Amendola A. Critical review. Is stress radiography necessary in the diagnosis of acute or chronic ankle instability? Clin J Sport Med 1999;9:40–45.

15. Funder V, Jorgensen JP, Andersen A, et al. Ruptures of the lateral ligaments of the ankle: clinical diagnosis. Acta Orthop Scand 1982;53:997–1000.

16. Garrick JG. The frequency of injury, mechanism of injury, and epidemiology of ankle sprains. Am J Sports Med 1977;5:242–247.

17. Hopkinson WJ, St Pierre P, Ryan JB, Wheeler JH. Syndesmotic sprains of the ankle. Foot Ankle 1990;10:325–330.

18. Inman VT. The Joints of the Ankle. Baltimore: Williams & Wilkins, 1976.

19. Kaikkonen A, Hyppanen E, Kannus P, et al. Long-term functional outcome after primary repair of the lateral ligaments of the ankle. Am J Sports Med 1997;25:150–155.

20. Kleiger B. The diagnosis and treatment of traumatic lateral ankle instability. NY State J Med 1954;54: 2573–2577.

21. Kumai T, Takakura Y, Rufai A, et al. The functional anatomy of the human anterior talofibular ligament in relation to the ankle sprains. J Anat 2002;200:457–465.

22. Landeros O, Frost H, Higgins CC. Post-traumatic anterior ankle instability. Clin Ortho Rel Res 1968; 56:169–178.

23. Lassiter TE, Malone TR, Garrett WE. Injury to the lateral ligaments of the ankle. Ortho Clin North Am 1989;20:629–640.

24. Lindstrand A. New aspects in the diagnosis of lateral ankle sprains. Ortho Clin North Am 1976;7:247–249.

25. Liu W, Maitland ME, Nigg BM. The effect of axial load on the in-vivo anterior drawer test of the ankle joint complex. Foot Ankle Int 2000;21:420–426.

26. Maffulli N. The clinical diagnosis of subcutaneous tear of the Achilles tendon: a prospective study in 174 patients. Am J Sports Med 1998;26:266–270.

27. Maisonneuve JG. Recherches sur la fracture du péroné. Arch Gen Méd 1840;165(1):433.

28. Mann RA. Principles of examination of the foot and ankle. In Mann RA, Coughlin MJ (eds), Surgery of the Foot and Ankle. St Louis: Mosby, 1993.

29. Manter JT. Movements of the subtalar and transverse tarsal joints. Anat Record 1941;80:397–410.

30. Matles AL. Rupture of the tendo Achilles: another diagnostic sign. Bull Hosp Joint Dis 1975;36:48–51.

31. Mazzone MF, McCue T. Common conditions of the Achilles tendon. Am Fam Phys 2002;65:1805–1810.

32. McCullough CJ, Burge PD. Rotatory stability of the load-bearing ankle: an experimental study. J Bone Joint Surg 1980;62B:460–464.

33. Monk CJE. Injuries to the tibio-fibular ligaments. J Bone Joint Surg 1969;51B:330–337.

34. Mulder JD. The causative mechanism in Morton's metatarsalgia. J Bone Joint Surg 1951;33B:94–95.

35. Mullins JF, Sallis JG. Recurrent sprain of the ankle joint with diastasis. J Bone Joint Surg 1958;40B:270–273.

36. O'Brien T. The needle test for complete rupture of the Achilles tendon. J Bone Joint Surg 1984; 66A:1099–1101.

37. Rosse C, Gaddum-Rosse P. The free lower limb: thigh, leg, and foot. In Rosse C, Gaddum-Rosse P, Hollinshead's Textbook of Anatomy, 5th edn. Philadelphia: Lippincott–Raven, 1997, pp. 337–418.

38. Rubin G, Witten M. The talar-tilt angle and the fibular collateral ligaments: a method for determination of talar tilt. J Bone Joint Surg 1960;42A:311–326.

39. Safran MR, Benedetti RS, Bartolozzi AR, et al. Lateral ankle sprains: a comprehensive review. I: Etiology, pathoanatomy, histopathogenesis, and diagnosis. Med Sci Sport Exer 1999;31(suppl. 7):S429–437.

40. Sammarco GJ, Burstein AH, Frankel VA. Biomechanics of the ankle: a kinematic study. Orthop Clin N Am 1973;4:75–96.

41. Scott BW, Al Chalabi A. How the Simmonds–Thompson test works. J Bone Joint Surg 1992;74B:314–315.

42. Siegler S, Block J, Schneck CD. The mechanical characteristics of the collateral ligaments of the ankle joint. Foot Ankle 1988;8:234–242.

43. Siegler S, Chen J, Schneck CD. The three-dimensional kinematics and flexibility characteristics of the human ankle and subtalar joints. I: Kinematics. J Biomech Eng 1988;110:364–373.

44. Siegler S, Chen J, Schneck CD. The effect of damage to the lateral collateral ligaments on the mechanical characteristics of the ankle joint: an in-vitro study. J Biomech Engng 1990;112(2):129–137.

45. Siegler S, Wnag D, Plasha E, et al. Technique for in-vivo measurement of the three-dimensional kinematics and laxity characteristics of the ankle joint complex. J Orthop Res 1994;12:421–431.

46. Simmonds FA. The diagnosis of the ruptured Achilles tendon. The Practitioner 1957;179:56–58.

47. Stiehl JB. Biomechanics of the ankle joint. In Stiehl JB (ed.), Inman's Joints of the Ankle, 2nd edn. Baltimore: Williams & Wilkins, 1991, pp. 39–63.

48. Stormont DM, Morrey BF, An D, et al. Stability of the loaded ankle: relation between articular restraint and primary and secondary static restraints. Am J Sport Med 1985;13:295–300.

49. Stricker PR, Spindler KP, Gautier KB. Prospective evaluation of history and physical examination: variables to determine radiography in acute ankle injuries. Clin J Sport Med 1998;8:209–214.

50. Taylor DC, Englehardt DL, Bassett FH. Syndesmosis sprains of the ankle: the influence of heterotopic ossification. Am J Sports Med 1992;20:146–150.

51. Teitz CC, Harrington RM. A biochemical analysis of the squeeze test for sprains of the syndesmotic ligaments of the ankle. Foot Ankle Int 1998;19:489–492.

52. Thompson TC, Doherty JH. Spontaneous rupture of tendon of Achilles: a new clinical diagnostic test. J Trauma 1962;2:126–129.

53. Thompson TC. A test for rupture of the tendo Achillis. Acta Orthop Scand 1962;32:461–465.

54. Title CI, Katchis SD. Traumatic foot and ankle injuries in the athlete: acute athletic trauma. Orthop Clin N Am 2002;33:587–598.

55. Tohyama H, Beynnon BD, Renstrom PA, et al. Biomechanical analysis of the ankle anterior drawer test for anterior talofibular ligament injuries. J Ortho Res 1995;13:609–614.

56. van Dijk CN, Lim LSL, Bossuyt PMM, et al. Physical examination is sufficient for the diagnosis of sprained ankles. J Bone Joint Surg [Br] 1996;78B:958–962.

57. Xenos JS, Hopkinson WJ, Mulligan ME, et al. The tibiofibular syndesmosis. J Bone Joint Surg 1995;77A:847–855.

I ndex

Page numbers in italic, e.g. *215*, refer to figures. Page numbers in bold, e.g. **191**, denote entries in tables.